OLAGOKE ADENIYI

MANAGEMENT OF HEALTH SERVICES

ARNOLD D. KALUZNY, M.H.A., Ph.D.
Department of Health Policy and Administration
School of Public Health
University of North Carolina, Chapel Hill

D. MICHAEL WARNER, M.H.A., Ph.D.
Department of Health Administration
Duke University Medical Center

DAVID G. WARREN, J.D.
Department of Health Administration
Duke University Medical Center

WILLIAM N. ZELMAN, Ph.D., C.P.A.
Department of Health Policy and Administration
School of Public Health
University of North Carolina, Chapel Hill

Prentice-Hall, Inc., Englewood Cliffs, New Jersey 07632

Library of Congress Cataloging in Publication Data
Main entry under title:

Management of health services.

    Bibliography: p.
    Includes index.
    1. Health facilities—Administration. 2. Health
services administration. I. Kaluzny, Arnold D.
[DNLM: 1. Health services—Organizations. W 84.1 M266]
RA971.M343   362.1'068   81-21129
ISBN 0-13-549469-9   AACR2

To Barbara, Polly, Marsha, and Janet

Editorial/production supervision by
  Leslie Nadell and Zita de Schauensee
Interior design by Leslie Nadell
Cover design by Edsal Enterprises
Manufacturing buyer: John Hall

Printed in the United States of America

10 9 8 7 6 5 4 3 2 1

ISBN 0-13-549469-9

Prentice-Hall International, Inc., *London*
Prentice-Hall of Australia Pty. Limited, *Sydney*
Prentice-Hall of Canada, Ltd., *Toronto*
Prentice-Hall of India Private Limited, *New Delhi*
Prentice-Hall of Japan, Inc., *Tokyo*
Prentice-Hall of Southeast Asia Pte. Ltd., *Singapore*
Whitehall Books Limited, *Wellington, New Zealand*

Contents

Preface

The effective and efficient delivery of health services challenges traditional concepts of management and management training. As increased attention is given to the management of health service organizations, it becomes obvious that management approaches developed in industrial organizations, while providing the general basis for much of the management necessary for health services delivery, are not directly transferable to health service organizations. Nor is the simple development of specialty areas within management sufficient to meet the challenge. Management of health services, like the management of industrial organizations, requires an integrated approach combining insights from several basic disciplines while accounting for the unique characteristics of health service organizations.

The objective of this book is to provide a survey of concepts and methodologies basic to the managerial disciplines of organizational behavior, operations research, financial management, and the law which are directly applicable to the management of health service organizations. Our aim is to define the managerial process and then to selectively identify concepts and methods from each area that fit into this process. Obviously, any attempt to survey an area so rich in content must sacrifice depth to attain an integrated view of the disciplines and methodologies relevant to health services management.

The book was planned to show the relevance of each of these disciplinary areas to the various steps of the managerial process. The process is defined as having three phases corresponding to the major sections of the book: planning and design, implementation and operations, and control and evaluation. Within each chapter relevant concepts are first introduced followed by specific methods and strategies appropriate to health service organizations. These are further illustrated by case studies and exercises from a variety of health service agencies.

In addition to the sections on the management process, the book has two other sections. The first provides an introduction to the managerial process and the basic characteristics of health service organizations. The concluding section describes the structure and function of the health service system, the social, political, and economic context within which it operates and speculates about the future issues facing health service managers. Readers with limited knowledge of health services may wish to begin with Chapter 13 to help make sense of the management of health service organizations.

The book is directed primarily to two major groups of readers. First, to undergraduate students in health administration, as well as business, social work, allied health, and nursing administration who have a developing interest in health services. The use of this book is considered an introductory effort upon which a student is encouraged to take additional course work in each of the disciplinary perspectives represented by this text.

A second group of potential readers is graduate students in social work/welfare, public health, pharmacy, allied health, nursing, and business administration who are required or who elect to take one course in health services administration. These students require an interdisciplinary perspective of the management process as well as an understanding of the context within which this process occurs.

ACKNOWLEDGMENTS

An introductory text in the management of health service organizations involving four authors representing different disciplines provides a wealth of resources. Different disciplinary insights, work style, and personality provided the challenge and comradery required to complete a book of this size and scope.

The reader is the ultimate judge of how well we utilized our resources; however, we would like to thank a number of people for their support, patience, and assistance. On the Chapel Hill side a very special thanks is given to Donna Cooper for her typing and overall organizational abilities. Typing what must have seemed endless drafts as well as keeping track of the various chapters in their various stages of development was greatly appreciated.

Thanks are also given to Shari Jones for typing drafts of the financial chapters as well as Jean Yates and Bruce Fried for their overall bibliographic assistance. A number of students made helpful comments and supplied material; these included Skip Singer, Nancy Tigar, Jerry Delaney, Wendy Bardet, and Ken Rethmeier. A special thanks is given to Barry Solomon for his efforts in preparing case study materials. Sagar Jain, the chairman of our department, provided resources and an intellectual climate within the department that encouraged writing activities.

On the Duke side thanks go to Harriett Carden for her patient typing and retyping of the legal and quantitative decision-making chapters. Our colleagues in the Department of Health Administration provided intellectual support and models for doing research and teaching in health administration, and they should be recognized, especially E. Harvey Estes, director of the **Division of Health Sciences Education at Duke.**

A special note of thanks is given to Joyce Wesolowski, Susan Bove, and Zita de Schauensee for their editorial efforts and to Beatrice Schall for her art work in Chapter 2. Thanks are also given to Dr. Mickey and his colleagues at the American College of Hospital Administrators for their permission to incorporate fellowship cases into the text.

Chapel Hill, North Carolina

Arnold D. Kaluzny
D. Michael Warner
David G. Warren
William N. Zelman

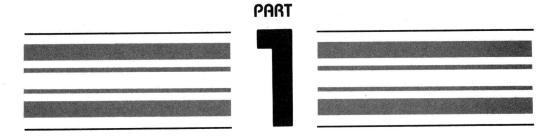

PART

1

INTRODUCTION

A man was walking along a winding road when suddenly his foot slipped and he fell down a cliff. There was one tree on the side of the cliff and, as he tumbled down, he managed to get hold of it. He was hanging there, one hand grabbing a limb of the tree thanking his lucky stars that it was there to stop his fall. After he had caught his breath he looked up and shouted "Is there anybody up there?" After a moment or two he heard a sepulchral voice intone, "Yes, my son. I'm always here." The man said, "Thank God. Tell me what to do." The voice replied, "Have faith and let go." Well, the man hung on a little bit longer, and then looked up again and shouted, "Is there anybody else up there?" [Sheps, 1981]

In the management of health services there are few, if any, authorities or "voices at the top." In many situations the best thing that managers can do is to have faith. The objective of this section is to give the basis for faith and to provide an overview of the managerial process and the organizational setting in which management occurs. Chapter 1 presents an introduction to the management process. It defines the various phases of the process and discusses the unique contributions of organizational behavior, operations research, financial management, and the law to the managerial process.

Chapter 2 operates on the assumption that just as a physician needs to understand human anatomy and physiology to function effectively, so the manager requires a basic understanding of the anatomy and physiology of organizations. The chapter discusses the components of performance, design, and environment and identifies unique characteristics of health service organizations.

1

Health Services Management

┌─────────────────────── **OVERVIEW** ───────────────────────┐

"Better management or the lack of it will determine the future of health services." To some this recognition is long overdue. To others it represents the beginning of "red tape," hassles, and barriers to achieving important health care objectives. Whether viewed as a panacea or as a hazard to the operations of health service delivery, the role of management must be understood by all people involved in health service organizations.

This chapter defines the managerial process and identifies three stages of that process: planning and design, implementation and operations, and control and evaluation. Attention is also focused on the relationship of management to the basic disciplines of organizational behavior, operations research, financial management, and the law. Each of these disciplines is defined and concepts unique to each are identified.

Two hypothetical cases will help illustrate some of the basic problems in planning and design, in implementation and operation, and in control and evaluation. The chapter concludes with a preview of remaining chapters of the book and their relationship to the managerial process.

└──┘

Dawton Dawson and the Memorial Hospital

Dawton Dawson, the administrator of Memorial Hospital, just left a meeting with the Health Affairs Committee of the Board of County Commissioners. The topic of discussion was the county's need for additional primary care services (doctors' offices, clinics, etc.), and what role the hospital might play in meeting that need. Dawson suggested that the hospital expand its primary care services by enlarging its existing outpatient clinic. The committee asked him to return with a complete proposal.

Memorial Hospital is a 250-bed voluntary general acute-care hospital under the ultimate authority of its board of trustees. The only hospital in Orange County, it provides most types of secondary medical services (general medicine, general surgery, pediatrics, obstetrics) but no tertiary or special services (for these patients are referred to University Hospital in an adjacent county). The hospital operates an emergency room 24 hours a day and a small general outpatient clinic three days a week.

To the casual observer, Memorial Hospital is an efficient, well-run institution—a monument to twentieth-century technology. A closer look reveals a number of problems. For example, the demand for outpatient clinic services has risen rapidly over the past three years. There are long waits by patients to get appointments, and long waits to be seen once they arrive. Moreover, there is general congestion; doctors and nurses who staff the clinic complain that there is not enough room, equipment, or personnel.

Another problem is that the clinic does not appear to operate as a unit. All the key professionals within the clinic report directly to their inpatient chiefs—medicine, surgery, ob-gyn, nursing—and each individual has only limited concern with the overall objectives of the clinic. Mr. Dawson is worried that this problem is affecting the quality of care provided by the clinic. Many patients are having incomplete diagnostic workups. Recently, several patients have returned to the clinic with advanced medical problems, problems that should have been diagnosed at the first visit.

The problem of quality is not restricted to clinic physicians. Several supervisory nurses have complained that nursing personnel are not following standard procedures. In fact, clinic personnel in general appear to be more interested in their own welfare than in the welfare of clinic patients.

Finally, the clinic is always losing money, even when there is a demand for its services. Accounts receivable is running three to four months behind schedule and, in fact, many accounts are never paid.

Dawson believes that both the expanding demand for services and the Board of Commissioners' interest in primary care indicate that he should "straighten out" the existing clinic and that he and the board should begin immediately to plan for a major expansion. He calls in Mr. Larson, one of two assistant administrators who is responsible for managing the clinic, the emergency room, and all ancillary services. Several alternatives are considered. First, Dawson and Larson consider the type of personnel that are needed to staff and expand the clinic. One idea is to employ a number of nurse practitioners because they require lower salaries than do full-time physicians. However, some question remains about what responsibilities they can assume because the state law is still ambiguous.

A second consideration is to change the relationships between the clinic and the various inpatient departments. Larson has been reading about "matrix design" in various hospital journals and suggests its use. Under this scheme a unit manager would be appointed to manage the operations of the clinic. The chiefs of service would retain a supportive role and be responsible for training their respective types of personnel and setting standards of performance. However, they would not be responsible for the day-to-day operations of the entire clinic.

A third possibility—and not a mutually exclusive one—is to establish a quality assurance program. Although such a program would be difficult to implement, sufficient work has occurred in the field to establish criteria for various types of diseases and thereby to determine whether results in treating them represent good or bad quality. Emphasis could be given to the process of care or even to a strategy that assesses diagnostic and therapeutic outcomes.

The manner in which these various changes are implemented must also be determined. Dawson and Larson want these changes to be implemented as smoothly as possible. Both recognize, however, that a number of personnel as well as members of the board may be upset with the various changes and in fact may sabotage both expansion and any reorganizational efforts.

Maxine Maxwell and the State Department
of Public Health

Maxine Maxwell is the director of local health services in the State Department of Public Health. For years she and her colleagues have been concerned about the limited, and in some communities the inadequate provision of primary care services to the residents of the state. Physicians are in short supply and the state's population falls below the national average on a number of well-accepted indicators of education, poverty, and health status.

After many years of working with various members of the state assembly and staff in the governor's office, the assembly passed legislation allocating funds to local health departments throughout the state to establish primary care programs. Maxine Maxwell and her colleagues were delighted and enthusiastic about the work ahead. The Department quickly invited local departments to submit program requests so that funds could be allocated and services provided to the residents in the state.

Their enthusiasm was short lived. Six months into the program only 20 of the expected 100 departments submitted proposals to establish primary care programs. Moreover, the program encountered a great deal of criticism from the state medical society. Meetings were held throughout the state and press releases characterized the program as "socialized medicine," "a government conspiracy," and "second-rate medical care." Essentially, the criticism centered around the cost, design, and the planned use of nurse practitioners in the program. It was argued that health departments were incapable of providing cost-effective primary care services regardless of elaborate reimbursement strategies with third-party payers; the departments, in limiting provision of services to normal operating hours, were not able to offer "true" primary care (defined by the medical society as "continuous care"); and that the existing program standards and guidelines for the supervision of physician extenders and nurse practitioners were "obscure and confusing . . . and could encourage such individuals to perform medical acts in violation of patient safety and state statutes."

The position taken by the medical society stimulated a great deal of debate over the program and culminated in the formation of a special Governor's Task Force on Primary Care. To assure that there was adequate representation of all interested parties, the task force was composed of representatives from the state medical society and state assembly, as well as personnel from the state and local health departments. The task force worked long and hard and within six months was able to formulate a set of comprehensive and meaningful recommendations regarding the program. To assure that these recommendations were ultimately accepted by the state medical society, the task force itself was chaired by a past president of the society who was actively involved in the initial critique of the primary care program.

The final report was completed and submitted to the medical society with full expectations that it would be endorsed. Although the task force left the original program intact, significant changes were recommended in the operational guidelines for the program. Special emphasis was given to promoting involvement of private physicians in the state primary care program.

Maxine Maxwell participated as a member of the task force. It was an exhausting six months, and although many concessions were made, she remained optimistic and pleased that the program was still operational. Despite these efforts, however, when the report was submitted to the medical society, the house of delegates voted merely to "file" rather than to endorse the report. The controversy continues.

DEFINING THE MANAGERIAL PROCESS

Obviously, Mr. Dawson and Ms. Maxwell are confronted—if not overwhelmed—with a vast array of problems.

Dawton Dawson

- What is wrong with the way the clinic is currently organized?
- What size staff (and rooms, and what equipment) is needed to meet current demands?
- What will future demand be?
- Why is the clinic losing money? (Is it really losing money, or is it just the way the books are kept?)
- How should the expanded organization be designed? Should the clinic be more free-standing from the hospital or more integrated? Who should be in charge?
- Once the clinic is expanded in its operations, how can anyone be sure that it is running properly?
- How should new programs and personnel be implemented so that they will be accepted by existing personnel in the clinic?

Maxine Maxwell

- Why was the need for primary care services not recognized by the state medical society?
- How can the need for primary care services be reconciled with the criticisms of the state medical society?
- Does the program make a difference in the health status of the communities being provided with such service?
- What is the likelihood that the state will continue the program given the opposition of the state medical society?
- What is the likelihood that local communities could assume the cost of the program once initiated?
- How can future programs be implemented to ensure the cooperation of the medical society?

At first glance these problems appear almost random, and the extent to which Mr. Dawson and Ms. Maxwell are able to resolve them may be attributed to their innate ability as managers. Yet a closer look at the problems re-

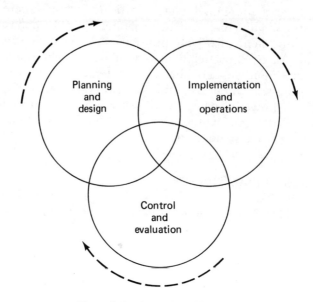

Figure 1-1 The managerial process.

veal a generic and sequential set of activities or phases, as illustrated in Figure 1-1. This set of activities or processes occurs at various levels of the organization and is defined as *management*.* The process itself is amenable to systematic analysis and is transferable as a set of concepts and skills.

Planning and Design

The planning and design phase of the managerial process is concerned primarily with the future, from several weeks or months to several years. During this phase, the manager determines what needs to be done and then decides what specific programs or activities can best meet the identified needs.

Planning and design decisions involve a wide variety of topics, from something as basic as "how many beds a hospital needs" and "how these beds are to be provided" to less basic but nevertheless important activities such as "when the annual Christmas party will be held" and "whether employees should exchange gifts." Within each of these topics is a great deal of future-oriented activity.

For example, to determine the need for a primary care program or the

---

*The terms "management" and "administration" are often used interchangeably. Historically, however, distinctions have been made. Individuals from a business orientation tend to refer to management as a higher-level activity within the organization and administration is described as a lower-level function of the managerial process. Conversely, individuals from a public administration perspective tend to use the term "administration" to describe the managerial process at a higher level within the organization and management as a lower-level function.

number of beds in a community requires forecasting the future age and sex distribution of the population, estimating how often the population will need or demand inpatient and outpatient services, estimating the length of stay, and deciding what other community hospitals and services will be operating in the future. This information must be translated into service programs as well as to the actual number of beds that will be needed to meet the estimated need and demand.

Other planning and design decisions involve the development of building and construction plans, determining funding sources for construction, and developing plans to assure approval by the appropriate regulatory agencies. In addition, expansion of services requires plans for staffing as well as methods to accommodate the needs of different types of personnel.

Any discussion of planning and design requires some clarification of the concept of *organizational goals*—a concept that has received a great deal of attention. Some authors suggest that organizations do not have goals toward which action proceeds (Weick, 1969), whereas others consider goals as the guide for actions and central to the basic questions of organizational effectiveness and efficiency (Mohr, 1973). The failure to arrive at operational definitions and the tendency to use terms such as "goals" and "objectives" interchangeably further complicates the issue.

Our approach considers goals as critical to the managerial process. Goals are developed and maintained by dominant groups within the organization and whether implicit or explicit, provide the basis for the managerial process. We also differentiate among goals, objectives, and activities as critical elements in the planning and design phase of the managerial process. Below are specific definitions and examples relevant to hospitals and the provision of drug treatment services.

- **Goal**—statement of general direction to be followed by the organization. *Example:* to provide high-quality patient care, education, and community service.
- **Objective**—desired ends that contribute toward goals. *Example:* the establishment of a crisis intervention service for the delivery of immediate help for a variety of drug, drug-related, or other crisis problems.
- **Activity**—activity/program undertaken by an organization. *Example:* providing intervention services; providing a "rap house" or walk-in center; providing a "hot line."

Implementation and Operations

The implementation and operations phase follows the activities of planning and design for the future and involves the day-to-day activities necessary to accomplish them. This phase is more present- than future-oriented and involves close contact with and influence upon the daily operations of the organization. Proposed programs and activities are actually implemented and the organization begins to feel the effect of decisions made during the planning and design phase.

To continue the example of designing and planning a new outpatient facility or primary care program, the implementation of the plan begins with obtaining approval from the appropriate boards and/or regulatory agencies, obtaining community support, and writing contracts with construction firms. Somewhat later, the implementation of the organizational changes begin, with perhaps new personnel, new job descriptions, and new line of authority and communications. During this time, management is monitoring the effects of the activities on a day-to-day basis, changing the implementation strategy where necessary, and sometimes even changing the overall plan.

Finally, the day-to-day operations of the organization require scheduling patients and personnel as well as monitoring and reporting current activities. Attention is also given to the endless and often unanticipated problems that somehow failed to be considered in the initial planning and design phase.

Control and Evaluation

The last phase of the managerial process focuses on both the present (concurrent control or evaluation) and on the past (retrospective control or evaluation) performance of the organization. In both cases, the major concern of this phase is whether or not the organization is meeting its planned activities, and if not, why not? To answer this question, management must have a clear idea of what the organization is trying to accomplish. A clear statement of goals and objectives makes it easier to control and evaluate an organization.

Control and evaluation requires that goals, objectives, and activities be translated into standards that provide the basis for comparing planned activities or programs with actual performance. Although the ultimate goal is to have quantifiable standards, many activities are not amenable to numerical control. Nevertheless, all organizations collect a great deal of information which provides the basis for comparing goals, objectives, and activities with actual performance. Data sources include daily reports on the number of admissions or visits to the hospital, hours worked by employees, informal and formal information on employee morale, the suggestion box, and financial reports on expenses and revenues.

Control and evaluation completes the managerial process. However, the process itself is never-ending. For the process to be successful, control and evaluation must lead to corrective action that identifies more goals, objectives, and activities.

RELATIONSHIPS AMONG MANAGERIAL ACTIVITIES

Two things should be clear from the foregoing description of managerial activities. First, there is considerable ambiguity among the respective activities and, in fact, they overlap to a large extent. A planning decision becomes an implementation process almost as soon as planning is initiated. Similarly, control activities are embedded in most operation activities.

Second, there is a great deal of interaction among the activities. Planning usually initiates implementation of the plan or design, but after the attempt to implement the plan, subsequent activities will require replanning or redesigning. The same is true with operations. Chronic problems involved in "fine tuning" the operation of an organization often initiate new planning and design efforts. Many planning and design efforts are initiated out of the control and evaluation phase, since the primary purpose of this phase is to identify problems that require planning and implementation. Some problems identified in control and evaluation require no new planning and design, but direct changes in the operation itself.

Even with the ambiguity and the interaction among the three managerial activities, it is extremely useful in the study of management to view it conceptually in these phases. Indeed, in this book, we define management as this three-stage process, and the chapters that follow will refer to these phases in describing the concepts and skills of management from several perspectives.

BEHAVIORAL VERSUS NORMATIVE MODELS

The managerial process described in the preceding pages represents a normative model. That is, it describes what managers *should do* in health service organizations—rather than what managers *actually do* in these organizations. While the model provides a useful framework for the administrative process as presented in management textbooks, it is equally important that we understand what managers actually do in organizations.

Mintzberg (1973, 1975) conducted a research study to measure what managers actually do. Through intensive case studies of five chief executives in different organizational settings (large urban hospital, consulting firm, research and development company, large suburban school system, and manufacturing company), he identified the existence of ten managerial roles. These roles represent a logical flow in which the development of a managerial position results in managers becoming involved in an extensive *interpersonal* set of relations. Through these interpersonal relations, managers become critical links in the *information* network. This affects their ultimate role in the *decision-making activities* of the organization. The interpersonal roles are:

- **Figurehead**—refers to the symbolic head of the organization obligated to perform a number of routine activities of a legal or social nature.
- **Liaison**—refers to interacting with peers and other people outside the organization to exchange information and favors.
- **Leader**—refers to interacting with subordinates to assure appropriate staffing, motivation, and training.

The information roles are:

- **Monitor**—refers to the seeking and receiving of current information and thereby achieving a thorough understanding of the organization.
- **Disseminator**—refers to the transmission of factual and interpreted information to subordinates.
- **Spokesperson**—refers to the transmission of information to outsiders about the organization's work plans and operating status.

The decisional roles are:

- **Entrepreneur**—refers to the initiation of change to enhance the operations of the organization.
- **Disturbance handler**—refers to corrective action when the organization faces important but unanticipated problems.
- **Resource allocator**—refers to allocation decisions regarding important resources, such as funds, equipment, and personnel.
- **Negotiator**—refers to the commitment of important resources in "real time."

A close inspection of the manner in which managers carry out these roles challenges some of the most cherished beliefs about managers and the managerial process. Table 1-1 presents four myths about the managerial job that fail to be supported by systematic observation of what managers actually do.

The empirical approach taken by Mintzberg has been applied directly to the study of managers in health service organizations. Two questions are critical in understanding the managerial role in health service organizations.

- Does the managerial role differ by type of health service organization?
- Are managerial activities performed by nonmanagerial personnel?

The first question recognizes the diversity of organizations in the health services field. The management of hospitals may be quite different from the management of community health centers, yet both are considered part of the general field of health services administration.

The second question recognizes the unique features of many health service agencies. That is, a significant portion of personnel within health service organizations are professionals and they represent an important force in the operations of the organization. It is important that we know whether these people are performing significant managerial functions in addition to their professional activities.

TABLE 1-1 *The Manager's Job: Fiction and Fact*

Fiction	Fact
The manager is a reflective, systematic planner.	Managers work at an unrelenting pace. Their activities are characterized by brevity, variety, and discontinuity; they are strongly oriented to action and dislike reflective activities.
The effective manager has no regular duties to perform.	In addition to handling exceptions, managerial work involves performing a number of regular duties, including ritual and ceremony, negotiations, and processing of soft information that link the organization with its environment.
The senior manager needs aggregate information, which a formal management information system provides best.	The manager strongly favors the verbal media: telephone calls and meetings.
Management is, or at least is quickly becoming, a science and a profession.	The manager's programs—to schedule time, process information, make decisions, and so on—remain locked deep inside his or her brains. To describe these programs, we use words such as judgment and intuition, seldom stopping to realize that they are mere labels for our ignorance.

SOURCE: Adapted from Mintzberg (1975).

Does the Managerial Role Differ by Type of Health Service Organization?

Forrest and Johnson (1980) attempted to answer this question by comparing a set of administrative activities performed by the chief executive officer in a national sample of hospitals with the activities of the chief executive officer in a sample of mental health/human service agencies in the state of Wisconsin. Analysis reveals that differences exist in both the number and the nature of tasks performed by managers in hospitals versus mental health/ human service agencies. Hospital administrators performed fewer tasks than their counterparts in the mental/human service agencies. Moreover, the nature of the tasks performed suggests that administrators in mental health/ human service agencies are more likely to perform tasks that are deeply involved in the operations of the organization and perform many tasks personally which are delegated to subordinates in the hospital setting.

Another investigation (Kuhl, 1977) compares the administrative activities performed by hospital administrators with activities performed by executives in prepaid health insurance plans. Although there are a significant number of activities which hospital and health plan executives share, there are also a significant number which they do not share. For example, the activities of hospital executives center around managing large numbers of people, whereas the primary activities of prepaid health plan executives center on the integration and maintenance of balance among major organizational components (financing, membership, and contracts with providing physicians). These differences reflect major characteristics of the two types of organizations and suggest that managers should be well aware of the nature of the organization within which they function.

Do Health Professionals Perform Managerial Functions?

A study of administrative personnel and public health professionals reveals that management activities are not confined to administrative personnel (Kaiser et al., 1980). The study of 16 local health departments, in which data were gathered from the director, the supervisor of nursing, the supervisor of environmental services, and a supervisor of the clerical staff as well as from a sample of all nonsupervisor personnel, clearly indicates that many personnel without administrative job titles and descriptions perform important administrative functions either through delegation or assumption of personal initiative. For example, a significant number of nonadministrative personnel, such as public health nurses and sanitarians, are involved with tasks normally thought to be the total purview of administrative personnel. These activities include determining salary and fringes for staff, improving access of health departments' services to the community, obtaining department insurance, improving efficiency and productivity, determining the number and type of health department staff, and maintaining liaison relationships with the general public and other health services facilities in the community.

Although these findings require additional analysis (with particular emphasis on assessing the intervening effects of organizational structure and style on role performance and organizational outcome), the available analysis has significant training implications. Training programs for health professionals *must* include the study of managerial theory and methods which are applied to health service institutions.

CONTRIBUTING DISCIPLINES TO THE MANAGERIAL PROCESS

The managerial process is built on the contributions of a number of applied disciplines. Although each discipline is important in itself, no single discipline is sufficient to meet the needs of management. Unfortunately, our educational process for managers in general, and health service managers in particular, has focused on disciplinary orientations rather than on the development of managers. As described by Mintzberg (1975):

> Our management schools have done an admirable job of training the organization's specialists, management scientists, marketing researchers, accountants, and organizational development specialists. For the most part they have not trained managers. Management schools will begin the serious training of managers when skill training takes a serious place next to cognitive learning. Cognitive learning is detached and informational, like reading a book or listening to a lecture. No doubt much important cognitive learning no more makes a manager than it does a swimmer. The latter will drown the first time he jumps into the water if his coach never takes him out of the lecture hall, gets him wet and gives him feedback on his performance. In other words we are taught a skill to practice plus feedback, whether in a real or simulated situation. Our management schools need to identify the skills managers use, select students who show potential in these skills, put the students into situations where these skills can be practiced, and then give them systematic feedback on the performance. (p. 61)

Figure 1-2 presents four disciplines or approaches which are major contributions to the managerial process.

Organizational Behavior

Organizational behavior may be defined as the analysis of individuals or groups and the structure of the behavior of organizations and, conversely, the effects of the operations of the total organization on the activities of individuals and groups within the organization. The application of this analysis to enhance individual, group, and overall organizational performance is known as *organizational development.*

Both organizational behavior and development are based on the social science disciplines of sociology, social psychology, psychology, and anthropology. Their primary focus is on the basic design of the organization and its interface with the environment and individuals within the organization. The management process has received important input from organizational behavior and development, including such concepts as role, structure, design, group process, change, and leadership.

Operations Research

Operations research may be viewed in several ways. In one sense, it is an approach to viewing the quantitative aspects of a wide variety of management decisions. As an approach, it involves building a conceptual model of the decision, determining which parts of the decision (or the model) can be quantified and which parts cannot, quantifying those parts that can be by using special techniques, and finally, using this information to help make a decision.

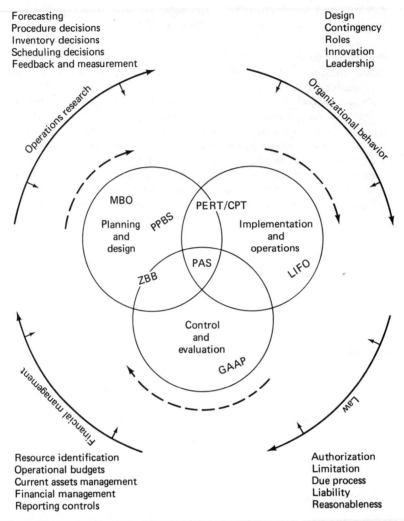

Forecasting
Procedure decisions
Inventory decisions
Scheduling decisions
Feedback and measurement

Design
Contingency
Roles
Innovation
Leadership

Operations research

Organizational behavior

MBO

Planning
and
design

PPBS

PERT/CPT

Implementation
and
operations

ZBB

PAS

LIFO

Control
and
evaluation

GAAP

Financial management

Law

Resource identification
Operational budgets
Current assets management
Financial management
Reporting controls

Authorization
Limitation
Due process
Liability
Reasonableness

Figure 1-2 Contribution of organizational behavior, operations research, financial management, and law to the management process.

Another view of operations research, although less powerful, is as a set of techniques used to quantify certain parts of the management decision-making process. Viewed either way, operations research often goes by the name of management science, quantitative techniques, or quantitative methods. All of these terms are considered to be the same for the purposes of this text.

Operations research can usually be applied to any management problem where quantification is involved, and it is especially useful in planning, in analysis and fine tuning of operations, and in control. Operations research is more powerful with some types of problems than with others.

Financial Management

Financial management is concerned with two major aspects of managing health care organizations. First, it focuses upon the best way to obtain funds so that the organization may carry out its plans. Once the funds are obtained, financial management is concerned in a very broad sense with the use of funds. In this regard, for example, it is concerned that all financial transactions are appropriately authorized, recorded, summarized, and reported; that the organization's assets are protected; that costs are contained, and reimbursement is maximized; and that financial obligations are anticipated and met.

Although financial management was once almost totally the province of accountants, it is now recognized as an integral part of managing a health care organization. Employees at all levels affect the use and well-being of the organization's resources, which in turn reflect upon the financial well-being of the organization. The pressures for good financial management come from both inside and outside the organization. With resources seeming increasingly scarce, it is in both the management's and the consumers' best interest to be as efficient as possible while providing quality care.

To accomplish the tasks listed above, a number of tools and techniques have been developed to help in the financial management of health organizations. These range from the design and implementation of accounting and reporting system and conventions to the use of quantitative techniques for managerial decision making.

Law

The law and its role in the management of health services may be described as either permissive or restrictive. In a real sense it serves both purposes simultaneously, providing the basis and the limits of management decision making in health services.

The traditional approach defines the law as "that which must be obeyed and followed by citizens, subject to sanctions or legal consequences . . . " (Black, 1979). But the broader definition of law claims that it is the agreed-upon set of rules that governs the actions and interactions of society. Law has historically provided not only the "game table" but also the "rules" for the whole range of societal endeavors from business to marital relations, including resolution of present disputes and planning for future public policy.

Law is the root of policy and the guide for its implementation. For example, consider the financing of health care for the aged. The national policy decision in 1965 to establish the Medicare Program was embodied in legislation that delegated the authority to develop rules and guidelines to the Social Security Administration (and now the Health Care Financing Administration). This program has resulted in an enormous accumulation of rules and conditions for institutional managers to cope with as part of their internal and external environment. Many health service managers view Medicare not only as a reliable source of reimbursement for services provided by the hospital but also as a source of restriction on the types of services that can be offered. Law in this form is both enabling and restrictive.

Law should also be viewed by health service administrators as a guide to effective and ethical decision making. Every manager is faced with hiring and firing employees, patient injuries and complaints, medical staff controversies, community relations (including dealing with the news media), planning, governance, and other daily issues that require legal and ethical guidance. Law, in the form of judicial precedent and legislation, provides a predictive mode for assessing the implications (and liabilities) in making decisions. In short, law is an essential consideration for managers of health care services in today's environment. It is a practical tool in evaluating the range of ethical and legal choices available to the decision maker in carrying out nearly every aspect of the job.

PLAN OF THIS BOOK

Figure 1-3 shows the basic structure of this book. The intent is not to make you an expert in either organizational behavior, financial management, operations research, or the law but to give future managers and health professionals a better understanding of the management process in health service organizations and the particular role that each of these basic disciplines has in that process.

Health service managers as well as health professionals operating within health service organizations need to understand the basic operations of these organizations. These elements and their relationships, that is, the basic anatomy and physiology of organizations, are presented in Chapter 2.

The next nine chapters outline the managerial process and are divided into three major phases: planning and design, implementation and operations, and control and evaluation. Chapters 3, 4, and 5 define selected aspects of planning: planning and design as it relates to organizational design characteristics (Chapter 3), planning as it relates to budgeting (Chapter 4), and planning as it relates to quantitative skills applied to the managerial process (Chapter 5).

Implementation and operations deals with the results of planning and design. Chapter 6 considers the operations (daily, weekly, monthly) of the organization, and emphasizes scheduling and other types of decisions initially planned and designed in Chapters 3, 4, and 5. Chapter 7 considers the acqui-

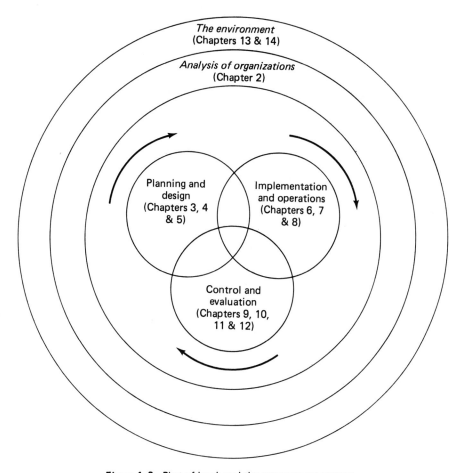

The environment
(Chapters 13 & 14)

Analysis of organizations
(Chapter 2)

Planning and
design
(Chapters 3, 4
& 5)

Implementation
and operations
(Chapters 6, 7
& 8)

Control and
evaluation
(Chapters 9, 10,
11 & 12)

Figure 1-3 Plan of book and the management process.

sition, protection, and use of financial assets to achieve organizational objectives. Chapter 8 considers the implementation of programs and activities generated during the planning phase of the managerial process.

Chapters 9, 10, 11, and 12 deal with various aspects of control and evaluation. Chapter 9 defines the concept of control and emphasizes the control of human resources within health service organizations. Chapter 10 introduces the concept and techniques of quantitative control and its use in the evaluation and maintenance of organizational operations. Chapter 11 considers the use of management information systems and managerial and formal reporting. Chapter 12 is the application of law and legal concepts to control.

The last section of the book looks beyond the management process and outside the health service organization. Chapter 13 defines the larger health services system within which various types of health service organizations operate. Here attention is given to the basic characteristics of the system and a review of the political, economic, and legal forces influencing the operations of the system. Chapter 14 considers the future of health services in the 1980s.

CASE 1

Long-Range Facility Planning*

In 1969, Trumbell Hospital completed a major building program. Many members of the board of trustees felt that the new facility would be adequate for many years, and no thought was given to developing a revised long-range plan for the hospital. The hospital experienced a rapid increase in volume of services, and considerable pressure was being exerted by the medical staff to provide additional space. The administration recognized that long-range planning, including master facility development, was vital to the continued successful operation of the hospital.

A major problem facing the administration was to convince the medical staff and the board of trustees that it was essential to start immediately to develop a long-range plan. The previous year the board of trustees had approved renovation projects totaling over $750,000, and many were of the opinion that hospital facilities were adequate. The medical staff executive committee was concerned with short-range problems of physician recruitment and physician coverage for in-house emergencies following the loss of the intern and residency educational programs. These were immediate problems they could recognize and it was difficult to convince them of the need for long-range planning.

Finally, responding to the recommendation of the administration, the board of trustees appointed a planning committee with the responsibility of exploring the need for a long-range plan. In October, a meeting of the committee was held with no consensus regarding the direction the hospital should follow. It was even suggested that the hospital's executive director should be able to define the problems that existed at the hospital and develop a long-range plan without the committee.

In November, a second meeting of the planning committee was held. The specific purpose of this meeting was to determine whether long-range planning should be accomplished internally by the board, medical staff, and administration, or externally utilizing a hospital consultant. After extensive discussion the committee was divided, with 12 members favoring and four members opposing a motion to recommend to the board of trustees that a consultant be hired.

A report of the deliberations of the planning committee was presented at the December meeting of the board of trustees. By that time the board saw that it was unreasonable to expect the executive director to develop a long-range plan and passed a resolution directing him to arrange interviews with qualified consulting organizations. This decision appeared to be a major step in the right direction as far as the management was concerned.

---

*Adapted from Johns (1978).

The administration arranged for representatives of six consulting firms to attend meetings of the planning committee. At this time the planning committee was composed of members of the board and representatives of the medical staff and the administration. By midyear a recommendation was made to the board that a consulting firm from New York City be retained. The purpose of their study was to review and evaluate existing health care programs in the community. They were to prepare a statement of mission for the hospital, including specific programs required to continue a position of hospital leadership in the community. This process consumed approximately six months and included the accumulation of information on the volume of services and interviews with a few physicians. Their report was presented to the planning committee and the board of trustees the following January. The report included 35 recommendations, many of them in areas that were known to be potentially controversial with the medical staff and the board of trustees.

Consulting Firm's Long-Range Plan Recommendations

1. Future growth of inpatient activity should be accommodated in the existing 498 beds.

2. The hospital should encourage the consolidation of pediatric and obstetric beds among the county hospitals.

3. The hospital should be prepared to reallocate its beds among the various services to optimize utilization.

4. The hospital should strengthen its program in discharge planning.

5. The hospital should encourage greater use of the rehabilitation hospital and home health care.

6. Plans for the provision of nonacute inpatient programs within the hospital should be developed.

7. The hospital should reinforce and intensify its program in utilization review.

8. The hospital should strengthen its psychiatric care programs by making greater use of the support available at the psychiatric receiving hospital.

9. The major thrust of the hospital's planning efforts should be to stimulate the growth of primary ambulatory care services.

10. The hospital should investigate the feasibility of establishing physicians' offices on the hospital site.

11. The hospital should act to encourage the formation of group practices.

12. The hospital should be prepared to establish a primary care program.

13. A subacute clinic should be established to supplement the hospital's emergency medical services.

14. The hospital's outpatient clinics may be phased out.

15. The hospital should consider expanding its new psychiatric program to provide ambulatory mental health services.

16. The hospital should encourage the development of shared services among the county's hospitals.

17. Diagnostic and treatment services should be strengthened to provide adequate support for the hospital's expanded programs.

18. The hospital should immediately limit its programs in physician training; longer term, the hospital should reestablish its house staff programs.

19. The hospital should seek an affiliation with a school of medicine.

20. The hospital should establish a summer training program for medical students.

21. The programs in continuing education should be strengthened.

22. Physicians on the medical staff that are currently board-eligible should be encouraged to obtain their certification.

23. Emphasis should be given to expand the hospital's program in paramedical education.

24. The school of nursing should phase out the nurses' dormitory.

25. The chiefs-of-service should be appointed by the board of trustees.

26. A full-time chief of medicine should be appointed as soon as possible and should also serve as the director of medical education.

27. Physician professional activities should be more in line with professional assignments within the medical staff organization.

28. Efforts should focus on developing an effective means of providing professional coverage of inpatients.

29. The hospital should make every attempt to continue to use its existing principal buildings.

30. The hospital should undertake an in-depth study of the movement of patients and supplies to identify opportunities to reduce operating inefficiencies and inconveniences.

31. Approximately 25,000 gross square feet of the existing nurses' residence should be converted into approximately 25 physician offices.

32. The hospital should plan to use phased-out clinic space for the subacute clinic and for emergency room use during peak hours.

33. Surface parking should continue to be used in place of structured parking for as long as possible.

34. The hospital should phase out and demolish residential houses and convert these sites to surface parking.

35. The hospital should develop a master facilities plan.

The immediate reaction of the medical staff was negative. Efforts were made to discredit the recommendations and accuse the administration of overly influencing the consultants. The generally negative reaction by the medical staff was a surprise to the administration because a good working relationship had existed. It became obvious very quickly that the board of trustees, reacting to the concerns of the medical staff, would not approve the recommendations as presented by the consultants. One of the concerns of the medical staff was that they had not been involved in the review or recommendation process.

Discussion Questions

1. *What is the role of management in the implementation of the consultants' recommendations?*

2. *What should management have done differently?*

3. *Select one of the recommendations and identify the critical questions associated with its planning and design, implementation and operations, and control and evaluation.*

CASE 2

Merger of the City and County Health Departments*

The public health needs of a medium-sized rural county were being served by three agencies. In addition to the city and county health departments, there was a 127-bed general acute-care hospital. The hospital operated a home health agency that was developed primarily to provide services to discharged patients covered under Medicare.

The hospital administrator was a member of the city council and chairman of the city finance committee. It was apparent to him that the city and county health departments lacked direction from the local and the state government as well as from the health officers. Because there were three agencies providing public health services, there appeared to be duplication of services. Combining the agencies could result in an economic saving to the residents of the county.

The existing public health offices were not conducive to providing a good atmosphere for the health workers, and it was felt that arrangements for space in or near the hospital might be more desirable.

To initiate the merger process, the city finance committee assessed its feasibility. For example, it was necessary to study the state code to be certain that it was legal to combine the city and county health departments.

The state health officer, the director of the nursing division of preventive health ser-

---

*Adapted from Hall (1978).

vices, and the director of business administration for the state health department were interviewed by the hospital administrator regarding this matter of a merger. Copies of the monthly reports for the previous year were examined, and the commonalities of the public health agencies were noted. The job descriptions for the nursing personnel were also reviewed.

The city and county health officers and the public health nurses were also interviewed to determine the interest and support for combining the health units. Their support was needed for the consolidation to become a reality. An attempt to identify unmet health needs was made by interviewing the two health officers. The county health officer replied: "The nurses are busy. As far as the doctors are concerned, it is questionable if more time and effort are necessary. One could go out and find something, but as far as I can see, things are functioning well." The city health officer said: "I think we're doing a fairly good job; you haven't heard any complaints, have you? I suppose that if there were someone working full-time, many more programs could be instituted." The county health nurse volunteered: "We need more skilled visits in the county. The problem is, we are limited as to how many visits we can make because of distance. We also need more public education about public health services. The people are unaware of what public health is. They think it is school health, immunization programs, and so on. We need more frequent immunization clinics. Only 42 to 46% of the children entering the first grade have had their shots."

Organizational charts were not available from either the county or the city health departments. Therefore, it was necessary to interview the nurses to determine the organizational structure of the agencies. They were asked to whom they were responsible or accountable. The county nurse responded: "Here's the way I see it. I think the county health officer is supposed to be my supervisor, but the county commissioners pay me. If the doctor has something he wants me to do, he will tell me, but I usually do what I want. The reports are submitted to the county commissioners. I guess I'd consider the commissioners my boss because the doctor doesn't give me the direction. The only time I really have any contact with him is at the immunization clinics. Several months can go by without talking to him. He has no contact with me as far as my programs are concerned."

One of the city public health nurses said: "I feel I am responsible to the following: city health officer, the mayor, chairman of the health committee, superintendent of schools, city auditor, and the state department of health." Another city nurse replied: "City health officer, state health department, and ourselves. We have to work it out our own way. Much of the time you don't know who you are accountable to."

The city health nurses stated they had very little contact with the chairman of the city's health committee. He did receive a copy of the monthly statistical report. One city nurse who had been employed for four years said: "I never see the city board of health. The only city health board meeting I've been to is the one when I was hired."

According to state law, the county board of health consists of the state's attorney, the county superintendent of schools, and the county health officer. The nurse employed as county nurse had been working in that capacity for approximately three years. She had stated that the county health board had not met since she had been employed, although according to state law the county health board was required to meet at least once every three months. The county nurse and both city nurses indicated that they had very limited contact with their respective health officers. They expressed concern about "bothering" them because they knew the doctors were busy.

Finally, a thorough study was made of the budget of the city and the county health departments, since the city council and the county commissioners were interested in the financial implications of combining the units. The issue was complex because of the laws regarding the state participating in local health units, combined health units, and health districts.

Neither the county courthouse nor the city hall had sufficient space for the combined departments, so it was necessary to look for a location for the city–county health department.

The results of the analysis were reported to the county commissioners and the city council. A joint function agreement was prepared and signed by the mayor and the chairman of the county commissioners. The hospital board of directors was responsive to the space needs of the combined health unit and approved the lower level of the south wing of the hospital for its use. Shortly after the combined city–county health board held its first meeting, the department moved into the hospital.

Discussion Questions

1. *Using the perspectives of organizational behavior, financial management, operations research, and the law, what are the respective managerial issues associated with the merger?*

2. *Using each of the perspectives, what are the managerial issues associated with the operations of the combined city–county department physically located in the community hospital?*

3. *What assumptions are made about the operations of the city department of public health, the county department of public health, and the county hospital when a merger is considered, using only the perspective of (a) organizational behavior, (b) operations research, (c) financial management, and (d) the law?*

FURTHER READING

ALLISON, R. F., W. L. DOWLING, and F. C. MUNSON. "The Role of the Health Services Administrator and Implications for Education." Commission on Education for Health Administration, *Education for Health Administration*, vol. II. Ann Arbor, Mich.: Health Administration Press, 1975, pp. 147–182.

ATWATER, J. B. "Must Local Health Officers Be Physicians?" *American Journal of Public Health* 70(1) (Jan. 1980): 11.

BELLIN, L., and L. WEEKS, eds. *Challenge of Administering Health Services.* Ann Arbor, Mich.: Health Administration Press, 1980.

CAMERON, C., and A. KOBYLARZ. "Nonphysician Directors of Local Health Departments: Results of a National Survey." *Public Health Reports* 95(4) (July–Aug. 1980): 386–391.

KOVNER, A., and D. NEUHAUSER, eds. *Health Services Management: Readings and Commentary.* Ann Arbor, Mich.: Health Administration Press, 1978.

LEVEY, S., and N. P. LOOMBA. *Health Care Administration: A Managerial Perspective.* Philadelphia: J. B. Lippincott, 1973.

LONGEST, B. "The Contemporary Hospital Chief Executive Officer." *Health Care Management Review* 3(2) (Spring 1978): 43–84.

McCOOL, B., and M. BROWN. *The Management Response: Conceptual, Technical and Human Skills of Health Administration.* Philadelphia: W. B. Saunders, 1977.

PFEFFER, J., and G. SALANCIK. "Organizational Context and the Characteristics and Tenure of Hospital Administrators." *Academy of Management Journal* 20 (1977): 79–88.

RAKICH, J. S., B. B. LONGEST, and T. R. O'DONOVAN. *Managing Health Care Organizations.* Philadelphia: W. B. Saunders, 1977.

WEAVER, J. L. *Conflict and Control in Health Care Administration,* Vol. 14. Sage Library of Social Research. Beverly Hills, Calif.: Sage, 1975.

2

The Analysis of Health Service Organizations

┌─────────────── **OVERVIEW** ───────────────┐

Just as a physician needs to understand human anatomy and physiology to function effectively, the manager requires a basic understanding of the anatomy and physiology of organizations. Although this understanding is just in the beginning stages, the basic concepts are available to provide a good start to understanding the important variables and their interrelationships. The objective of this chapter is to consider the important organizational components, their interrelationships, and the way these components characterize the various types of health service organizations in the health system. Specific attention is given to the unique characteristics of health service organizations.

└───┘

KEY ORGANIZATIONAL CONCEPTS

Health service organizations come in a wide variety of shapes and sizes, including private medical practice, health maintenance organizations, local health departments, hospitals, community-based drug action programs, and multi-hospital systems. Although it is easy to be overwhelmed by the differences, it is important to stress the similarities among these different types of organizations. All organizations are composed of two or more individuals who attempt to coordinate their activities toward achieving a set of goals or objectives.

To understand these coordinating activities further, organizations are viewed as interacting with the environment and are termed *open systems*. Three components are important to understanding the system and its operations: environment, design, and performance. Figure 2–1 presents the major components of the organization and their interrelationships.

PERFORMANCE COMPONENTS

The ultimate payoff of organizations is performance. What has the organization accomplished? In fact, from a managerial perspective, performance is the most critical component to which all other components relate.

Two general models have been developed to help understand the basic variables defining organizational performance: the goal model and the systems model.* The goal model views organizations as instruments for achiev-

_____

*For a discussion of specific models and criteria, see Steers (1975) and Campbell (1977).

28

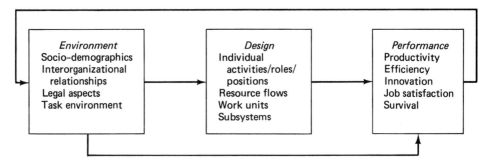

Figure 2-1 Organizational components.

ing some a priori specified set of goals or objectives. Performance is defined by the organization's ability to meet the stated goals or objectives. The systems model emphasizes the interface with organization's environment and its ability to survive in a changing environment.

The distinction between the goal and systems model is somewhat arbitrary and artificial. Organizations are concerned with both goal achievement and survival. A useful scheme to integrating the goal and system model is to consider various aspects of performance along a time continuum (Gibson et al., 1976). Under this formulation, goal-directed activities such as productivity and efficiency are considered together with more systematic activities, such as job satisfaction, innovation, and survival itself. An important feature of this scheme is the relationship of time to various performance variables. What may be effective in the short term may or may not be effective in intermediate- or long-term considerations. For example, in the short run it may be possible to increase various aspects of productivity and efficiency. However, this may be done to the detriment of job satisfaction or organizational adaptation and to the longer-term considerations of organizational survival. Below is a discussion of each of these performance components.

Productivity

Productivity refers to the quantity and quality of services provided by the organization. Quantitative productivity is measured by counting the number of people served by the organization. Measures may include such things as the number of patients using a particular service during a given period of time: for example, the number of x-rays done or the number of transfusions given.

Qualitative productivity is a far more difficult concept. It generally refers to the organization's ability to provide services according to accepted professional standards and in a manner that is acceptable to the patient. The methods used to measure quality center on three basic approaches

(Donabedian, 1966): structural measures, process measures, and outcome measures.* Structural measures focus on the internal characteristics of the organization and its personnel. Illustrations of structural measures include the presence of personnel with specific qualifications (e.g., board-certified or eligible physicians, and licensed administrators), the presence of certain committees, and the presence of various policy statements, such as manuals, forms, and contracts required by accrediting commissions.

Process measures focus on whether the activities within organizations are being appropriately conducted. This is usually determined by using a medical or nursing audit in which criteria of care are established for various diagnostic conditions against which actual activities are compared.† Criteria may be established either by a consensus of best judgment or, where data are already available, on an empirical assessment of patterns of care provided in other similar institutions.

Outcome measures are the most challenging aspect of qualitative productivity and refer to whether the services provided by the organization make any difference to the health status of the population.‡ Since outcome is influenced by a wide range of environmental factors beyond the control of the organization, administrators are often content to measure qualitative performance in structural or process terms. They simply assume that services provided in sufficient quantity and under appropriate structural and process conditions will have desirable outcomes.

Where outcomes *are* considered, a common approach is to use mortality and morbidity statistics. These statistics have limited value, however, because they provide no useful information on the level of health (Miles, 1977) and involve a time frame (i.e., between the onset of a program or set of activities and their effect on morbidity and mortality indices) that is of limited use to the manager in the allocation of resources. An alternative approach is to measure the physical functioning of people during a number of activities by using a survey questionnaire. Several measures have been developed to assess individual behavior patterns under various conditions (*Health Services Research*, 1976). For example, individuals are considered functioning at the highest level in their normal social role if they hold jobs without health-related limitations. Individuals forced to stay in bed are functioning at a lower level. Similarly, individuals having difficulty climbing stairs or walking would be classified at a lower functional level.

---

*For a more detailed discussion of quality assessment methodologies, see Vanagunas (1979), Green (1976), and Brook et al. (1977).

†For procedures to establish criteria, see Williamson (1978a,b), Payne et al. (1976), and Romm and Hulka (1979).

‡For an excellent review of quality assessment focusing on outcome, see Brook et al. (1977), and McAuliffe (1978).

Efficiency

Efficiency refers to the ratio between resources allocated to accomplish a given task or activity and the total task or activity to be accomplished. Measures of efficiency include such things as cost per unit of output (cost per pound of laundry, housekeeping cost per unit of floor space, laboratory cost per test performed), manpower per occupied bed (ratio of full-time equivalence personnel per occupied bed), and occupancy rates (average occupied beds as a percentage of total beds).

Innovation

Innovation refers to the ability of the organization to adapt to changes that are either internally or externally induced. This aspect of performance presents an intermediate time perspective and it emphasizes that the organization is operating within a constantly changing environment. Organizations may be highly productive and efficient in the short run, but unless they are innovative in a changing environment, their overall performance will decline.

Innovation is viewed as a process having a series of stages (Zaltman et al., 1973). These stages are generally classified as problem recognition, identification, implementation, and adoption or acceptance by organizational personnel. Except for implementation, which may be measured by the actual presence of different programs or technologies, measures of recognition, identification, and adoption are provided by responses to questionnaires given to organizational personnel.

Job Satisfaction

Job satisfaction refers to the degree to which organizational personnel have positive attitudes toward various aspects of organizational activities. Like innovation, this aspect of performance presents an intermediate time perspective. However, unlike innovation, the emphasis is on the human quality of organizational activities. This aspect is particularly important in health service organizations, where service activities are conducted through the interactions between clients and organizational personnel. Again, it is possible to be effective in the short run, but failure to consider the satisfaction of organizational personnel will have detrimental effects on the organization's long-term performance. Measures of satisfaction include employee attitudes toward their job or organization, turnover rates, tardiness, and the number of grievances reported by personnel.

Survival

Survival refers to the ultimate ability of the organization to function and emphasizes a long-term perspective. Although this measure of performance is often thought of as having limited value to administrators because many organizations continue for long periods of time, many health service organizations are, in fact, currently facing the possibility of extinction, at least in their current form. For example, 25% of the medical groups operating in 1969 were disbanded by 1975 (Goodman et al., 1976; Freshnock and Goodman, 1979). Similarly, the very survival of many hospitals (Hernandez and Kaluzny, 1981) and local health departments (Blendon, 1981; Terris, 1976; Bellin, 1977) is currently in question. Moreover, emergent organizations such as HMOs and community-based action programs have similar concerns with survival during the early phases of their development.

DESIGN COMPONENTS

Organizational design, as the overall configuration of the organization, is an important determinant of organizational performance. What are the critical elements and relationships involved in design?

Figure 2-2 presents a model of the major elements and relationships important to organizational design. The key features of the figure are the resource flows of interlocking people, funds, clients or patients, equipment, and information. These flows represent an ongoing set of transactions to which all activities, roles, and positions relate, and from which emerge work groups and subsystems unique to a particular organization. The work groups and subsystems occur in several ways. First, the type of activity or tasks affecting the resource flows determines the existence and relationship of basic organizational subsystems of production, maintenance, adaptation, and management (Katz and Kahn, 1978). As will be described later, the presence of the subsystems determines the overall level and character of the organization's development.

Second, the clustering of activities creates organizational roles. The concept of role is particularly important to understanding design since it links individuals who have their own set of values, attitudes, and abilities into the ongoing activities of the organization. The clustering of roles intended for a single person represents an organizational position. These positions or offices and their interrelationships determine the basic work groups of the organization as characterized by the degree of vertical/horizontal differentiation, integration, and stratification.

Finally, the interaction of work groups and subsystems permits the classification of four organizational types. Building on the work of Mintzberg (1979), these types are simple structure, machine structure, professional structure, and divisionalized structure.

Our model, like any model, is a caricature of reality. We cannot prove the cause-and-effect relationships, and its particular formulation has not been unequivocally supported by empirical research. Nevertheless, the model

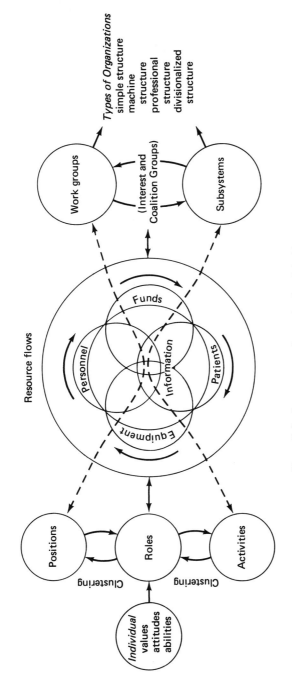

Figure 2-2 Components of organizational design.

provides a mechanism to present a complex set of variables affecting the managerial process as well as a framework so that managers can make sense of the situations within which they function. Each of the major design elements and relationships is presented below.

Roles

Roles refer to a set of activities or expected behaviors of an individual within the organization (Katz and Kahn, 1978). Roles are the building blocks of organizations. They serve to link an individual's activities to the activities of others in the organization. As seen in Figure 2–3, roles form a network of expectations guiding individual behavior.

At the simplest level, an individual is expected to perform and actually

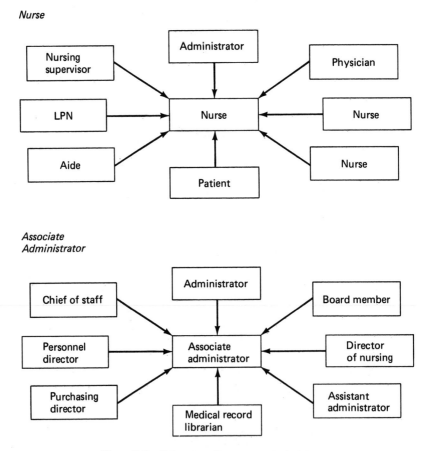

Figure 2-3 Role networks: nurse and administrator.

does perform a set of related activities. For example, a nurse is expected to routinely distribute medications, order certain procedures, and monitor the overall process of patient care. Individuals, however, often play multiple roles. For example, the nurse may be responsible for planning work assignments, chairing staff meetings, and evaluating the performance of other nursing personnel in addition to performing clinical activities. The greater the number of roles, the more likely the individual is to experience conflict among the roles. This problem is further complicated by the fact that roles played within organizations are only a small part of the total roles played by the individual.

Boundary roles refers to a special type of role where individuals from one organization interact with constituents in their own organizations as well as with other individuals from other organizations who similarly have a set of constituents with whom they interact (Adams, 1976). Figure 2-4 symbolizes the relationships between two boundary role positions.

Many individuals within health service organizations occupy boundary role positions. For example, social workers or nurses who are involved with discharge planning interact with individuals in their own organization as well as with their counterparts in various types of long-term care facilities. Similarly, hospital planners or administrators represent boundary role positions interacting with their own colleagues as well as with their counterparts in other organizations.

Individuals occupying boundary role positions experience different expectations and problems from individuals not involved in such activities

ENVIRONMENT

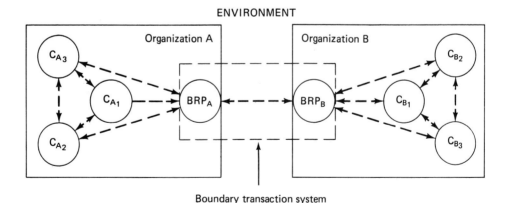

Boundary transaction system

Figure 2-4 Boundary role relationships. Structural model of organization boundary systems. [J. Stacy Adams, "The Structure and Dynamics of Behavior in Organizational Boundary Rules." In M. D. Dunnette (ed.), *Handbook of Industrial and Organizational Psychology* (Chicago: Rand McNally, 1976), p. 1180.]

(Adams, 1976). Boundary role people are charged with the responsibility of representing, if not presenting, the "image" of the organization to outsiders. It is through the boundary role person that outsiders develop their views and their expectations of the organization.

Another distinguishing characteristic is that individuals in boundary role positions are often more closely involved in the organization's environment and are psychologically if not physically distant to the organization. These relationships may potentially weaken their identity within the organization, generating suspicion among colleagues about their loyalty.

Finally, the person in a boundary role position can expect a great deal of conflict and ambiguity. Conflict and ambiguity generated by the unstable nature of the relationships among the various boundary role positions are further complicated by the expectations of various constituents.

A number of factors are thought to affect the activities of the boundary role person. These include the norms of the organization, the visibility of the boundary role person to constituents, the time frame within which the boundary role person is operating, the perceived effectiveness of the overall organization, and the credibility of the boundary role person to constituents. The exact nature of these relationships and their direction to boundary role operations are still unresolved issues and are areas of current research interest. For example, a study assessing the intermediate affects of constituent trust on boundary role behavior suggests that once constituent distrust exists, a chain reaction occurs (Adams, 1976). Constituent distrust results in increased monitoring of the boundary role position. The boundary role person is aware of the monitoring and proceeds to toughen negotiations with counterpart boundary role persons. Tougher negotiations may lead to a decrease in organizational effectiveness. This results in further substantiation of constituent distrust and a further increase of boundary role monitoring.

Positions

Positions refers to a cluster of roles intended for one individual. The idea of office or organizational position locates the individual in organizational space. In the simplest case, a set of activities defines one role in one position. For example, the position of a staff nurse may involve solely clinical activities. This represents the situation of one role in one position. Nurse involvement with clinical as well as managerial activities illustrates multiple roles in a single position.

Activities and Resource Flows

Activities and resource flows refer to the specific tasks within any given role affecting personnel, patients, funds, equipment, and information. These flows provide the basic substance of the organization to which all activities are directed (Forrester, 1961).

- Personnel refers to countable individuals in the organization.
- Capital equipment refers to physical space, tools, and equipment necessary for the processing of patients or clients.
- Patients or clients refers to actual patients receiving services within the organization.
- Money refers to the actual cash flow within an organization as well as between organizations.
- Information refers to data generated about any of the other networks.

The patterning of the elements results in the development of work groups and subsystems. For example, a group of nurses who regularly perform general physical examinations of children, exchange information about their children, use equipment, and are paid for these activities are said to constitute a specific work unit. Multiple work units performing similar tasks involving an exchange of resource flows constitute subsystems. Work units and subsystems are described below.

Work Groups

Work groups refer to the clustering of positions within the organization to achieve some objective. Specifically, a group is any number of people who (1) interact with one another, (2) are psychologically aware of one another, (3) perceive themselves to be a group (Schein, 1970), and (4) work toward a common goal (Hamner and Organ, 1978). Within organizations there are three kinds of groups: work groups, interest groups, and coalitions. Work groups are composed of individuals who participate in the group because participation is part of the individual's organizational role. The health services manager and his or her administrative assistants and the surgical team that does open-heart surgery are examples of work groups.

The interrelationship of positions within and between work groups provide the basis of organizational structure. This structure (viewed as a relatively fixed set of relationships among positions within the organization) may be characterized by the following features:

1. Vertical differentiation refers to the number of hierarchical levels in the organization. Here we are concerned with "stacking" of organizational offices or positions. The higher the stack, the greater the degree of vertical differentiation. Using this concept, organizations are often characterized as being "flat" or "tall," depending upon the height of the stack.

   A related structural characteristic describing the hierarchical arrangement of offices is *span of control.* This characteristic describes a number of positions at one level of the organization that relate to a single office at a higher level within the organization. This characteristic has received attention as researchers and managers attempt to describe the optimal number of offices that may efficiently and effectively report to one single office. Although there is little agreement on the exact number, there is general consensus that the diversity of activities or the number of roles involved in any particular office greatly affect the span of control. The less diverse the activity or the fewer the number of roles within any given office, the greater the span of control.

2. Horizontal differentiation refers to the clustering of positions into functional groupings or departments. Clustering may be done in terms of purpose, function, place, or type of clientele.

   a. *Clustering by purpose* means that all relevant offices are grouped together to accomplish some objective. For example, most emergency units in large metropolitan hospitals require a purposefully differentiated organization, since the unit contains many relevant skills to deal with the process of providing emergency care. Thus within the emergency unit the individuals involved in various positions will represent a fairly comprehensive spectrum of relevant skills.

   b. *Clustering by function* requires grouping by similar activities. For example, the department of surgery is an excellent illustration of a functional department since it groups all surgical activities together.

   c. *Clustering by place* recognizes the importance of location in grouping activities. For example, a hospital may have a number of satellite clinics, and the nature of their location represents a basis for clustering positions.

   d. Finally, clustering may occur on the basis of *type of client.* Within a general acute hospital, roles are clustered on the basis of providing services primarily to children (pediatrics) or on the basis of sex (ob-gyn) or further divisions of surgical wards by male or female.

In reality, all four bases of differentiation are used within the organization. As discussed in Chapter 3, many of the bases are used in combination to create alternative organizational designs.

Integration refers to the degree of collaboration that exists among differentiated units within the organization. The greater the differentiation among the units, the greater the need for integration. Integration may be achieved through a number of mechanisms, including specifically designed units or teams to coordinate differentiated departments or functional groupings, coordinating roles as well as managerial plans and procedures directed at achieving coordination (Lorsch, 1970; Lawrence and Lorsch, 1969a,b).

Stratification refers to the social distance that separates offices or positions within the organization. Depending upon the organization or the particular functional grouping within the organization, the amount of social distance may vary greatly. For example, surgical wards have a higher degree of stratification than do medical wards (Seeman and Evans, 1961).

In addition to formal work groups, organizations have a mosaic of interlocking interest groups and coalitions (Bacharach and Lawler, 1980). Interest groups are composed of individuals who are aware of the commonality of their goals and their common fate beyond their interdependence in work activities. Coalitions are defined as a grouping of interest groups who are committed to achieving a common goal. These types of groups are elusive because they pervade the organization yet are constantly shifting as various groups compete for resources.

Subsystems

Subsystems refer to the particular and recurrent pattern of activities affecting the resource flows and the interrelationships among work groups in the organization (Katz and Kahn, 1978). These subsystems are described below:

- *Production subsystem* refers to the activities comprising the major functions of the organization. In the case of health service organizations the production subsystem involves those recurring activities concerned with patient care.

- *Maintenance subsystem* refers to those activities concerned with assuring the predictability and stability of the operations of the organization. For example, the development of a personnel department represents a cluster of activities concerned with assuring the recruitment, training, and maintenance of personnel for the organization.

- *Adaptive subsystem* refers to activities concerned with assuring that the organization adapts to the changing demands and expectations of the environment. For example, the health services research component within a health care organization represents an attempt at systematic evaluation of changes in disease patterns and in the expectations of the population toward health services as well as evaluation of the available technology and programs for dealing with the health services needs and demands of a community. Unfortunately, most health service organizations have not developed adaptive subsystems to evaluate environmental changes or systematic programs and technologies to accommodate these changes.

- *Managerial subsystem* refers to those activities that are concerned with coordinating and controlling the activities involved in the other subsystems. Ideally, the managerial subsystem cuts across all other subsystems and provides the basic integrity for the entire organization. However, as we shall see, the particular stage of organizational development and the manner of linking various subsystems within the organization greatly affect the ability of the managerial subsystem to function within the organization.

Development of Subsystems

Although four subsystems have been identified, their actual presence varies among health service organizations. In some organizations it is possible to identify the subsystems easily; in others, many of the subsystems are embryonic or nonexistent.

Katz and Kahn (1978) have proposed a developmental sequence or "stages of growth" involving various subsystems. Figures 2-5 presents the stages of development.

Organizations begin as a result of environmental problems interacting with the needs and abilities of the population. This interaction results in a set of cooperative activities to resolve various environmental problems. This cooperative activity represents a primitive production subsystem and is illustrated by various types of self-help groups and community-based drug treatment or rape crisis centers.

As the production subsystem functions over time, a need develops to acquire increased reliability of performance. The pressure for reliability results in the development of managerial and maintenance subsystems. The managerial subsystem provides a mechanism for formulating and enforcing rules to assure that activities are performed in a predictable manner. Activities are no longer a simple response to environmental demands; they represent a predetermined set of activities to accomplish some objective.

To assure continued predictability it is important that individuals are recruited and socialized into the organization and that rewards and sanctions are administered in a predictable fashion. This predictability is accomplished by a set of specialized activities that focus on personnel. This set of activities is called the maintenance subsystem.

The final stage is the organization's need to accommodate changes in the environment. Shifting populations, changing disease patterns, and funding sources illustrate important environmental factors that must be constantly monitored if the health service organization is to function effectively over time. This monitoring is accomplished through the development of an adaptive subsystem. Organizations that fail to develop adaptive subsystems may find that there is no demand or need for their services.

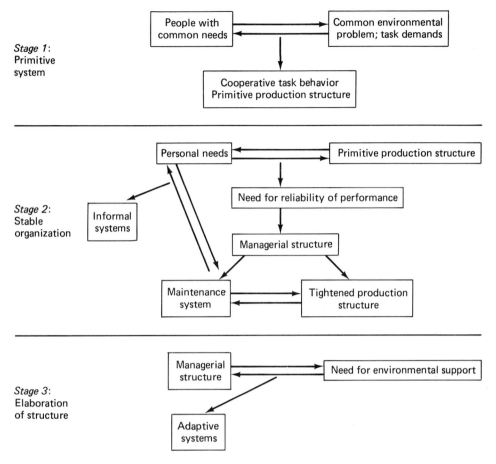

Figure 2-5 Stages in development of organizational structures/subsystems. [D. Katz and R. Kahn, *The Social Psychology of Organizations,* 2nd ed. (New York: Wiley, 1978)]

The sequential development of various subsystems has important implications to understanding health service organizations. First, health service organizations are often at different stages of the developmental sequence. Failure to recognize the stage of development can result in unrealistic expectations. For example, many community health service organizations are at stage 1 in the developmental sequence, yet external funding agencies assume that the organizations are operating at stage 2 or 3 with a fully developed managerial subsystem. As we will discuss, the problem is further complicated by the nature of the relationships among the subsystems.

Second, many health service agencies fail to develop any adaptive mechanism. As described above, disease patterns change and political contingencies shift, presenting problems to the survival of the organization. This is easily demonstrated by the plight of many local public health agencies (Shonick and Price, 1977) and small hospitals (McNeil and Williams, 1978).

Linking Subsystems

The relationship among the subsystems is as problematic as their development. Just as we assume that most health service organizations are operating with a fully developed set of subsystems, we also assume that the subsystems that exist are tightly related to each other and represent an integrated whole. As Karl Weick (1976) points out, many organizations are "loosely coupled." The various subsystems are tenuously related and although they are "somehow attached," each retains some identity and separateness. The attachment may be circumscribed, infrequent, weak in mutual affects, unimportant, or slow in response.

In health service organizations this type of relationship is most commonly seen between the production and managerial subsystems. Production activities associated with patient care are based on a highly specialized technology requiring extensive and specialized training. The subsystem tends to be both self-limiting and self-controlling and is organized around its own technical requirements and activities. The managerial subsystem, although fully developed, has only a tangential relationship with production activities. This limits its overall impact.

Subsystems and Groups as the Basis of Organizational Types

The degree of structure, subsystem development and linkage, and nature of groups provide the basis for understanding the various types of health service organizations. Figures 2-6 through 2-9 illustrate the conventional and symbolic relationships among the various subsystems as characterizing four basic types of health service organizations.*

Simple Structure

Many health service organizations are best described as simple structures. These organizations have a fairly well developed production subsystem and an emergent managerial subsystem which may or may not be loosely coupled to the production subsystem.

Positions within the simple structure are characterized by limited vertical and horizontal differentiation. That is, there are few hierarchical levels and few departmental divisions. The degree of stratification will depend upon

---

*See Mintzberg (1979) for a similar but expanded classification scheme applicable to all types of organizations. An application of the proposed classification scheme to various types of primary care programs is presented in Kaluzny and Konrad (1981).

the organization; however, most simple health service structures have limited stratification. Groups tend to follow positional lines and there is probably considerable overlap among formal and informal groups. Integration is achieved through hierarchical relationships, but the entire structure is characterized by an overall commitment to achieving some end.

The major advantage of the simple structure is that it provides a mechanism to achieve a single objective. Our earlier discussion of a stage 1 type of organization is an example of a simple structure. Under this structure individuals can easily identify with the task and achieve a great deal of satisfaction, since they play a critical role in meeting the organization's objectives. Moreover, its simplicity limits the effect of structure on aspects of performance. For example, Hage and Dewar (1973), in a study of community-based health and welfare organizations, report that the single most important predictor of innovation is the values of the elites in the organization. If the elites, that is, the executive director and all those who regularly participate in important decisions, have positive values toward change, the agency will have a high rate of program innovation.

The obvious disadvantage of the simple structure is that its entire managerial activity is centered on one (or a few) individuals. As stated by Mintzberg (1979): "One heart attack can literally wipe out the organization's prime coordinating mechanism." The second limitation is that the individual in the managing position, particularly in a "tightly coupled" structure, can abuse the position. Subordinates in this situation have no alternatives or recourse except to leave the organization.

Physician solo or group practice illustrates a simple structure with an embryonic and loosely coupled managerial subsystem. Visiting nurses associations are examples of simple structures with a more fully developed and tightly coupled managerial subsystem. Figure 2-6(a) presents a symbolic diagram of the structure, subsystems, and groups characterizing a visiting nurses' association. Figure 2-6(b) presents a more conventional diagram of the visiting nurses' association and a group practice.

Machine Structure

Organizations in which all subsystems are developed and tightly related approximate our understanding of bureaucratic organizations. Positions are characterized by a high degree of vertical and horizontal differentiation and a high level of stratification. As in the simple structure, groups tend to follow positional lines. However, because of the size and complexity of the structure, interest groups emerge throughout the organization. These interest groups may serve to facilitate or impede the formal activities of the organization. Integration occurs primarily through hierarchical relationships as well as formalized plans and procedures.

The major advantage of the machine structure is its ability to assure

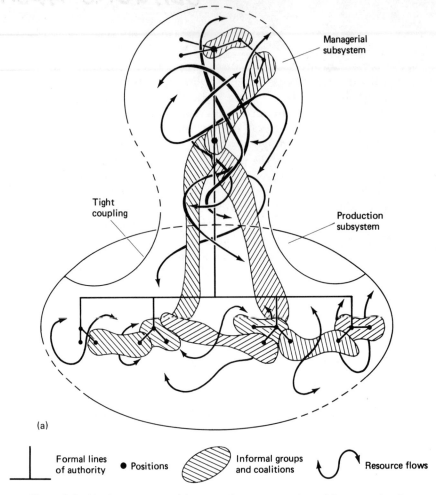

Managerial
subsystem

Tight
coupling

Production
subsystem

(a)

| Formal lines of authority | ● Positions | Informal groups and coalitions | Resource flows |

Figure 2-6 Simple structure: (a) symbolic representation; (b) conventional representation.

accountability in its use of resources and predictability in its activities. The development of four subsystems, the dominance of the managerial subsystem, and their "tight coupling" assure a high level of control within the structure.

Accountability and predictability are not achieved without cost. First, the structure appears to operate without recognizing the unique contribution of individuals. Individuals are often used as interchangeable parts and appear as "cogs within the system." Second, the quest for predictability often makes it difficult for machine structures to meet the varying needs of the clients and patients it was developed to serve. The problems of people often do not conform to the structural requirements for accountability and predictability. Although the problem is often mitigated by the ability of individual personnel to go beyond the prescribed role and activities, this may require extra effort from already overwhelmed personnel.

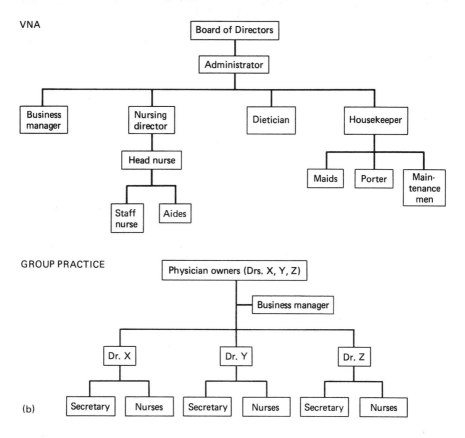

VNA

GROUP PRACTICE

(b)

In health services the machine structure is best illustrated by a state health department. Figure 2-7(a) and (b) present a symbolic and conventional diagram of a machine structure.

Professional Structure

Hospitals best illustrate the professional structure. The production system is well developed along with the managerial and maintenance subsystems, and in some cases there exists an adaptive subsystem. Although the subsystems may be well developed, they are characterized by their loose coupling. The production subsystem dominates the structure, and although the managerial subsystem is present, it is often isolated from the power base of the organization.

Positions within the structure are characterized by limited vertical differentiation and a high degree of horizonal differentiation. That is, the structure has relatively few layers even though there are many units within the organization reflecting its complexity and overall level of specialization. Moreover, the dominance of professionals tends to result in a high level of stratification among positions.

Integration is extremely difficult in professional structures. Professionals have little patience or interest in coordinating the organization, since their interest lies in specific tasks and the autonomy to complete these tasks. Data

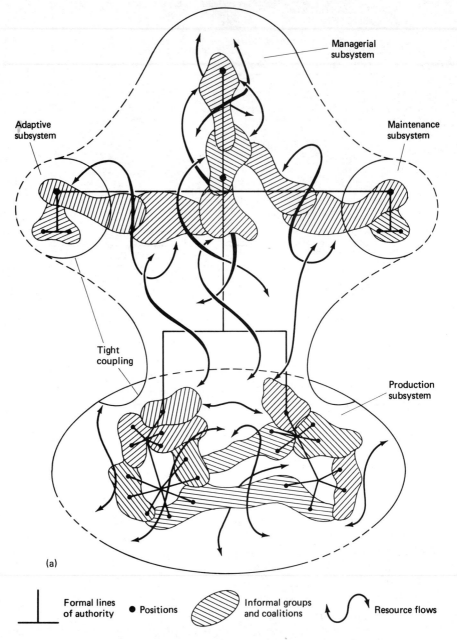

Managerial
subsystem

Maintenance
subsystem

Adaptive
subsystem

Tight
coupling

Production
subsystem

(a)

⊥ Formal lines of authority	● Positions	⬭ Informal groups and coalitions	⟿ Resource flows

Figure 2-7 Machine bureaucracy: (a) symbolic representation; (b) conventional
representation.

based on a study of community hospitals revealed that unlike industrial
organizations, which use structural integrative departments with specific
responsibility for promoting collaboration between various differentiated
departments, hospitals use few such structural mechanisms (Baldwin, 1972).

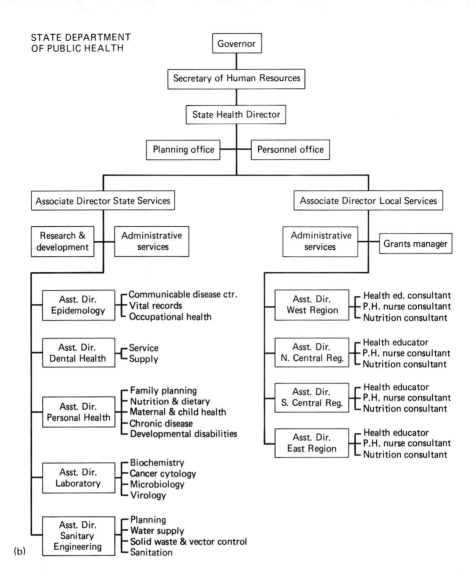

STATE DEPARTMENT
OF PUBLIC HEALTH

Governor

Secretary of Human Resources

State Health Director

Planning office — Personnel office

Associate Director State Services

Associate Director Local Services

Research & development — Administrative services

Administrative services — Grants manager

Asst. Dir. Epidemology
- Communicable disease ctr.
- Vital records
- Occupational health

Asst. Dir. West Region
- Health ed. consultant
- P.H. nurse consultant
- Nutrition consultant

Asst. Dir. Dental Health
- Service
- Supply

Asst. Dir. N. Central Reg.
- Health educator
- P.H. nurse consultant
- Nutrition consultant

Asst. Dir. Personal Health
- Family planning
- Nutrition & dietary
- Maternal & child health
- Chronic disease
- Developmental disabilities

Asst. Dir. S. Central Reg.
- Health educator
- P.H. nurse consultant
- Nutrition consultant

Asst. Dir. Laboratory
- Biochemistry
- Cancer cytology
- Microbiology
- Virology

Asst. Dir. East Region
- Health educator
- P.H. nurse consultant
- Nutrition consultant

Asst. Dir. Sanitary Engineering
- Planning
- Water supply
- Solid waste & vector control
- Sanitation

(b)

Instead, the most frequent form of integration was the inclusion of integrative activities as part of the overall managerial function.

Managers are able to provide integration by helping professionals negotiate the structure within which they operate. For example, managers are able to develop a great deal of credibility among professionals by negotiating programs or projects through "the system" and thereby enhance their ability to integrate and control the operations of the professional structure. As described by Mintzberg (1979):

> He [the professional] depends on the full-time administrator to help him negotiate his project through the system. For one thing, the administrator has time to worry about such matters—after all, administration is his job; he no longer practices the profession. For another, the administrator has a full knowledge of the administrative committee system as well as many personal

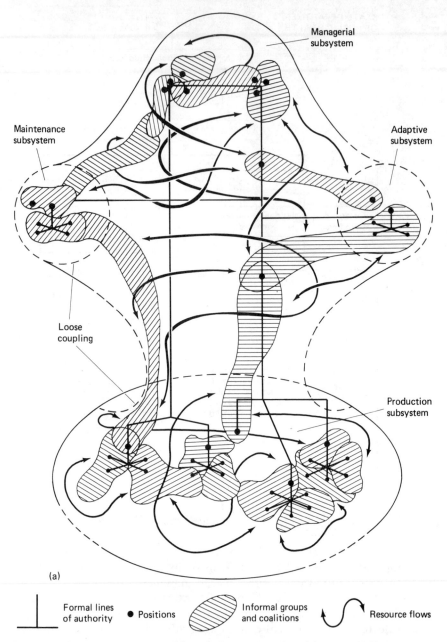

Managerial
subsystem

Maintenance
subsystem

Adaptive
subsystem

Loose
coupling

Production
subsystem

(a)

| | Formal lines of authority | ● Positions | Informal groups and coalitions | Resource flows |

Figure 2-8 Professional structure: (a) symbolic representation; (b) conventional representation.

contacts within it, both of which are necessary to see project through it. The administrator deals with the system every day; the professional entrepreneur may promote only one new project in his entire career. Finally, the administrator is more likely to have the requisite managerial skills, for example, those of negotiation and persuasion.

HOSPITAL

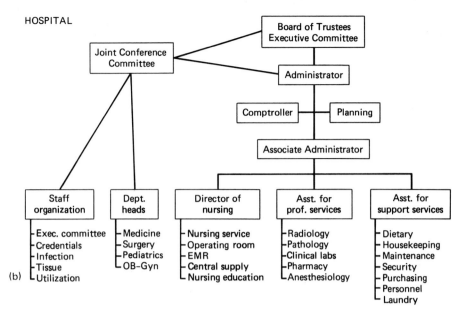

(b)

But the power of the effective administrator to influence strategy goes beyond helping the professionals. Every good manager seeks to change his organization in his own way, to alter its strategies to make it more effective. In the Professional Bureaucracy, this translates into a set of strategic initiatives that the administrator himself wishes to take. But in these structures— in principle bottom up—the administrator cannot impose his will on the professionals of the operating core. Instead, he must rely on his informal power, and apply it subtly. Knowing that the professionals want nothing more than to be left alone, the administrator moves carefully—in incremental steps, each one hardly discernible. In this way, he may achieve over time changes that the professionals would have rejected out of hand had they been proposed all at once.

A distinguishing characteristic of professional structures and a factor limiting integration are the groups within the organization. Unlike the simple and machine structures wherein groups tend to follow positional relationships, many groups in professional structures represent a loose amalgamation of vested interests which are constantly shifting as various groups compete for scarce resources (Bucher and Strauss, 1961). The creation of temporary alliances and coalitions to gain resources, as well as the loose coupling among the various subsystems, greatly confound the managerial process.

Despite these features the professional structure provides the mechanism for dealing with complex activities. It provides the operating setting for the function of professionals who have the special expertise to deal with complex and difficult problems.

The structure, however, is under increasing criticism for being unresponsive and unaccountable. Since professionals are free to define reality to fit their respective disciplines, it is increasingly obvious that problems fall between the cracks or problems are distorted to fit artificial categories. For

49

example: "The human body is treated not so much as one integrated system with interdependent parts, as a collection of loosely coupled organs that correspond to the different specialities" (Mintzberg, 1979).

Similarly, the autonomous nature of professionals within the structure makes it difficult to achieve programmatic innovation that cuts across disciplinary lines. Since each group is competing for resources, it is easy for the groups to cancel out each other's efforts (Wilson, 1966).

Finally, the failure of the structure to respond to reality has given the image to those outside that structure (clients, managers from machine structures, and governmental representatives) that it is out of control and no longer accountable. This has resulted in great pressure to adopt managerial approaches more consistent with machine structure: for example, direct supervision and the use of formal rules and regulations.

Figure 2–8(a) and (b) illustrates these relationships in symbolic and more conventional terms.

Divisionalized Structure

A developing form of health service organization, particularly among hospitals, is a divisionalized form of the professional structure. In this form a larger corporate structure is superimposed on a number of operating professional structures to create a multi-hospital system, as illustrated in Figure 2–9(a) and (b).

Positions are characterized by a high degree of vertical and horizontal differentiation and a great deal of stratification. Groups between divisions tend to follow positional lines; but within divisions, groups tend to be characterized by shifting coalitions typical of more professional structures. Integration is highly formalized and represented by specific departments or positions designated to coordinate activities at the corporate level as well as by role activities and formal procedures at the local hospital level.

Little is known about the potential or the problems of this type of structure in health services. As we discuss in Chapter 3, there are great expectations that this structure will combine many of the economic, manpower, and organizational benefits of the machine and professional structures.

ENVIRONMENTAL COMPONENTS

Performance and design components need to be understood within the context of the organization's environment. Environment potentially represents every event in the world that has any effect on the activities of the organization (Osburn and Hunt, 1974; Pfeffer and Salancik, 1978). These include the basic characteristics of the larger health system described in Chapter 13 as well as the basic cultural context of the larger society. In reality, however, every event confronting an organization does not affect it; thus it is important to define environmental factors that directly influence the goal-setting activities in daily operations of the organization. These factors constitute the organization's task environment and influence the organization's ability to obtain necessary resources, convert these resources into products and services, and dispose of the products and services within the organization's larger environment (Shortell, 1977). Components of the task environment include competing organizations, clients or customers, suppliers, labor markets, regulatory agencies, governmental bodies, and technological and legislative changes. Attempts to categorize the task environment have included fairly simple dichotomies along two dimensions, such as complexity and stability to more sophisticated classification schemes that attempt to differentiate complexity, diversity, stability, and uncertainty. These schemes are discussed in Chapter 3; however, at this point, it is important to emphasize that the character of the task environment varies among work groups and subsystems in the organization (Charns and Schaefer, 1982: Van de Ven and Morgan, 1980). Health service organizations as a totality do not function in an environment that can be specified as a single point on any dimension. Organizations have multiple work groups, each with its own task environment. For example, hospital dietary or maintenance departments may be characterized as relatively simple and stable environments, whereas emergency room and social work departments operate in more complex and unstable environments.

UNIQUE CHARACTERISTICS OF HEALTH SERVICE ORGANIZATIONS

Now that we have some basic understanding of the anatomy of physiology of health service organizations, it is important to call attention to some of their unique characteristics. Hasenfeld and English (1977b) specify the following features:

- *The raw materials of health service organizations are human beings.*

Although there are many similarities between health service organizations and industrial organizations, perhaps the most dramatic difference is the fact that health service organizations process human beings. As stated by Elliot Friedson (1975):

> In the human services of medicine, education, welfare, and law, the aim is not merely to "turn out" some measured product of a given quality at a given cost but to serve human beings in need of help. In manufacturing we do not concern ourselves with the tortures through which fibers, plastics, materials, or the like are put in the course of the production process. In the human services we are concerned that the course of providing help includes some sensitive recognition of and responsiveness to the human quality of the structure of flesh and bone being processed. Responsiveness and recognition themselves

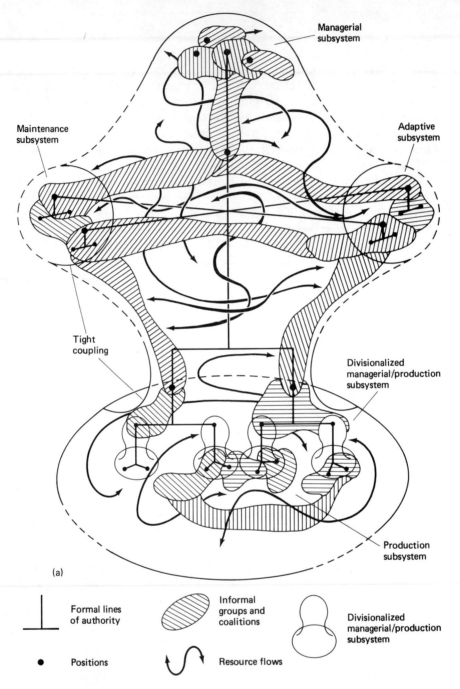

Managerial
subsystem

Adaptive
subsystem

Maintenance
subsystem

Tight
coupling

Divisionalized
managerial/production
subsystem

Production
subsystem

(a)

| ⊥ | Formal lines of authority | ⬭ (hatched) | Informal groups and coalitions | ⬯ (figure-8 shape) | Divisionalized managerial/production subsystem |

● Positions

↝ Resource flows

Figure 2-9 Divisionalized structure: (a) symbolic representation; (b) conventional representation.

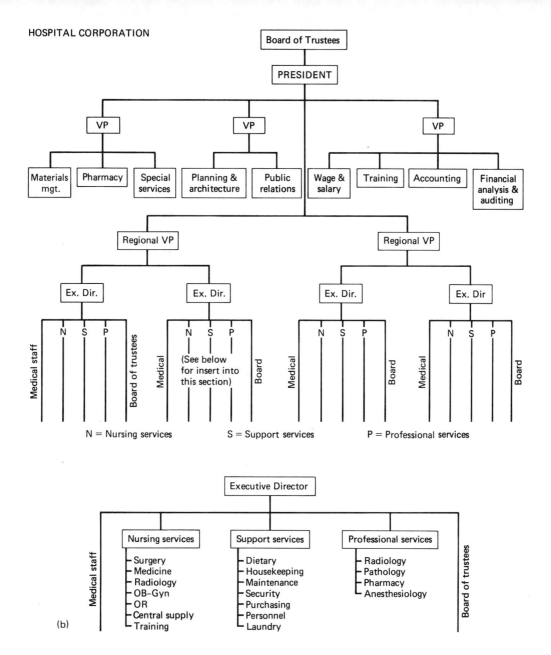

N = Nursing services   S = Support services   P = Professional services

N = Nursing services

(b)

may constitute the service and its benefit: without it the encounter is dead and the service provided to a mere object albeit not one of fiber, plastic or metal.

This difference has several important implications for the management of health service organizations. First, the organization is constrained in the application of its technology by a larger set of values within which the organization operates. The effects of these values are especially evident in areas where rapid advances in science and technology have challenged the nature of social and individual life. Developments in such areas as genetic technology have forced governmental and community agencies to question the limits of the scientific enterprise. This had led not only to sustained methods of monitoring such research, but also in imposing moritoria when public and political values appear to be jeopardized. This is well illustrated by the development of institutional review boards charged with the responsibility of protecting the rights of human subjects (U.S. DHEW, 1974; National Commission, 1978a,b). These federally mandated and locally administered boards are required to review all research and determine whether human subjects are involved, and if involved, whether they are at risk to potential physical or psychological harm. If subjects are judged to be at risk, the board must determine whether the benefits of the proposed research outweigh the risks, whether the risks can be minimized, and whether the subject is given adequate information to provide full and informed consent to participate in the research (U.S. DHEW, 1974; National Commission, 1978a,b).

Second, the human subjects processed by the organization have social identities that influence the process itself. Although health service organizations try to dehumanize (and many patients say they succeed) the entire process, organizations must recognize the social status of patients or clients in that process. It is well documented that organizational personnel react differently to individuals of different social status (Walsh and Elling, 1968; Duff and Hollingshead, 1968).

- *Goal definitions are problematical and ambiguous.*

Whereas industrial organizations can easily define their primary objective as obtaining the greatest return on investment, the goal of meeting the health needs of a community is a far more difficult concept. The idea of health is ideological in nature (Hastings Center, 1973). Each individual, whether internal or external to the organization, has his or her own definition of what constitutes an acceptable level of health. This degree of diversity makes it extremely difficult to arrive at any consensus. So the organization must either define its goals in extremely abstract terms and thereby arrive at consensus, or develop multiple goals to appease the various interests involved in the organization.

Another problem is that even when goals are defined, the activities of the organization may resemble a bargaining arena rather than a cooperative system guided by official goals. As a bargaining arena, the group in power determines the operational goals and activities of the organization. These activities may be more critical to the overall survival of the organization than providing quality service to patients or clients. Examples include providing employment opportunities in communities where business and industry cannot generate enough jobs, segregating and controlling people who are defined as deviant, and providing economic opportunities for individual business interests (Perrow, 1977).

- *Technology is indeterminant.*

A popular belief about health services technology is that it is proven to be safe and effective. Although the technology has been effective in many situations, much of accepted technology is being challenged.* For example, surgical procedures such as tonsillectomies, hysterectomies, and other technologies, such as intensive care (Russell, 1979) and electronic fetal monitoring (Banta and Thacker, n.d.), are increasingly criticized as being ineffective, overly expensive, and occasionally dangerous. Emphasis has been placed on the need for assessment, yet the guidelines are unclear. At least three types of assessment have been suggested (Greer, 1981): assessment of effectiveness and safety, assessment of cost, and assessment of social consequences. Each type of assessment is politically and methodologically complex, and it is likely that much of the technology will remain indeterminant for the foreseeable future (Banta and Sanes, 1978). In addition, the failure to make significant inroads on well-accepted health status indicators such as maternal and child morbidity and mortality rates as well as other pressing public health problems will continue to raise serious doubts about existing technology (Cochrane, 1972; McCarthy, 1980; Banta and Sanes, 1978).

- *Staff/client/patient relationships are coactivities.*

Despite an expanding technology, health service organizations are characterized by the amount of interpersonal interaction between patients and staff. The technology is not simply applied but applied through a pattern of human interaction.

Historically, the pattern of interaction characterized the client as being relatively passive vis-à-vis the role of health service providers. This relationship has changed and has significant implications for the management of health service organizations. First, the more aggressive role of the patient or client has undermined the authoritative and presumably expert position of the staff. Procedures are no longer taken for granted and staff and professional personnel are often required to explain them and participate in meaningful dialogue with clients and patients. Moreover, recent data suggest a greater tendency for patients to change doctors because of dissatisfaction with this aspect of care (Kasteler et al., 1976). Both technical competence and socioemotional factors in the doctor–patient relationship were cited as important determinants of change.

Second, the more active role of consumers has increased the vulnerability of organizations to external influences and counterpressure groups. This results in an increased diversion of crucial resources from service functions to management and somewhat political functions. For example, it is increasingly difficult for health officers in local health departments simply to present a

---

*See U.S. Congress, 1978; Council of Wage and Price Stability, 1976; Urban Institute, 1978; Altman and Blendon, 1979; National Research Council, 1979.

budget to the county commissioners on the basis of their professional advice. Although their professional advice may be accepted, successful negotiations occur only when this advice is supplemented by well-reasoned and documented requests for funds as well as built-in evaluation components.

• *Important role of professional staff.*

Professionals represent a powerful force within most health service organizations. Many professionals are trained outside the specific service organization and bring to the organization a set of expectations different from those of the employing agency. These differences often result in a conflict between professional autonomy and bureaucratic accountability. For example, professional staff request greater flexibility and more freedom at the same time that administrative personnel are requesting greater monitoring of staff and client relationships to assure increased accountability.

• *Lack of reliable and valid measures of effectiveness.*

Although health service organizations are increasingly under pressure for accountability, it is difficult, if not impossible, to develop reliable and valid measures of their effectiveness. The organization's inability to define goals precisely, the indeterminant nature of the technology, and the inability to design evaluation studies result in a chronic inability to demonstrate program or organizational effectiveness. Lack of an operational definition of desired outcomes results in an emphasis on input and process standards and considerable faith that the organization is doing "good work."

Even when it is possible to present data challenging our underlying faith in technology, faith usually prevails. Cochrane (1972), in an evaluation of home care versus intensive care for cardiac patient, reports:

> The first report after a few months of the trial showed a slightly greater death-rate in those treated in hospital than in those treated at home. Someone reversed the figures and showed them to a CCU enthusiast who immediately declared that the trial was unethical, and must be stopped at once. When, however, he was shown the table the correct way round he could not be persuaded to declare CCUs unethical!

CASE 1

Effectiveness of a Student Health Service

In an effort to secure greater understanding of, and funding for, the student health service, Harry Piedmont, president of the state university, requested the commissioner of education to contract with a consulting firm to evaluate the student health services at the six state colleges governed by the statewide board of trustees. The current state of the economy and a growing hostility toward the university system stemming from recent disclosures of drug and alcohol arrests of students, as well as news reports that birth control and abortion referral services were being provided by student health services, has resulted in increasing concern about the effectiveness and future role of student health services. The commissioner agreed with President Piedmont that a consulting report which emphasized the value and economies of student health services would enhance its image and assure a sustained high level of funding. Thus the commissioner contracted with a national consulting firm for preparation of the desired report. It was agreed that this report would be submitted to the legislature during budgetary hearings.

The student health services on the six campuses varied in structure and program content. All were funded through a combination of state tax funds, student fees, and charges to students for services rendered. In addition, some of the student health services received grants from private and governmental agencies, as well as contributions from university departments, such as the athletic department for services rendered to athletes, and from academic departments in which health science students received training.

After six weeks of investigation, the consulting firm presented its report to the commissioner. It was quite detailed and included the following findings:

1. That there was no central policy establishing objectives or programs for student health services. This was confirmed in discussions with the commissioner, each of the presidents, and the respective directors of student health services. The legislature has refrained from setting such policy, since this would be interpreted as interference with academic freedoms. It was noted that, where written policies existed, such policies were ill defined and provide poor direction as guidelines for the management of these programs.

2. At times funds were utilized for conflicting objectives. For example, legislatively generated tax revenues included an explicit prohibition against providing family planning services, while the same institutions accepted grants for the provision of such services.

3. Where campuses had the same program, there was inconsistency in the quality of the services. For example, laboratory services were provided on all campuses; however, some were under the jurisdiction of poorly qualified technologists and physicians not trained in pathology, whereas on other campuses services were provided by highly qualified pathologists and technologists. Moreover, there was considerable cost discrepancy among the programs. This in part is the result of inadequate data-gathering and accounting procedures as well as failure to use basic definitions of service units.

4. Student health services tended to be guided by broader institutional objectives rather than health objectives derived from examination and identification of student health needs. There were no standards upon which to measure the effectiveness of the student health services program.

President Piedmont was obviously disturbed when presented with the consulting report by the commissioner. Instead of supporting his case before the legislature, this report would probably serve to induce the legislature to reduce expenditures further. The report appeared well done and exhaustive. Although he had been aware of some of the problems reported, he personally believed that the program has had and continues to have a positive effect on student health. Moreover, personal conversation with various student groups revealed a general consensus that the program was providing an essential service at minimal cost.

Discussion Questions

1. *Was President Piedmont in error in requesting consultation? Was there another method to influence the legislature?*

2. *Why is a student health service so difficult to evaluate? Why had there not been stated goals and objectives? How would you establish these goals and objectives?*

3. *What are researchable goals and objectives for a student health service? How can these be measured?*

4. *What should the president recommend to the commissioner regarding the use of the consulting report? What other evidence can the commissioner use to avoid legislative cutbacks?*

CASE 2

A Hospital Consortium*

The Metropolitan Northwest Detroit Hospitals Corporation was officially incorporated four years ago under state law and consists of four general acute-care community hospitals. Since the initial development of the corporation, the organization has been successful in establishing consolidated obstetrical and pediatric programs, a consortium rehabilitation program, an areawide pediatric–psychiatry program, several primary care satellite facilities, and combined medical education programs, in the areas of pediatrics, obstetrics, urology, plastic surgery, orthopedics, and oral and maxillofacial surgery.

The consortium (see Exhibit A) is governed by a board of trustees comprised of 16 persons who are appointed to the corporation by the member institutions for a one-year term. Officers are elected from the board for a two-year term. The trustees include four chief executive officers of the hospitals, four medical staff representatives, four members of the board of trustees of the member institutions, and four community representatives at large. The board of trustees meets approximately four times a year, and according to state corporation law and bylaw requirements, an annual meeting is held within 90 days of the close of the fiscal year.

The function of the board of trustees is to elect officers, to establish corporate policies, to supervise affairs of the corporation, and to carry out the expressed purposes of the bylaws. The occupational background of the trustees reflects the composition of the

---

Adapted from Popoli (1978).

EXHIBIT A: HOSPITAL CONSORTIUM

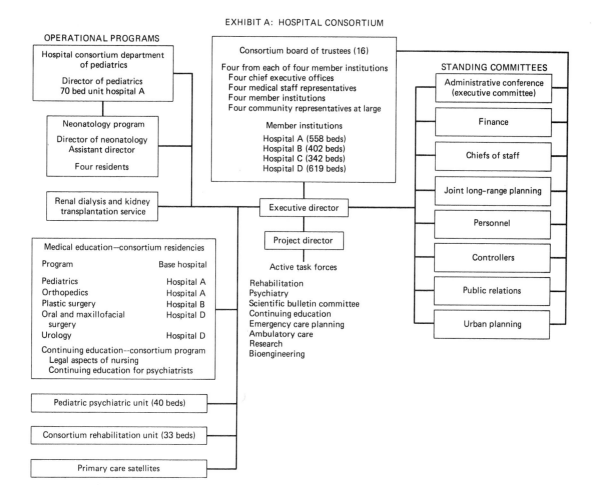

OPERATIONAL PROGRAMS

Hospital consortium department of pediatrics

Director of pediatrics
70 bed unit hospital A

Neonatology program

Director of neonatology
Assistant director

Four residents

Renal dialysis and kidney transplantation service

Medical education—consortium residencies

Program	Base hospital
Pediatrics	Hospital A
Orthopedics	Hospital A
Plastic surgery	Hospital B
Oral and maxillofacial surgery	Hospital D
Urology	Hospital D

Continuing education—consortium program
Legal aspects of nursing
Continuing education for psychiatrists

Pediatric psychiatric unit (40 beds)

Consortium rehabilitation unit (33 beds)

Primary care satellites

Consortium board of trustees (16)

Four from each of four member institutions
Four chief executive offices
Four medical staff representatives
Four member institutions
Four community representatives at large

Member institutions

Hospital A (558 beds)
Hospital B (402 beds)
Hospital C (342 beds)
Hospital D (619 beds)

Executive director

Project director

Active task forces

Rehabilitation
Psychiatry
Scientific bulletin committee
Continuing education
Emergency care planning
Ambulatory care
Research
Bioengineering

STANDING COMMITTEES

Administrative conference
(executive committee)

Finance

Chiefs of staff

Joint long-range planning

Personnel

Controllers

Public relations

Urban planning

individual hospital boards to a reasonable extent—a clothing retailer, a corporation lawyer, a former president of a utilities company, an insurance executive, four hospital administrators, four physicians, two religious sisters, and a retired businessman.

There are four standing committees of the board of trustees:

1. The *administrative conference committee* functions essentially as the executive committee for the board of trustees. As a general rule, the committee reviews all matters brought before the board. The committee consists of the chief executives and operating officers of each of the hospitals. The executive director of the consortium prepares agenda material and makes presentations before this group. In an effort to relate the activities of the corporation to the local planning organizations, representatives of areawide planning agencies are frequently invited guests to this

committee. Also, from time to time, various individuals are invited to make presentations to this committee.

2. The *finance committee* consists of one representative from each of the member institutions. The function of the finance committee is to supervise corporate budgets and various project budgets that are a part of the corporation's financial structure.

3. The *chiefs of staff* is equivalent to a joint conference committee in a hospital setting. The purpose of this committee is to bring the chiefs of staff of the member institutions together and explore subjects of mutual interest (medical staff privileges, common education programs, and so on) and to encourage communication and cooperation between the respective medical staffs of the institutions.

4. The *urban planning committee* is appointed by the member hospitals and represents a mix of trustees and hospital administrators. The function of this committee is to examine the extent of urban blight in the consortium service area and to establish a planning process that will enable the member institutions to identify various options that will permit the hospitals to resolve some of their problems.

In addition to the standing committees listed above, there also exist a number of ad hoc committees in the following areas: long-range planning committee, personnel administrators committee, controllers committee, and public relations committee. These committees are convened by the executive director and meet as required, depending on the intensity of the planning effort involved. Briefly, the functions of these committees are as follows:

1. The purpose of the *long-range planning committee* is to relate the long-range planning effort of the individual institutions, one to another, and to encourage the sharing of program planning, hospital information, and hospital statistics among the participating hospitals. The individuals are usually assistant administrators who have the internal responsibility for long-range planning and program development.

2. The *personnel committee* is comprised of the personnel directors of four institutions. The committee meets monthly and shares manpower information, wage and salary data, and labor relations activities. In addition, the committee supervises a consortium joint advertising program that has been operational for several years.

3. The *controllers committee* is staffed by the financial managers of the member institutions. Its function is to share financial and policy information that affects the member institutions (e.g., Blue Cross, Medicare, and Medicaid policies and regulations). Also, this committee negotiates contractual arrangements (corporation budget, neonatology, and medical education residency programs) between the consortium hospitals.

4. The *public relations committee* is comprised of the directors of public relations in the respective institutions. Its function is to aid the corporate office in the prepa-

ration of an annual report and to facilitate consortium communications within the member hospitals as well as with the general public.

Also, there are a number of task force committees whose composition varies, depending on the subject matter, and whose purposes may generally be to (1) stimulate shared service programs with the consortium, (2) foster communications, and (3) initiate a specific proposal or action by the consortium. The task forces at this time involve rehabilitative medicine, psychiatry, emergency care planning, scientific bulletin, continuing education, ambulatory care, medical research, and bioengineering. The status of these activities varies from preliminary planning to that of actual implementation.

In terms of specific operating programs, there exists the consortium department of pediatrics, which is centrally administered from one hospital.

The director of pediatrics is responsible for the clinical and educational activities of this department as well as the regional neonatology program, which is directed by full-time neonatologists. The director of pediatrics is responsible to the four member institutions. As a practical matter, the consortium department of pediatrics is represented in the executive committee of each of the institutions by a pediatrician coordinator who is a member of that hospital's staff.

In terms of medical education, five consortium programs exist in the areas of pediatrics, orthopedics, plastic surgery, oral and maxillofacial surgery, and urology. Pediatrics and orthopedics are based at hospital A, plastic surgery at hospital B, and oral and maxillofacial surgery and urology are at hospital C. Appropriate representatives are appointed in each of the hospitals for the purpose of coordinating the educational activities at that institution. Generally, the chiefs of services perform this function.

Also, there are educational activities in continuing education. For example, "Legal Aspects of Nursing" is a four-hospital educational program directed by the heads of the departments of nursing, and "Continuing Education for Psychiatrists" involves organized teaching programs for psychiatrists from the member institutions as well as a state and private hospital and a neighboring community general hospital.

The method of financing consortium programs involves two general approaches: the first is equal cost sharing. The second involves pro rata cost allocating. An example of the first method involves the distribution of the corporate office expenses among the member institutions. The corporate budget is about $150,000 per year and includes such items as three full-time equivalent personnel, supplies, services, and other expenses. These costs are allocated to the member institutions on a direct one-fourth-share basis. This approach acknowledges that the member institutions are equal partners in the corporation. Accordingly, each institution is expected to pay an equal share of the operating expenses of the corporation. As the end of each fiscal year approaches, a decision is made to reserve unexpended balances or to credit excessive revenues against next year's budget. At the end of the first year of operation, unspent funds were reallocated against the second year of operations. At the end of the second year, the policy was changed to permit the buildup of an unspent reserve of approximately $50,000. The change in policy was made to permit a cash reserve that could be used to support approved programs or to use the funds for program development.

The second method involves the financing of specific projects using the pro rata approach. An example using this method is the financing of the neonatology program. In this instance there were 11 full-time equivalent employees in the program projected in the next fiscal year, all of whom represented a combined salary of approximately $195,000. It was recognized between the consortium hospitals that the distribution of the personnel among the various institutions is unequal. Accordingly, the cost distribution is allocated on a time-and-effort basis.

The hospitals agreed to simplify the accounting system by using an all-inclusive rate (25% of salaries) for calculating the overhead distribution to each institution. Accordingly, the neonatology program costs $194,240 in direct personnel costs, 25% for overhead and fringe benefits amounting to $48,560, and $4800 for administrative services, for a total program cost of $247,600.

This method is used to distribute costs for each of the residency training programs as well. The system works well because the costs are fully reimbursed by Blue Cross and because the consortium hospitals agreed to a prenegotiated rate for fringe benefits and administrative overhead costs. The method avoids a costly and duplicate system of determining actual and true costs.

Another area of cost allocation deals with capital costs for programs that have consortium orientation, for example, the development of a neonatal intensive care unit and the addition of 40 pediatric beds in the psychiatry program. In these instances, the neonatal intensive care unit costs were borne directly by the host institution, hospital A, and the costs of the pediatric–psychiatry program were borne partially by the host institution. The corporate office prepared a grant proposal to a national foundation and received support for the balance. In the case of the development of the rehabilitation program, funds were expected to be forthcoming from the local United Fund agency.

There is no commonly prescribed pattern of obtaining capital construction costs, and funds are usually sought from whatever source is available.

The function of the executive director has been to:

1. Prepare and manage budgets that relate to corporation activities.

2. Organize and coordinate the activities of various shared services task forces. This work involves the selection of task force members, defining the charge to the committee, convening and coordinating the actual work of the task force, preparation of minutes, and where necessary, the collection of data and the preparation of task force reports. In some instances the documents are submitted to areawide planning organizations and state agencies as required under the state's certificate of need law.

3. Prepare grant applications to various federal and state agencies and national foundations involving consortium programs.

4. Act as liaison with community groups, individuals, and public agencies. Such organizations include the health systems agency, the local area hospital council, and the community interagency group, which consists of some 25 to 30 neighborhood organizations, city and state officials, and hospital consultants engaged by the member institutions.

In a broad sense, the relationship with these groups varies depending on the nature of the activity under review, but generally it may be defined as sharing of data, program planning, and community organization. It may also include involvement of these groups individually in the program activities of the consortium to a degree appropriate under given circumstances.

It should be noted that in addition to this general liaison activity with community groups, the executive director is also a member of the board of trustees of the health systems agency, and is a member of community task forces such as the shared services committee of the hospital council. As a consequence of this involvement, the corporation has a positive relationship with these organizations and has a voice in their policies and program decisions.

5. Act as a spokesman in the community for the consortium hospitals. An example of this activity might be that the executive director provided testimony to the house public health committee of the state concerning a health facilities bill that would affect the number and availability of health services throughout the state.

6. Provide technical planning support to the hospitals, usually through those individuals in the member institutions who are responsible for long-range planning.

7. Develop a direct service capability to the member hospitals. For example, it is anticipated that by next year the consortium central office will provide direct bioengineering services to three of the four member institutions. As the service becomes operational and is well received, additional programs are contemplated, such as centralized continuing education programs and group purchasing.

8. The corporate office provides an important communications function through the executive director among the member institutions.

Discussion Questions

1. *Evaluate the consortium as a social system. Given the available information in the case, characterize (a) the performance component, (b) the design component, and (c) the environmental component.*

2. *What subsystems are developed within the consortium? Are the subsystems loosely or tightly coupled?*

3. *Is the consortium structure best characterized as a simple, bureaucratic, professional, or decentralized structure?*

4. *What are the skill requirements of the executive director? As a boundary role position, what type of problems is he or she likely to encounter, and how might these be solved?*

FURTHER READING

DONABEDIAN, A. *The Definition of Quality and Approaches to Its Assessment.* Vol. 1. Ann Arbor, Mich.: Health Administration Press, 1980.

GEORGOPOULOS, B. ed. *Organization Research on Health Institutions.* Ann Arbor, Mich.: Institute for Social Research, 1972.

GRIFFITH, J. *Measuring Hospital Performance. An Inquiry Book.* Chicago: Blue Cross Association, 1978.

HASENFELD, Y., and R. ENGLISH, eds. *Human Service Organizations.* Ann Arbor, Mich.: University of Michigan Press, 1977.

KALUZNY, A. D., and J. E. VENEY. *Health Service Organizations: A Guide to Research and Assessment.* Berkeley, Calif.: McCutchan, 1980.

SCOTT, W. R. et al. "Organizational Determinants of Services, Quality and Cost of Care in Hospitals," *Milbank Memorial Fund Quarterly/Health and Society,* 57(2) (Spring 1979): 234-64.

SHORTELL, S. "Measuring Hospital Medical Staff Organization Structure." *Health Services Research* 14(2) (Summer 1979).

SHORTELL, S., and M. BROWN, eds. *Organizational Research in Hospitals. An Inquiry Book.* Chicago: Blue Cross Association, 1976.

PART

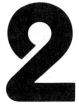

PLANNING
AND
DESIGN

> *Picture a pasture open to all. It is to be expected that each herdsman will try to keep as many cattle as possible on the commons. Such an arrangement may work reasonably satisfactorily for centuries because tribal wars, poaching, and disease keep the numbers of both man and beast well below the carrying capacity of the land. Finally, however, comes the day of reckoning, that is, the day when the long-desired goal of social stability becomes a reality. At this point, the inherent logic of the commons remorselessly generates tragedy.*
>
> *As a rational being, each herdsman seeks to maximize his gain. Explicitly or implicitly, more or less consciously, he asks, "What is the utility to me of adding one more animal to my herd?" This utility has one negative and one positive component.*
>
> *The positive component is a function of the increment of one animal. Since the herdsman receives all the proceeds from the sale of the additional animal, the positive utility is nearly +1.*
>
> *The negative component is a function of the additional overgrazing created by one more animal. Since, however, the effects of overgrazing are shared by all the herdsmen, the negative utility for any particular decision-making herdsman is only a fraction of –1.*
>
> *Adding together the component partial utilities, the rational herdsman concludes that the only sensible course for him to pursue is to add another animal to his herd. And another; and another. . . . But this is the conclusion reached by each and every rational herdsman sharing a commons. Therein is the tragedy. Each man is locked into a system that compels him to increase his herd without limit—in a world that is limited. Ruin is the destination toward which all men rush, each pursuing his own best interest in a society that believes in the freedom of the commons. Freedom in a commons brings ruin to all. [Hardin, 1968]*

As with the commons, resources in health service organizations are limited. To maximize the use of organizational resources, it is important to consider planning. The objective of this section is to describe various facets of the planning and design phase of the management process. Chapter 3 presents the concept of organizational design. It defines alternative design perspectives and describes various design strategies appropriate to health service organizations.

Chapter 4 focuses on the acquisition and use of resources to assure that an organization fulfills its service mission and financial responsibilities. The chapter considers some of the major financial activities associated with the management process.

Chapter 5 considers the manner in which basic resources are allocated. The chapter describes various quantitative tools appropriate to planning and health service organizations.

3

Designing Effective Organizations

┌─────────────────── OVERVIEW ───────────────────┐
│   │
│ Sooner or later most managers confront the issue of designing │
│ new departments of existing organizations, or in a few instances, │
│ designing the operation of a totally new organization. In both │
│ situations managers expect a well-developed set of principles and │
│ guidelines to help deal with the task. Although this may be ex- │
│ pected, the manager often confronts confusion verging on chaos. │
│ The objective of this chapter is to define organizational design, │
│ assess its importance and its limitations, and describe several │
│ design theories from which managers may choose to guide their │
│ decisions. The chapter concludes with a discussion of design │
│ strategies appropriate to health service organizations. │
│   │
└───┘

WHAT IS ORGANIZATIONAL DESIGN?

Organizational design is the arrangement and the process of arranging activities, roles, or positions in the organization to coordinate effectively the interdependencies that exist (Pfeffer, 1978) and to improve the efficiency, effectiveness, and adaptability of the organization (Kilmann, 1977). As described by Simon (1969):

> Everyone designs who devises courses of action aimed at changing exist-
> ing situations into preferred ones. The intellectual activity that produces
> material artifacts is no different fundamentally from the one that prescribes
> remedies for sick patients or the one that devises a new sales plan for com-
> pany or social welfare policy for a state. Design, so construed, is the core of
> all professional training; it is the principal mark that distinguishes the pro-
> fessions from the scientists. Schools of engineering as well as schools of
> architecture, business, education and law and medicine are all centrally con-
> cerned with the process of design.

Although most health service managers pride themselves in their pragmatic orientation, their design efforts occur within an uncertain environment—forcing them to adopt or develop, often through a process of trial and error, some theory or model to explain the internal workings of their organization (Elmore, 1978). In essence, these are the models of the design process and depending upon which model is implicitly or explicitly selected leads to different perceptions and conclusions. As described by Graham Allison (1971): "What we see and judge to be important depends not only on the evidence but also on the 'conceptual lens' through which we look at the evidence."

Several "conceptual lenses" or models are currently available to guide the design process in health care organizations. Each model provides a somewhat different explanation or highlights different design issues and emphasizes different factors important to the resolution of these issues. Design may be viewed from one of three perspectives:

1. Design is a conscious attempt to enhance some aspect of organizational performance. From a *rational* perspective, the process of organizational design attempts to derive some fit between environmental and organizational characteristics or between individual and organizational characteristics. Where this fit occurs, there is an expected positive effect on the overall performance of the individual, work group, or organization.

2. Design is a result of an unfolding of larger events within the environment. From an *ecological* perspective the design of the organization is a function of the nature and distribution of resources in the organization's environment. Emphasis is not given to short-run changes but rather to understanding the long-run transformations. Unlike the rational perspective, there is no implication that the interface of the environment and organization results in a better organization (Aldrich, 1979).

3. Design is the result of an ongoing evolutionary process internal to the organization. From an *evolutionary* perspective the design of the organization is less determined by outside factors than it is by the organization's unfolding history and stage of overall development. Emphasis is given to size and age as critical factors influencing design (Greiner, 1972; Adizes, 1979).

WHY IS DESIGN IMPORTANT?

Regardless of the perspective, why should managers be concerned about design? Why not simply assume that the design is a constant, and attempt to manipulate dollars, information, materials, or individuals in order to enhance overall organizational performance? Part of the importance of design stems from the increasing evidence within health service organizations that design characteristics are important predictors of organizational performance.

A summary of selected studies contrasting the differential effects of organizational design characteristics and personal characteristics of physicians on organizational performance is presented in Table 3-1. A review of the studies suggests several points. First, it suggests that organizational design characteristics are extremely important in affecting measures of organizational performance. In fact, in all the studies the design characteristics were the primary predictors of performance. Differences among physicians

TABLE 3-1 *Selected Studies of Organizational Design and Physician Characteristics: Performance/Effects*

Researcher	Physician Characteristics	Design Characteristics	Measures/ Performance	Primary Predictors
Rhee (1976, 1977)	Specialization, type of medical school, time in practice	Type of ambulatory care setting[a] Type of hospital	M.D. compliance with explicit criteria	Design
Flood and Scott (1978)	Length of training, years in practice, specialization	Size, teaching status, staff organization variable[b]	Post surgical— morbidity/mortality	Design
Roemer and Friedman (1971)	Training	Medical staff structure[c]	Severity adjusted death rate	Design

[a]*Type of ambulatory care setting included the following categories: solo practice, small single-specialty groups with no prepayment, small multi-specialty groups with no prepayment, medium multi-specialty groups with no prepayment, medium multi-specialty groups with some prepayment, and large multi-specialty groups without respect to payment methods. Types of hospitals include the following categories: small rural community hospitals, small urban community hospitals, large urban community hospitals, teaching hospitals, and Kaiser Foundation hospitals.*
[b]*Staff organization variables included perceived influence exercised by various groups once given a set of decisions (e.g., hire staff nurse, purchase contract services, add clinical services, terminate personnel); degree of centralization of decision making with surgical staff; and formalization of rules (e.g., strictness of admission requirements for new members).*
[c]*Medical staff structure was based on a weighted score involving seven features of medical staff relations: composition of this staff, appointment procedures, commitment, departmentalization, control committees, documentation, and informal dynamics.*

could not account for as much variance in various indicators of performance as could the organizational design variables.

Second, the review suggests several methodological problems limiting our complete interpretation of the effect that design characteristics have on organizational performance. Perhaps most apparent is that the overall pattern of relationships among the various design variables is not known, since no single study incorporates all the variables. Thus, our understanding is indeterminant and it is impossible to assess the full impact of such factors as the type of practice (e.g., group versus solo) or other design variables, such as differentiation and integration, on organizational performance.

A related problem is the lack of a standardization in the measurement of design variables. Researchers tend to use the same measures for quite different theoretical constructs. For example, occupancy rate may be used by different investigators as measuring such design concepts as organizational slack and coordination as well as measuring organizational efficiency (Neuhauser and Anderson, 1972).

Yet, the findings are sufficient to document the importance of design as well as to suggest implications for administrators. As applied to quality assurance, Palmer and Reilly (1979) have suggested that:

> Changing the process of care at the individual level is not the only nor necessarily the best means of improving quality of care. To the extent that struc-

tural characteristics (design characteristics) determine the quality of care, efforts to improve care in the long run through changing the structure of care (design) may prove to be more cost effective than short run, quality assurance programs.

A second reason for the importance of organizational design stems from the evolutionary perspective. As outlined above, this perspective does not emphasize the relationship of design and performance but suggests that the design reflects the unfolding history and stage of organizational development. Thus design provides a map for the manager which reflects the outcomes of past power struggles and provides a clue for the future course of events.

A final reason why design is important is that a firm understanding of the design sets realistic limits within which the manager operates. The ecological as well as the evolutionary perspective suggests that managers are more reactive than proactive in designing organizations and that many of the basic design questions are often beyond their control. That is, basic design features are functions of the evolutionary spiral through which all organizations pass or they are functions of larger external factors affecting the design characteristics of the organization. Recognizing these relationships provides administrators with a healthy insight into their own roles, and their own potential and limitations, and in the long run prevents the development of unrealistic expectations and the subsequent effects of "organizational/administrative burnout."

LIMITS OF DESIGN

It has been difficult to develop a set of guidelines to help health service managers confront problems of organizational design. Several reasons can be cited. First, there is little agreement on what constitutes the variables and conditions of organizational effectiveness. In an extensive review of the available models of effectiveness, Steers (1975) concludes:

> From the findings to date, it appears that either the effectiveness construct is invalid or that there may indeed be such a valid construct for which the relevant observable criteria have not yet been discovered. Optimistically, one would argue for the latter position; that is that a great deal more work is necessary to discover the set of variables and conditions that constitute an integrated construct that may be termed organizational effectiveness. Until the construct can be explained, however, it will be difficult to make meaningful recommendations to managers about steps to improve effectiveness in their organization. [p. 552]

This problem is complicated further by the distinctive characteristics of health service organizations (Hasenfeld and English, 1977b). As outlined in

Chapter 2, the ambiguity and problematical nature of goal definitions, the fact that raw materials in health service organizations are human beings, and the fact that the technology of health service organizations is indeterminant and largely dictated by interpersonal relations confound an already difficult situation.

A second reason we are unable to provide a well-developed set of design principles and guidelines is that the systematic study of organizational design characteristics, particularly their role in health service organizations, is a relatively recent phenomenon. Traditionally, design characteristics were considered assumptions or constraints within which administrators functioned. Under these constraints the primary focus was to manipulate information, dollars, materials, or people and thereby enhance various aspects of organizational performance.

A third reason inhibiting attempts at design is our simple inability to maintain the creativity required for design (Leavitt, 1976) and to organize the skills necessary to encompass design activities. Design implies a creative process, yet the training programs for most managerial and professional personnel increase students' ability to analyze situations while negatively affecting their ability to generate creative solutions. Furthermore, the concept of design encompasses so many factors (technological, sociological, political, and psychological) that it is unlikely that many individuals will be able to develop the necessary skills to perform the task. This situation is further confounded by the lack of a common conceptual framework to provide a basic language for development of a general theory of organizational design.

THEORIES OF DESIGN

Although managers pride themselves on their pragmatic orientation as well as their ability to control events, most are victims of the past. As perceived by Keynes (1936) many years ago:

> Practical men, who believe themselves to be quite exempt from any intellectual influences, are usually the slaves of some defunct economist. Men in authority, who hear voices in the air, are distilling their frenzy from some academic scribbler of a few years back.

Below are descriptions of several major organizational design models, in part generated by voices in the air and in part generated by empirical research. In both cases the models are an important influence on the activities of health service administrators and their organizations.

Rational Perspective

Managers may choose between two approaches to the rational design of organizations. The first approach is usually termed *universal theories,* since it outlines a single "best way" to enhance organizational performance. The second approach, termed a *contingency approach,* attempts to match selected design characteristics of the organization with selected factors in the environment such as technology and selected environmental differences. Below are descriptions of the major contributors to each approach.

Universal Approach

Much of what has traditionally been taught to health managers as well as what appears in trade and professional literature represents a prescriptive approach to organizational design. Two general approaches are most often presented and they have had a significant impact on the design of most health service organizations. They are the classical theory and the behavior theory.

Classical Theory. Most managers deny that their actions are based on classical themes, yet their actions suggest that this type of approach is well accepted. Using this approach, the manager is well equipped with a set of prescriptions that can be applied universally. A few of the most commonly advocated prescriptions are (Hanlon, 1974):

1. An organization should have a hierarchy, sometimes referred to as the "scalar process," wherein lines of authority and responsibility run upward and downward through several levels with a broad functional base at the bottom and a single executive head at the apex.

2. Every unit and person in the organization without exception should be answerable ultimately to the chief executive officer who occupies the supreme position in the hierarchy.

3. The principal subdivisions on the level immediately under the chief executive officer ordinarily should consist of activities grouped into divisions or bureaus on the basis of function or general purpose.

4. The number of these departments should be small enough to permit the chief executive to have an effective "span of control," yet large enough to provide effective contact with all the major functions of the organization.

5. Each of these departments should be self-contained insofar as this does not interfere with the necessity of integration and coordination.

6. Provisions should be made for staff services, both general and auxili-

ary in nature, to facilitate overall management of the organization as a whole and coordination and function of its component divisions.

7. In organizations large enough to warrant it, staff involved in certain auxiliary activities, such as personnel and finances, should be directly under the chief executive officer and should work closely with similar units in each of the line departments.

8. The distinction between staff and line activities and personnel should be recognized as an operating principle and be made clearly understood to all concerned.

The indiscriminate application of these principles results in several problems. First, the approach oversimplifies the characteristics of individuals and in fact usually ignores the interaction of individual attitudes, values, and abilities with the basic design characteristics of the organization. A second limitation is the failure of the approach to consider some of the unanticipated consequences. Several researchers have attempted to document these consequences.

Use of rules and standard procedures: Organizations require predictability to assure that services are provided in a predictable manner, that rules and standard procedures are implemented, and that personnel policies are designed to ensure role compliance among organizational personnel. The unanticipated consequences of this dependence on rules are that (1) the rules become an end in themselves, and (2) the rules are applied indiscriminately without any attention to the unique circumstances in which the rules are being applied (Merton, 1957).

In health service organizations it is impossible to develop rules to cover all situations. A mindless employee following the rules can do a great deal of damage or at least destroy the illusion that the organization is concerned with the welfare of the community and its citizens.

Delegation of authority: As organizations expand, managers often find it necessary to create subunits and delegate authority for the management of these subunits (Selznik, 1949). Unfortunately, there is a risk that the unit will develop its own dynamic and set of objectives independent of the overall goals of the organization. Under this process, termed *suboptimization,* the subunit activities begin to take precedence over the larger goals of the organization.

Use of impersonal rules to guide performance: The presence of managers closely supervising organizational personnel may have a detrimental effect on their overall performance. To minimize this effect, managers are often encouraged to develop guidelines or standards for the behavior/performance of employees. The unanticipated consequence is that the standards become the minimal accepted level of behavior. As managers become aware of this behavior, they respond by developing additional rules, procedures, and standards that create an increasing spiral of tension between managers and their personnel (Gouldner, 1954).

Behavioral Theory. As a reaction against the simplistic assumptions about individuals as well as the unanticipated consequences of many of the classical principles, social and behavioral scientists have attempted to design organizations that acknowledge the characteristics of individuals.* Perhaps the best developed of these behavioral approaches is illustrated by Likert's model (1961, 1967). Under this model of organizational design Likert tries to capitalize on the growing literature of behavioral science. The model that was eventually developed was based on four guiding principles:

- Group processes maximize motivation.
- Motivations need to be channeled—therefore, the need for clustering in small groups or families.
- An individual is a member of two work units.
- Communication feedback loops are short.

Based on these assumptions, Likert argued that organizations can be described in terms of eight dimensions, each of which is on a continuum with classical design organizations at one extreme (system 1) and the ideal (system 4) at the other extreme. The eight dimensions and their extreme points are presented in Table 3-2.

This approach provides a conceptualization of organizational design as illustrated in Figure 3-1. The figure shows that organizations are composed of families tied together through common members acting as "linking pins." Through the organizational families as well as the membership of supervisors in more than one family, the basic design features of the organization capitalize on basic group processes within the organization, maximizing motivation and channeling it to ensure fulfillment of organizational goals.

The model has been tested extensively in various industrial settings and its supporters believe that the approach is universally applicable. Advantages cited for the approach are listed below (Katz and Kahn, 1978):

- Resolves the potential clash between the informal or primary group structures, and the formal or secondary structures. The primary

---

*Historically, the social scientists questioned neither the appropriateness of the rules nor the conceptual framework of the classical approach but only the behavioral assumptions implicit in the approach. The behavioral approach was able to coexist with the classical approach by (1) defining the phases as different (i.e., the classical deals with macro aspects of organizations, whereas social scientists deal with micro aspects of organizations), and (2) differentiating between formal and informal organizations with the latter being the province of the social scientist (Woodward, 1965).

TABLE 3-2   *Classical Design and System 4 Organization*

Classical Design Organization	System 4 Organization
1. *Leadership process* includes no perceived confidence and trust. Subordinates do not feel free to discuss job problems with their superiors, who in turn do not solicit their ideas and opinions.	1. *Leadership process* includes perceived confidence and trust between superiors and subordinates in all matters. Subordinates feel free to discuss job problems with their superiors, who in turn solicit their ideas and opinions.
2. *Motivational process* taps only physical, security, and economic motives through the use of fear and sanctions. Unfavorable attitudes toward the organization prevail among employees.	2. *Motivational process* taps a full range of motives through participatory methods. Attitudes are favorable toward the organization and its goals.
3. *Communication process* is such that information flows downward and tends to be distorted, inaccurate, and viewed with suspicion by subordinates.	3. *Communication process* is such that information flows freely throughout the organization—upward, downward, and laterally. The information is accurate and undistorted.
4. *Interaction process* is closed and restricted; subordinates have little effect on departmental goals, methods, and activities.	4. *Interaction process* is open and extensive; both superiors and subordinates are able to affect departmental goals, methods, and activities.
5. *Decision process* occurs only at the top of the organization; it is relatively centralized.	5. *Decision process* occurs at all levels through group process; it is relatively decentralized.
6. *Goal-setting process* is located at the top of the organization, discourages group participation.	6. *Goal-setting process* encourages group participation in setting high, realistic objectives.
7. *Control process* is centralized and emphasizes fixing of blame for mistakes.	7. *Control process* is dispersed throughout the organization and emphasizes self-control and problem solving.
8. *Performance goals* are low and passively sought by managers who make no commitment to developing the human resources of the organization.	8. *Performance goals* are high and actively sought by superiors, who recognize the necessity for making a full commitment to developing, through training, the human resources of the organization.

SOURCE: Adapted from R. Likert, *The Human Organization* (New York, McGraw-Hill, 1967), pp. 192–211.

group now functions to move toward organizational goals, not to set limits on organizational performance.

• Minimizes the internal organizational conflicts between competing officers and competing units. The head of a unit cannot rely on private lines to the supervisor but must work together with his or her coordinates in a group that includes the superior officer. Moreover, the supervisor cannot manipulate subordinates by maintaining separate

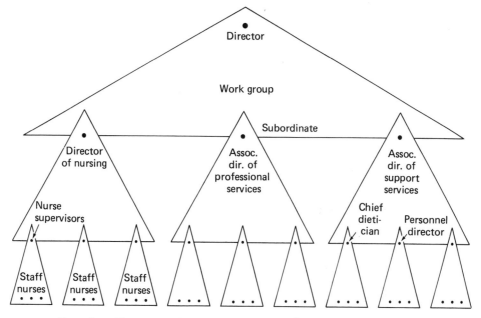

Figure 3-1 Work groups forming an organization. [Adapted from R. Likert, *The Human Organization* (New York, McGraw-Hill, 1967), p. 50.]

vertical lines of communication. Horizontal communication is maintained at the appropriate group level, thereby minimizing the need to maneuver for a more favorable position, or spend time gathering privileged pieces of information from upper levels of the organization.

- Increases the effective flow of information and removes the barriers to communication. There may not be a greater total exchange of information, but the information exchanged will be more functional for the organization. Upward communication is enhanced by the fact that it is not only the privilege of the unit head to talk about the problems of his or her own group, but it is normal and required. Downward communication is facilitated by the fact that the members who leave their "upper" group to interpret policy to their subordinates really understand and appreciate the decisions because they have been involved in them.

- More effective utilization of the skills and motivations of organizational members.

- More effective implementation of decisions, since they were often made by the same group. As Maier (1952) has demonstrated, there is a built-in acceptance of group decisions, which are in a sense the group member's own decisions.

The approach is not without limitations. Below is a list of limitations that need to be given consideration (Katz and Kahn, 1978):

- The voice of the rank-and-file personnel is greatly attenuated in its representation up the line. By the time the ordinary member's voice is reinterpreted through several levels of the organizational structure, it may be so faint as to be ghostlike.

- Specifically, the Likert model is directed primarily at the technical and task problems of the organization. The interest group conflicts in organizations over the distribution of rewards, privileges, and perquisites between hierarchical levels are difficult to meet in a system of organizational families.

- One consequence of this limitation is the need for personnel to have external representation. Overlapping hierarchical groups cannot substitute for the labor union, which cuts across all organizational families at the rank-and-file level and is still the workers' best chance of gaining representation of their interests. Legitimate differences in interests between groups may in fact be obscured by an application of the Likert model.

- The determination of the area of decision making for each organizational family is not automatically solved by the criterion of relevance to a given sector of organizational space. Decisions about specific tasks are perhaps not difficult to handle by this criterion, but decisions about the distribution of rewards, about the impact of the decision of one organizational family on another, remain difficult.

- A group process that is kept to a limited set of decisions, especially when the limits are imposed on the group, can prove unsatisfactory. Personnel may prefer their own representatives, where officers are elected and must stand for reelection on the basis of their performance, to work groups in where they do not elect their leaders and have only a remote voice in larger issues. Group process generates its own dynamic and people involved go beyond their limited directives.

Contingency Approach

Although the universal approach remains the basic orientation for many practicing administrators, it has been challenged. The contingency approach does not require that we abandon the ideas and insights gained by the classical approach, only that we understand the conditions for their application. In a sense, a new set of variables has been added in selecting the appropriate design for the organization: the nature of the organization technology and/or differences in the environment of the organization.

Below are descriptions of some of the more popular contingency theories and their relationship to the design of health service organizations. Although each contingency approach presents the same general set of relationships, each is unique in specifying the exact nature of factors upon which an organizational design is contingent. Below is a selection of models that emphasize environmental, technological, and information-processing factors as important contingencies to the design of organizations.

Task Environmental Model. The task environmental model begins with an attempt to characterize the set of environmental factors directly influencing the goal-setting activities and daily operations of the organization. These factors influence the organization's ability to obtain necessary resources, convert resources into products and services, and sell these products and services in the marketplace (Shortell, 1977).

Task environment has been defined and measured in a number of different ways. Two formulations have been applied to health service organizations.

Lawrence and Lorsch (1969b) formulation: Task environment is considered to vary along two dimensions: certainty or uncertainty of the environment and its diversity or homogeneity. Since an organization has many facets and interacts with many aspects of the environment ranging in degrees of uncertainty and diversity, two central concepts characterize the design aspects of the organization: differentiation and integration. *Differentiation* is defined as the differences in cognitive and emotional orientation among managers in different function departments and the differences in formal structure among these departments. Therefore, in an organization in which the task environment is characterized by a high degree of uncertainty and diversity, a highly differentiated organization can be expected.

A second concept associated with design is what Lawrence and Lorsch term *integration,* that is, the quality of the state of collaboration that exists among departments required to achieve unity of effort by the environment. In a highly differentiated organization, high performance is achieved to the extent to which the differentiating units are integrated.

Empirical data for the study of various industrial organizations tend to support these general relationships (Lawrence and Lorsch, 1969b). Moreover, where the approach has been used in the study of hospitals, data reveal that the greater the degree of differentiation and integration, the higher the organizational performance. The one variation in hospitals is that differentiation is more significant to organizational performance than integrative activity (Baldwin, 1972).

Shortell's (1977) formulation: A two-dimensional view of the task environment is an oversimplification. Several efforts have been made to define the principal dimensions of the organizational task environment. Below is one formulation.

- Complexity refers to the number of external factors with which an organization has to contend. Complexity may vary from high to low.

- Diversity refers to the extent to which the external factors are different from each other in the nature of the problems that they pose for the organization. Diversity may vary from high to low.

- Instability refers to the rapidity with which external factors change over time. Instability may vary from a situation in which changes occur rapidly to a situation in which changes occur very slowly or hardly at all.

- Uncertainty (unpredictability) refers to the extent to which (1) the occurrence of external factors can be predicted, and (2) the nature of the problem or content of the event can be predicted. Each dimension of uncertainty may vary from high to low.

For the sake of simplicity in considering relationships with various design characteristics and thereby deriving propositions, these four dimensions are reduced to two. Organizations operating within highly complex, diverse, unstable, and uncertain environments are said to be operating in an intense environment; those operating in simple, homogeneous, stable, and certain environments are said to be operating in less intense or tranquil environments. The approach goes on to relate various dimensions of the task environment to specific design variables, such as work specification, decision making, reward systems, coordination mechanisms, and control systems. Below are two illustrative contingency hypotheses representing the extreme ideal types.

> **Hypothesis 1.** Organizations operating in low-intensity environments are likely to experience greater efficiency and effectiveness by employing a relatively high degree of work specification, centralized-nonparticipative decision-making structures, undifferentiated reward systems, and programmed coordination and control mechanisms.

> **Hypothesis 2.** Organizations operating in highly intense environments are likely to experience greater efficiency and effectiveness by employing a relatively low degree of work specification, decentralized-participative decision making, differentiated reward systems, and nonprogrammed mechanisms of coordination and control.

In addition to dealing with ideal types, the approach offers a number of hypotheses by which design characteristics vary with the nature of the task environment. For example:

> **Hypothesis 3.** Organizations operating in relatively low-intensity environments but with low ability to predict the content of future changes are likely to experience greater efficiency and effectiveness by employing a somewhat more participative decision-making structure than organizations operating in hypothesis 1.

Hypothesis 4. Organizations operating in relatively low-intensity environments but with a high rate of environmental change are likely to experience greater efficiency and effectiveness by employing a somewhat more decentralized decision-making structure than organizations operating in hypothesis 1. [Shortell, 1977, pp. 288-291]

Each hypothesis identifies different design variables that relate to particular aspects of the task environment. Hypothesis 3 focuses on the relationship between low predictability and participative decision making. The rationale is that through more participative decision making, a wider range of knowledge may be drawn upon to adapt to the consequences of the change. Similarly, hypothesis 4 focuses on the relationship between the rate of environmental change and decentralized decision making. According to this hypothesis, decentralized decision making provides greater flexibility and thereby permits the organization to adapt quickly to frequently occurring changes.

The testing of an application of this formulation is incomplete. However, one study has presented partial support. A study of 33 proprietary nursing homes finds that efficiencies are associated with nondifferentiated rewards, a centralized decision-making structure, and formal rules for coordinating work in low-intensity task environments. There is no significant relationship for nursing homes operating in high-intensity environments (Smith et al., 1979).

Information-Processing Model. In this model the contingent variable is the uncertainty of the task (Galbraith, 1973, 1977). The underlying proposition is that the greater the uncertainty of the task, the greater the amount of information that has to be processed by decision makers. *Uncertainty* is defined as the difference between the amount of information required to perform the task and the amount of information already possessed by the organization.

The model outlines the types of design strategies that are possible. Given limited or moderate uncertainty, the organization is able to coordinate activities successfully by setting goals, applying prescribed rules and regulations, and relying on the basic hierarchy of the organization. However, as task uncertainty increases, these design strategies prove ineffective and new approaches are required. Two approaches are outlined which can increase organizational capacity and enable the organization to handle more information. The first two methods reduce the need for information and the latter two methods increase the information-processing capacity of the organization.

Reducing the need for information is achieved through creating slack resources in the organization or through creating self-contained tasks. The creation of slack resources through a reduction in expected performance levels reduces the amount of information required to perform at an acceptable level. For example, limiting the comprehensiveness and continuity of care provided in a hospital to specific episodic diseases reduces the number of exceptions that must be considered on an individual basis. This reduces the amount of information that must be processed.

The creation of self-contained tasks also reduces the need for information. Under this approach, work groups have all the resources necessary to function, thereby reducing the amount of information that must be processed.

Increasing the capacity to process information is achieved through the development of vertical information systems and the creation of lateral relations. Vertical information systems refers to computers and decision algorithms to provide mechanisms for processing information without overloading hierarchical communication channels. Patient scheduling schemes and management information systems are illustrations of vertical information systems.

Finally, the creation of lateral relations provides a mechanism for decision making across lines of authority. Using this approach, decisions are made at the level where information is available rather than transmitting information to a central point for decision. Lateral relations may involve direct contact of individuals from separate departments attempting to resolve the same problem. More complex types of lateral relations include task forces, coordinating roles, and matrix designs.

Technology Model. One variable given special attention within the organization's environment and its impact on design characteristics is technology. Although the term "technology" has been used in a number of ways, it is not our purpose to view the various meanings but rather to isolate the critical context of the term. At the simplest level, technology is what the organization uses to convert human and material resources into some product or service. This conversion process may be characterized by predictability of the search for the appropriate technology or by complexity of the conversion process.

With technology as a critical contingency variable, several relationships may be hypothesized. For example (Scott et al., 1976):

- When the complexity of the technology is high, the greater the differentiation of structure, the better the quality of care.
- When the complexity of technology is high, the higher the staff qualifications, the better the quality of care.
- When the uncertainty of the technology is high, the greater the formalization of procedures, the poorer the quality of care.

Theoretical interest in technology and its effect on design variables will continue. Research in the relationship of technology to design in nonhealth service organizations suggests that it is not the sole determinant of design characteristics. Its exact role in health service organizations, however, needs further investigation.

Organizational/Individual Relationships. The final contingency model involves the interface between the individual and the design characteristics of the organization. This model assumes that motivation of individuals is a function of the development of the individuals and the nature of the current organizational design (Lorsch, 1973). Motivation may be enhanced by attempting to affect the individual sets of values and perceptions to fit better the design characteristics of the organization, or designing the organization to fit better the characteristics of the individual. Individuals may be influenced by motivational training and through criteria selection for promotion of individuals. These approaches and relevant conceptual models are discussed in Chapter 9.

Organizations can be affected by altering the task or the grouping of task roles and activities to fit the expectations of the individual. For example, in an organization where individuals are characterized by high needs for achievement and affiliation, it is important that design characteristics meet both these expectations. Structure that places great emphasis on standards, and a management style in which administrators act as coaches, increase expectations that the needs for achievement and affiliation will be satisfied. Although this approach is a contingency-based theory of organizational design, it has received only limited attention in the organizational literature and no attention in the health services literature. It obviously needs to be tested before it receives the same respect as the other contingency models.

Ecological Perspective

A growing criticism of the contingency model in both industrial and health service organizations is that the relationships involving the environment, the organization, or the individual are tautological (Meyer, 1978). That is, the idea of fit between design and environment and between design and individual characteristics is in principle, if not in practice, closely related to effectiveness.

An alternative view that retains the role of environment but not the tautological relationship to performance is the ecological approach to organizations. This approach suggests that design characteristics are a function of the organization's environment, and although the organization is, over time, moving toward a better fit with its environment, the approach makes no judgment as to whether this fit represents a better organization. The ecological model does not intend to account for short-run changes in design but instead accounts for long-run transformation in the design characteristics. The model is intellectually based on the natural selection model of biological ecology. It explains design as well as the emergence of new types of organizations with their own design characteristics by examining the nature and distribution of resources in the organization's environment (Aldrich, 1979).

This model can be easily applied to understanding various design developments in health service organizations. For example, Longest (1979) reviews the development of various design strategies that resulted as hospital environment changed from a supportive to a less supportive environment over a 30-year period. Using indicators of political and economic resources to characterize the hospital's environment, significant design changes can be noted. In more supportive environments (1950–1969) hospitals expanded in traditional areas and maintained their traditional design characteristics. That is, the period recorded an increase in the number of community hospitals, the number of community hospital beds, and an increase in inpatient days and full-time equivalent inpatient medical–surgical personnel.

The period between 1967 and 1977 began the transfer from a highly supportive to a less supportive environment. Although resources and demand continued to expand during this period, there were already signs of an increasingly hostile environment. That is, hospitals were confronted with an increasing array of control mechanisms and the development of alternatives to hospitals, such as health maintenance organizations. This is reflected in the slowing rate of growth in traditional areas of service, increased diversification, and increased coalition among community hospitals.

Finally, in nonsupportive environments (1977–present) where resources are limited, hospital growth rates slowed significantly. To accommodate this change, hospitals underwent major redesign efforts, such as mergers, the development of shared services, and the use of contract management.

Evolutionary Perspective

Whereas the ecological and contingency perspectives look to the outside to explain design characteristics, the evolutionary perspective looks to the internal dynamics of the organization. Two variations of this perspective are relevant to the design of health service organizations.

Power Perspective

Organizational design may attempt to maximize various indices of effectiveness, or it may reflect the nature and distribution of resources in the organization's environment. An alternative view is that design is simply a mirror of the preference and interests of those served by the organization. From this perspective, technology becomes a tool in the design rather than a determinant of it. Actually, the cause and effect of relationships are reversed. Social power groups affect organizational structure; in turn, structure affects which technology is used. For example, the success of scientific management approaches has been inversely related to the power of the groups to whom the method has been applied. The difficulty encountered in attempting to get physicians to use standardized computer records is greater than that encountered in training laundry workers to use automated equipment. Groups that have power jealously guard their domain (Smith and Kaluzny, 1975).

Phasing Perspective

A final view of design suggests that future design will be determined less by external factors or by internal power distributions and more by the logical unfolding of the organization's history. Under this perspective, critical design issues can be predicted by knowing the age and size of the organization (Greiner, 1972; Adizes, 1979).

As illustrated in Figure 3-2, organizations go through a series of specific phases of evolution and revolution, with each evolutionary period creating its own revolution. Each evolutionary period is characterized by the dominant management style used to achieve growth, whereas the revolutionary period is characterized by the dominant management problem that must be solved for organizational development to occur. For example, in the early stages of growth through creativity, a crisis of leadership occurs. This crisis requires some type of managerial solution to determine whether the organization will move forward to the next stage of evolutionary growth. Health service organizations are at various phases of development. It is important for managers to recognize the current phase of development and to realize that this stage will end only with certain specific solutions. They must also recognize that these solutions are different from those applied to preceding evolutionary periods.

DESIGN STRATEGIES

Whether managers choose the rather deterministic views of the ecological and evolutionary models or feel more comfortable with the more active views of the contingency theory, they are expected to participate in design activities. Below are samples of strategies that have appeared in the health services field.

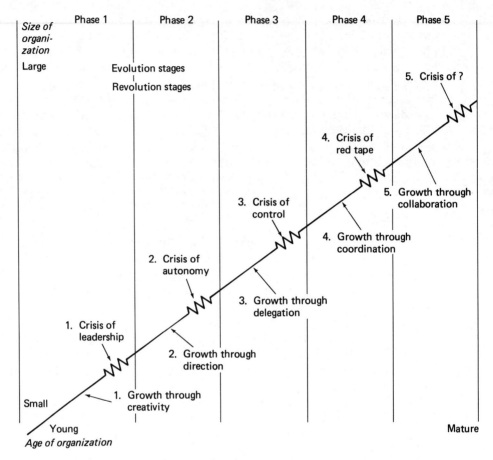

Figure 3-2 The five phases of growth. [Reprinted by permission of the Harvard Business Review. Exhibit from "Evolution and Revolution as Organizations Grow" by Larry E. Greiner (July–August 1922). Copyright 1972 by the President and Fellows of Harvard College. All rights reserved.]

Environmental Manipulation

One approach is to maintain the basic design features of the organization but to attempt to influence the environment, thereby making the environment more congruent with the existing design. This approach has been termed "strategic choice" and suggests that the environment, rather than posing structural imperatives on the design of the organization, is mediated by important decisions made by persons having the power to initiate actions (Child, 1972).

The ability to manipulate the environment successfully is extremely difficult. However, in the health services area there are many illustrations of "strategic choice." For example, the very development of Blue Cross as a third-party financing mechanism for hospitals illustrates a "strategic choice."

Blue Cross provided a vehicle for the continuation of financial resources without requiring any modification on the basic design of hospitals or the health services system. As described by Sylvia Law (1976):

> Hospitals were hard hit by the depression. In one year, 1929 to 1930, the average hospital receipts per patient fell from $236.12 to $59.26. Average percent of occupancy fell from 71.28% to 64.1%. Average deficits as a percentage of disbursements rose from 15.2% to 20.6%. The hospitals had an immediate interest in developing a stable source of payment for services and also had the technical and financial resources to create such a program. Of 39 Blue Cross plans established in the early 1930s, 22 obtained all of their initial funds from hospitals; five were partially financed by hospitals.

Hospitals and their relationship with Blue Cross are not unique. Paul Feldstein (1977), in an extensive study of health professional organizations (including health manpower associations representing physicians, dentists, and registered nurses) and nonprofit health institutions (associations representing voluntary hospitals, Blue Cross, and medical and dental schools) assesses the demand for health care legislation supportive of their own activities as a way in which organizations influence their environment. Analyses reveal that the associations varied in their ability to develop legislation to their own benefit. Nevertheless, all groups actively participated and the process has important, but not always positive, implications for the larger health services system and the consumers of its services.

"Strategic choice" also occurs among more direct service providers. Perhaps the classic illustration is among drug companies. These organizations were able to control effectively three aspects of their environment: pricing and distribution, patent and copyright laws, and their relationships with other relevant organizations (Hirsch, 1975). For example, in the area of pricing and distribution, drug manufacturers (through the formation of the National Pharmaceutical Council) were able to redefine the term "substitution" at the retail level. Its initial definition prohibited the provision of different types of drugs from those prescribed by the physician. However, under redefinition "substitution" prohibits the druggist from substituting one manufacturer's brand name for another.

Similarly, in the area of copyright and patent laws, drug companies were able to extend patent protection to all new drug discoveries under the premise that patent protection was necessary to encourage new research and to develop new drugs. Although it may have encouraged some new research, the primary effect was to increase the number of patents awarded to variations of existing drugs.

Finally, the control of the environment requires coalition formations with important organizations such as the American Medical Association. Hirsch (1975) nicely documents the drug companies' ability to affect the change in the American Medical Association drug advertisement policy. Before 1950 the AMA acted as a major gatekeeper, permitting only the originating drug company to advertise in its journals by brand name. All other drug companies could advertise only by generic name until the particular drug was evaluated by the AMA's own Council on Drugs. After 1950 all drug companies could advertise by brand name if certified by the Federal Drug Administration. This alliance brought increased revenues for both the AMA and the drug companies.

Multi-Organizational Networks

An increasingly popular form of organizational design is the development of networks among a set of hospitals. These networks take many forms, ranging from the simple sharing of clinical or administrative services to a formal merger of previously separate organizational entities. Four basic types of multi-institutional design have emerged (Reynolds and Stunden, 1978).

The consortium model is usually the first step in the development of a multi-institutional network. Under this arrangement the hospital retains individual autonomy, and efforts are devoted primarily to the voluntary coordination or implementation of various types of shared service arrangements. The sharing of services or coordination of activities usually begins with service departments (e.g., purchasing and coordinated home care arrangements) and slowly moves to the coordination or sharing of major clinical departments, such as radiology or laboratory services.

The overlapping board model is a further formalization of the consortium approach. Here there is consolidation of respective hospital boards into an integrated governing board with representation from each of the participating institutions. The integrated governing board has substantially more authority over the operations of the respective institutions than do the boards in the consortium model.

The holding company model presents a formalized effort at design of an overall system, yet it retains some of the autonomy of the respective institutions. Each hospital retains its own individual board and management; however, overall operations within the corporate structure are governed by the corporate board and its management.

The final model in the development of a multi-hospital system is the corporate approach. Under this arrangement the corporate board and its management are directly responsible for the operations of the respective hospitals, whereas the operations of the respective institutions are totally directed by corporate policies.

Contract Management

A particular form of multi-organizational networks is known as contract management. Under this design, one entity manages the organization with ownership residing with someone else.

A management contract usually contains the following elements (Brown and Money, 1976).

- The board of directors of the managed hospital controls policy and retains legal responsibility for and ownership of the facility.

- The managing organization appoints an administrator, subject to board approval, and pays the administrator's salary.

- The administrator manages the operation of the facility under a budget approved by the board of directors and obtains approval of key decisions from the board.

- Specialized services and personnel are provided to the managed hospital by the managing corporation. The administrator may implement new management systems, conduct assessment studies, suggest changes in services, and take daily managerial responsibility for the institution. All major changes and operations or activities are typically performed with the approval of the board of directors.

The approach offers several advantages. First and perhaps most critical is that it provides the contracting institution with backup resources that otherwise would not be available. Thus it is possible for the organization to benefit from standardized procedures and obtain better prices through group purchasing. Second, contract management provides stability in managerial positions, since administrators operating under the contract are replaced by the managing corporation. This is particularly important in small rural hospitals, where it is difficult to recruit and retain qualified management personnel.

Supporting Research: How Effective Are Multi-Institutional Networks? There is considerable debate over the relative effectiveness of multi-institutional systems. The debate centers on a number of critical questions. For example, are multi-institutional arrangements able to benefit from the economies of scale? Are multi-institutional arrangements able to attract better personnel or expand service areas? What are the benefits to the organization versus the community?

In an extensive review of available research, the results are mixed (Zuckerman, 1979; Zuckerman and Weeks, 1979). The review concludes that the economies of scale evidently do appear; however, they are limited to supporting and hotel-type service activities. There also appears to be improved access, availability, and scope of hospital services, primarily in underserved areas. Finally, there appears to be an increased ability to successfully recruit and retain clinical personnel. The overall impact of economic benefits for patient care and medical service areas remains to be determined, together with the differential effect on aspects of organizational and community activities.

The debate, as well as the expansion of multi-institutional systems, will undoubtedly continue for the next decade. However, much can be learned from other industries which have already experienced consolidation and merger activity. In a recent review (Schramm, 1980) of several for-profit sector industries (banking, transportation, and retail groceries), experience suggests that mergers do not always result in expected operating efficiencies or other envisioned reductions of per unit price. As stated by Schramm (1980):

> Consolidation undertaken on the rationale that the resulting institution will be more efficient, generally sounder economically, more able to accrue operating surpluses or more ready to meet the demands of the future may be ill advised. The process of engineering a consolidation of two firms is complicated, costly and never certain of success. Those contemplating mergers should recall that the return-to-scale efficiencies expected of many mergers never are realized. Further, long after the institution has been consolidated, the new entity may be subject to scrutiny for the actions of one of the pre-existing firms which were allegedly violative of established rules of conduct. [P. 61]

He goes on to state:

> Mergers are complicated and difficult to execute in large measure because of conflicting interest of trustees/owners. . . . While government may encourage mergers among hospitals, the lesson from other industries seems to indicate that if a significant number of hospital consolidations take place, increased government regulation of the industry is likely to follow. [P. 73]

Matrix Design

Health service organizations are faced with two simultaneous structural problems. The first is how to differentiate personnel and functions into specialty areas, or how to create a division of labor among personnel. The second problem is how to integrate the various specialized tasks into a meaningful whole. The matrix design provides a mechanism for providing integration and specialization at the same time (Davis and Lawrence, 1977).

Matrix design has been the primary design for many health service organizations. However, until legitimized by the aerospace industry, it was always considered an anomaly.

An example of a matrix organization is presented in Figure 3–3. In this arrangement there is the traditional vertical or hierarchical control within the respective departments, but there is also the lateral or horizontal control generated by the interaction with the medical staff through patient care teams and various committees.

This general concept has been formalized with the development of the service unit manager. This approach has shifted a set of traditional nursing

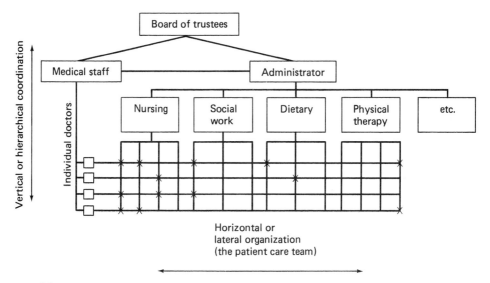

(X) Indicates a member of both a department and a patient care team.

Figure 3-3 Hospitals and matrix design. (D. Neuhauser, "The Hospital as a Matrix Organization," *Hospital Administration* (Fall 1972), 20.]

activities, such as nonprofessional patient services, unit service activities, informational and reporting activities, and coordination activities with other patient care departments, to a service unit manager. Nursing activities can then focus on professional patient care, such as patient teaching, patient monitoring, preparation of patient care plans, and patient care activities that require professional judgment (Munson, 1973).

This approach has been used in a number of inpatient as well as outpatient activities. Figure 3-4 illustrates a matrix design using a unit manager in an inpatient setting. As seen from the figure, individuals in the work groups are responsible both to the unit manager (representing a task or purpose formulation) and to their respective functional supervisors, such as nursing, internal medicine, pediatrics, and social work. This particular design forces decision making to the most relevant unit and at the same time provides professional personnel with necessary identification and support from their respective functional or professional colleagues.

The approach, however, is not without problems. Perhaps the most critical is the inability of individuals to reconcile the potentially conflicting expectations of both professional or functional personnel and the expectations of service unit managers.

Other difficulties include a misconception of the actual operation of the matrix design (Davis and Lawrence, 1977). For example, it is easy to confuse the matrix design with group decision making. This is a form of "groupitis"

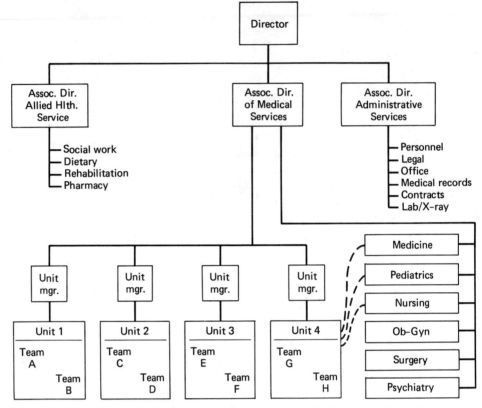

Figure 3-4 Inpatient unit manager. [Adapted from I. M. Rusin et al., *Managing Human Resources in Health Care Organizations: An Applied Approach* (Reston, Va.: Reston, 1978), p. 283.]

in which there is a mistaken idea that all decisions must be hammered out in group meetings. This misconception eventually results in the strangulation of the entire decision-making process and in personnel spending many hours discussing rather than resolving problems.

Another problem is the preoccupation with the internal dynamics of the matrix instead of dealing with the substantive problems of service delivery. In this situation the service unit manager tends to get absorbed in the internal interpersonal relations at the expense of service delivery and the welfare of patients being served. All of these problems can be resolved or prevented if individuals are aware of the functions as well as the limitations of the matrix design.

Job Enlargement and Enrichment

At the most basic level of design, managers need to be concerned with the content and arrangement of activities within roles and positions. Two concepts, job enlargement (the horizontal expansion of activities within the organization) and job enrichment (the vertical enlargement of activities), are critical and need to be understood. Job enlargement involves little modification in the distribution of power within the organization. It has been severely criticized because it represents a mechanism for merely adding disagreeable tasks to already beleaguered personnel. On the other hand, job enrichment involves substantive task modifications and thereby some redistribution of power among personnel.

Since health service personnel are highly professionalized, job enrichment and enlargement activities have had only limited effect in health service organizations. Perhaps the significant exception is the development of the nurse practitioner as an expansion of traditional nursing activities. Although nurses are traditionally taught to assess the health status of clients and their families, the assessment skills of nurse practitioners have been expanded to enhance their expertise in data collection and in defining health and developmental problems. Based on their own judgment, practitioners have the authority to initiate specific diagnostic and treatment procedures. The nurse practitioner often assumes responsibility for the total management of a client's care, including the initiation and coordination of services provided by other health care professionals.

How this expanded role is accepted by patients and other health professionals is an area of current research. The findings suggest that nurse practitioners are generally accepted by the community. However, it is unlikely that they will develop a status of an independent, authoritative expert in the eyes of the public (Breslau, 1977). Physicians, on the other hand, have reported mixed feelings. They tend to endorse the concept of a nurse practitioner and have been willing to work with nurse practitioners in a supportive role, but a significant number of physicians would not hire one for their own practice (Lawrence et al., 1977). Similarly, health care administrators report mixed feelings, and in general there is a great deal of uncertainty, confusion, and lack of information about the nurse practitioner (Fottler and Pinchoff, 1976). The implication of these findings is that despite significant job-enrichment efforts, ultimate acceptance of expanded activities is not an easy task.

CASE 1

The Administrative Physician: An Integrative Mechanism?*

Saint Joseph Hospital is a 475-bed general nonprofit church-sponsored hospital which has been in operation since 1889. The hospital and similar hospitals in the community serve a low-growth urban area in a county that has a population of approximately 800,000.

---

*Adapted from Harris (1979b).

In the past five years St. Joseph, like other health care institutions, found itself overwhelmed with governmental and third-party rules and regulations which resulted in increasing pressures and demands on the administrative staff. Particular concern was given to the ability of the administrator and associate administrator to deal with the medical staff. To meet these concerns, the hospital considered employing a full-time physician to function as a member of the administrative staff.

The board and administration were enthusiastic about the position, but they still had the formidable task of obtaining approval and support from the medical staff. Previous experience with the medical staff had demonstrated their attitude of "hands-off, the medical staff will govern its own."

At a special meeting of the executive committee, Mr. Smith, the administrator, presented the concept of an administrative physician. The main reason cited for the position was that "with the rapidly changing concepts of delivery of health care and the ever-increasing limitations and controls being set by government and other outside parties, the expertise and judgment of a professional to assist the administrative staff is becoming more and more a necessity." The following were other reasons given for adding the position:

1. Increasing legal implications for institutions providing health care.
2. Society's and government's implication that comprehensive health care is a right.
3. Time demands of private practitioners.
4. Extension of prepaid health care.
5. Rapid increases in technology.
6. Significant concern about health care expenses.
7. Rapidly changing concepts of delivery of health care.
8. Obligations to share planning with the public and other agencies.
9. Increasing involvement of government in the delivery of and reimbursement for medical care.

As predicted, members of the executive committee were skeptical of the concept of "medical director," primarily because of the two principles of authority and responsibility. They feared that the "medical director" would be accountable to the chief executive officer for managing and supervising all medical staff functions and that, in effect, he or she would serve as a full-time, paid chief of staff.

Administration assured the committee that the job description would show the position in a staff relationship only and the title of "administrative physician" would be used instead of "medical director." The elected chief of staff would continue to be in charge of all medical staff affairs and responsible for the effective discharge of the medical staff organizational functions as set forth in the Bylaws, Rules, and Regulations of the medical staff.

After considerable deliberation the executive committee responded favorably, but they made several stipulations which were incorporated in the following job description.

Job Description

This position constitutes an employer-employee relationship designed to engage the services of a licensed physician to assist the hospital administrator in medico-administrative matters and to provide the organized medical staff with administrative assistance in its efforts to fulfill responsibilities imposed by its Bylaws, Rules, and Regulations. The incumbent in this position has no authority over individual medical staff members, other than whatever authority is granted, in written form, by the organized medical staff through its chief of staff. The incumbent shall be under the direction of the hospital administrator.

The credentials of candidates for this position may be submitted by the hospital administrator for review and recommendation to the Joint Conference Committee.

Incumbents in this position may obtain privileges for private consultative practice, subject to such privilege being recommended by the Executive Committee and approved by the Board of Trustees. In any instance where such privileges are granted, the time available for such endeavor shall be subject to limitations established by the administrator, prior to their being granted. Any activities of this nature shall be understood as being outside the scope and responsibility of the position of administrative physician.

Duties

1. To maintain external relationships by representing the hospital at local, state, and national conferences and with professional organizations.

2. To assist in continuing education programs for medical staff, nursing staff, and paramedical personnel, and to aid in furthering programs for patient/public education within and without the hospital.

3. To represent the hospital, when directed, in matters involving governmental or private third-party reimbursement and regulations.

4. To aid in the coordination efforts required by the establishment of professional educational affiliations.

5. To offer specific administrative assistance in expediting the processing of applications for medical staff memberships or reappointments.

6. To maintain professional liaison with the nursing department and medical staff to ensure that patient care needs are effectively met.

7. To assist in budget preparations, both capital and operational.

8. To assist, as requested, medical staff committees in the performing and carrying out of their functions in the appraisal of medical care rendered.

9. To serve, when directed, as an ex-officio member of medical staff committees.

10. To consult on the nature, progress, and effects of the hospital's employee health program.

11. To assist, when indicated, in specific problems identified by the hospital's social service unit.

12. To recommend specific research efforts designed to promote more effective and efficient internal or external systems of care.

13. To assist in policy development concerning the operation of a professional office facility as an adjunct to Saint Joseph Hospital.

14. To perform specific studies which might be requested by the medical staff's Executive Committee.

15. To serve on hospital committees when so requested by the Administrator.

16. To prepare reports for the administrator, as directed.

17. To study and report on significant changes in technology which might be of concern or interest to the medical staff or the administrator.

Discussion Questions

1. *What are the advantages and disadvantages of the administrative physician position?*

2. *Why is the administrative physician considered an integrative mechanism?*

3. *What problems might an administrative physician experience with physician colleagues? With administrative colleagues?*

4. *In what sense is the administrative physician a boundary role?*

CASE 2

The Design of a Local Health Center*

A local health center began operations to provide comprehensive family-centered health care services for a neighborhood where low-income families represent the significant element of the population. The particular area served by the local health center in this major city is inhabited primarily by blacks, Puerto Ricans, and elderly Jews. There are at present 12,000 families in the area, representing a total of 45,000 people to be served.

The social innovation that distinguishes the local health center is the utilization of health teams as the primary vehicle for providing "comprehensive family-centered health care." The crucial element in the philosophy of health teams is that an *entire family* becomes the patient. For example, Mrs. Jones comes to the center because she thinks she is pregnant. In addition to attending to the pregnancy, a complete diagnosis (medical, social, economic) is done of the *entire Jones family situation;* the Jones family with all its problems now becomes the concern of the health team.

---

*Adapted from Rubin, Fry, and Plovnick. *Managing Human Resources in Health Care*, 1978, chapter 3, exercise 2. Reprinted with permission of Reston Publishing Co. Inc., a Prentice-Hall Co.

The Health Team

Generally, a health team consists of approximately 12 people. The three salient roles within a health team are doctors, nurses, and family health workers. A team would then consist of one internist, one pediatrician, three nurses, six family health workers, and a part-time psychiatrist and dentist. (Several teams share each dentist and psychiatrist). Ob-gyn is a backup service for all teams but is not represented on each team.

The typical family health worker is a female who resides in the neighborhood being served by the local health center. In many ways, she is typical of the average resident—little, if any, formal education, married but her husband may not live with her, two or three children. In preparation for her role as a family health worker, she received six months of formal training as a generalist in home nursing, health education, and the like. Family health workers have no separate supervisor at the local health center and report to the nursing director.

In addition to being responsible for supervising the family health worker, practicing well-baby care, pre- and post-natal care, and so on, the nursing director is the *team coordinator*. As coordinator, the director is theoretically responsible for pulling together all the team's efforts with all its families. Nurses at the local health center report to the nursing director.

The physicians (internist, pediatrician) have typically been hospital trained to deal with acutely ill patients. Their orientation toward the center is not one of rampant idealism—"the poor people of the world need medicine." For some minority physicians (female, foreign-trained, etc.), working in the local health center is one of the better opportunities available. Each type of M.D. at the local health center reports to a specialty chief (i.e., internist, pediatrician, psychiatrist).

The basic teams, of which there are presently eight serving 1500 families each, are backed up by necessary support services. Six teams are housed in the center. The remaining two teams are housed at a satellite center near the main complex.

Two teams form a unit and share a team office, so that space is optimally utilized (while one team is having clinic hours, the other team members are involved in their outreach, record-keeping, and follow-up activities). A family record is kept with each note recorded sequentially according to problem. All material referring to the family is kept in the inner leaf of the family folder, which contains all the individual folders. The nurses and physicians practice side by side in the center. One-fourth of the nurse's time is spent on home visits, usually in conjunction with the family workers. The family health workers work primarily in the field. The nurse and family health worker meet daily. Informal communication occurs throughout the day in the team office, the team area, over the telephone, or in the cafeteria.

Once a week all team members meet for one and a half hours over lunch. The team conference originally aimed to review the health plan of all families, review multi-problem families or "prototype" families, or to use the time for organizational or administrative issues. In addition to the team conference, the internists, pediatricians, nurses, and family health workers hold their own respective weekly meetings.

The delivery of comprehensive family health care (the center's mission) via this concept of health teams (the social innovation) does not fit any existing models of traditional medical care. Doctors, for example, given their hospital experiences, are not used to dealing with family and social issues. Doctors are trained to work as loners, and when not alone they expect to be the "unchallenged boss." On a local health center health team, in some areas of work they are to report to a nurse. For reasons like these, they often experience "culture shock."

Nurses, too, are trained in a hospital. Unlike the doctors, however, they have been trained to be submissive. Those attracted to the local health center have rejected the authoritarian structure of the hospital, but some of the "protoplasm" remains. Coordinating doctors is not part of their blood. Supervising the family health workers, who are often older, from different social and ethnic backgrounds, and who understand the community far better than they, adds to the strangeness of the nurses' role on a health team.

Family health workers are asked to develop colleague relationships with internists, for example, as the team tries to understand and treat a *family* as its patient. They are from the community, live in the community, but may want to get out of the community.

Major Problems as Viewed by the Director

In a recent conversation, the director of the local health center described the major problems as follows:

> Health care is delivered to the families in the community through health teams composed of physicians, nurses, and community-based and center-trained family health workers. We are having a lot of difficulties in the operation of the health teams.
>
> We have problems with the role of the public health nurses on the teams. They are assigned as the coordinators and leaders of the health teams, but this is a very strange role for them.
>
> We have a lot of communication difficulties between the community-oriented family health workers and the professionally trained physicians and nurses.
>
> We are having a number of problems with supervision, particularly with first-line supervisors (e.g., medical records supervisor, training supervisor), who are mostly community residents whom we have trained.
>
> We're having a lot of difficulty around information flow and record-keeping. Patient records are often incomplete and in the wrong place at the wrong time. A number of referrals get lost between departments and between the center and the hospital.
>
> Another problem for me is that the top team doesn't function very much as a team. Each functional department head, such as pediatrics or obstetrics, has functional counterparts on the delivery team reporting to him or her and tends, naturally, to be more concerned with his own functional area than with the overall management of the center. This makes it difficult to get the best decisions for the whole organization.

Present Organization Structure

The present organization structure of the local health center is presented in Exhibit A. This structure outlines the various departments and functions currently comprising the health center.

EXHIBIT A: ORGANIZATIONAL STRUCTURE

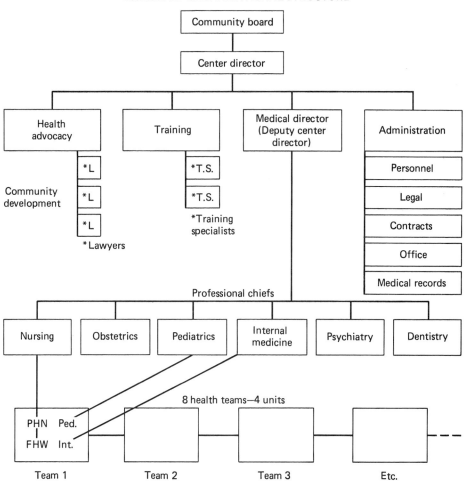

Revised Organization Structure

To help resolve some of the problems associated with the original structure, a modified matrix was proposed. Under this design, the chiefs of service were removed from the role of the primary and only supervisors of health care delivery personnel to a role of providing functional support (e.g., providing screening, in-service training, chairing monthly functional group meetings, setting professional standards, and providing functional input into the local health center policy/operations decisions). The health services director, through unit managers, became the primary operations manager of the team—a single coordinating chain of command (see Exhibit B).

EXHIBIT B: REVISED STRUCTURE

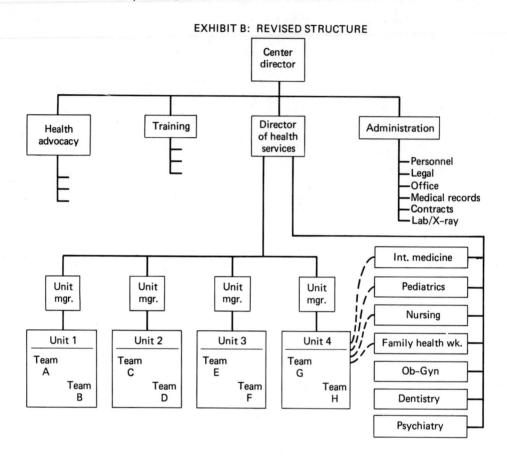

Discussion Questions

1. *What are the major problems caused by the original design of the local health center?*

2. *How does the introduction of unit managers resolve these problems? What new problems are created?*

3. *Why is the revised structure considered a* modified *matrix?*

4. *How does the development of the senior health worker position in the revised structure illustrate the differentiation-integrative process?*

FURTHER READING

BLOOM, J. R. "Team Care: Solution for Hospital Oncology Units." *Health Care Management Review* 4(4) (Fall 1979): 23–30.

CHARNS, M., and M. SCHAEFER. *Managing the Dynamics of Health Care Organizations.* Englewood Cliffs, N.J.: Prentice-Hall, 1981.

GEORGOPOULOS, B. S. *Hospital Organization Research: Review and Source Book.* Philadelphia: W. B. Saunders, 1975.

KALUZNY, A., and T. KONRAD. "Organizational Design and the Provision of Primary Care." In G. Bisbee, eds., *Innovation in Ambulatory Primary Care.* Chicago: Hospital Research and Educational Trust, 1981.

NEUHAUSER, D., and A. KOVNER, eds. *Health Services Management: Readings and Commentary.* Health Administration Press, 1978.

SMITH, D. B., and A. D. KALUZNY. *The White Labyrinth: Understanding the Organization of Health Care.* Berkeley, Calif.: McCutchan, 1975.

WEISBORD, M., P. LAWRENCE, and M. CHARNS. "The Dilemmas of Academic Medical Centers." *The Journal of Applied Behavioral Science* (July–Aug.–Sept. 1978).

4

Planning
and Budgeting

An important step in the planning and design phase of the management process is the acquisition and use of resources to assure that an organization fulfills its service mission and its financial goals. The acquisition and use of financial resources pervades all aspects of the organization. Modern health care providers recognize that a prudent use of resources is an integral part of both the day-to-day and long-range management of health care organizations. The objective of this chapter is to consider some of the major financial activities associated with the planning and design phase of the management process. Figure 4-1 provides an overview of these activities.

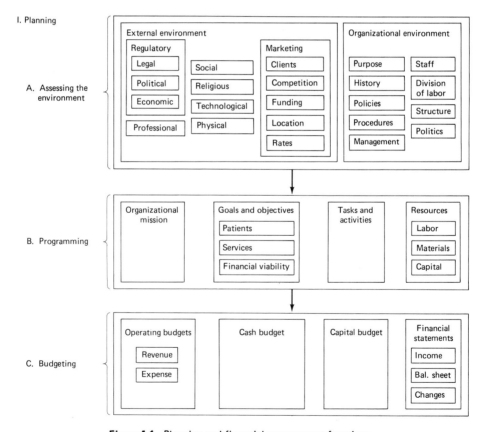

Figure 4-1 Planning and financial management functions.

The acquisition and use of resources begins with a basic understanding and constant monitoring of the environment in which the manager functions (American Hospital Association, 1973).

As described in Chapters 2 and 3, the entire managerial process functions within a larger organizational and environmental context. This context sets the limits as well as the opportunities for acquiring and using resources.

Before describing the specific environmental constraints and opportunities, it is important to distinguish two types of planning activities as they directly affect financial resources: proactive and reactive planning.

As presented in Table 4-1, *proactive* planning attempts to avoid or minimize a set of problems in the future by either influencing the change process and/or planning organizational responses to possible environmental changes. For example, local health department directors and directors of mental health centers are engaged in proactive financial planning when they lobby to change the funding patterns by which states and/or local governmental units provide money to their organizations. Similarly, health departments and mental health centers are engaging in proactive planning when they attempt to assess the impact of proposed legislation upon their health care organizations and to anticipate various organizational responses depending upon the final content of the legislation and subsequent regulations.

In practice, however, much of financial planning is limited to responding to changes that have already occurred. The problem is already at hand and the organization has to determine how to cope with the situation. This type of planning is called *reactive* planning. Examples of reactive planning include: planning how to reorganize a medical records office in response to federal edicts regarding quality assurance activities; planning to change cost accounting methods to take advantage of modification in third-party reporting guidelines for reimbursement; and planning new facilities to take advantage of changes in federal funding policies.

Whether proactive or reactive, planning begins with recognizing a problem and then trying to solve the problem in the context of the organization's environment (Vraciu, 1979). In order to develop reasonable courses of

TABLE 4-1 *Possible Organizational Planning Responses to the Change Process*

	Influences Environmental Change	Planning Responses to Environmental Change
Proactive	Attempts to influence the change process	Plans organizational responses to *possible* or impending changes
Reactive	Does *not* attempt to influence the change process	Plans organizational responses after changes have occurred

financial action, the organization must take into account its external and internal environments.

External Components

As seen in Figure 4-1, the external environment includes regulatory, professional, social, religious, marketing, technological, and physical components. Complicating the situation for health care providers is the fact that these external components are interdependent on each other as well as with those within the organization (internal environment). As a result, changes in one component affect each of the others, and often in ways that are not completely predictable. Below is a description of some of the environmental factors that must be considered in financial planning.

Regulatory Component

The regulatory component can be viewed as the economic, political, and legal factors operating at national, state, and local levels. The main effects of the regulatory component upon the financial management of a health care organization are on the amount and use of services offered and the amount and use of resources available to provide those services. Many of the effects of changes in the regulatory component on local providers stem from the passage of Medicare and Medicaid legislation. The decision of Congress to fund Medicare and Medicaid changed forever the pattern of health care funding as well as the internal management techniques employed by many health care organizations (Kinzer, 1977).

The involvement of government in reimbursement brought with it a complex set of regulations affecting all aspects of the managerial process. Figure 4-2 illustrates how the regulatory component affects major aspects of service delivery, including facilities and equipment, health manpower, and aspects of the service itself.

Many of these regulations were brought about as a result of social and political concerns with the cost of health care. The health care administrator must be knowledgeable of the various changes in the regulatory component as well as of the political context in which they take place. Even seemingly small changes in this area may have a significant effect on the policies, procedures, and resource needs of the health care organization.

The administrator must keep up with numerous regulatory activities and become familiar with various power groups and community, state, and national leaders, all of which can be helpful (or harmful) under different circumstances. Such political–social ties should be cultivated as an integral part of running a health care organization.

In addition, the general economic climate operating outside the formal regulatory system must also be monitored. For instance, deteriorating

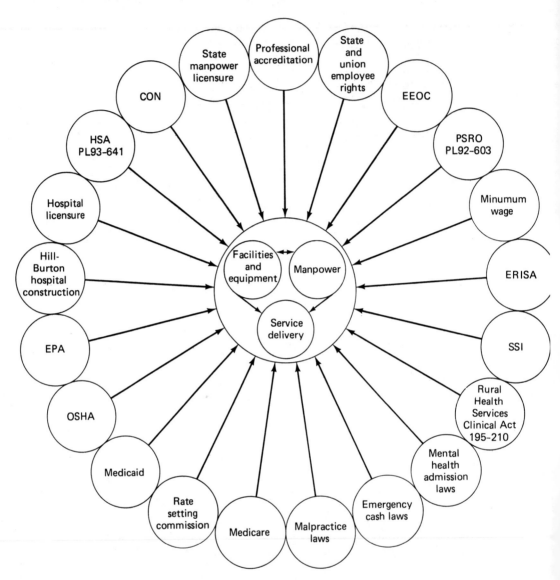

Figure 4-2 Examples of regulatory constraints on the financial management of health care organizations.

economic conditions can doubly affect the health care provider. On the one hand, poor economic conditions may result in less money available to spend on health care. On the other hand, there may be an increased demand for services due to the direct and indirect effects of the economy on the physical and mental health of the population. The combination of less money to spend and increased need for health services can pose severe financial constraints on a health care organization. Such conditions must be considered in any planning endeavor.

Professional Component

The professional component affects health care organizations in two ways: accreditation and certification. In the *accreditation process,* professional groups attest to the fact that a health care organization conforms to certain standards regarding such factors as physical safety and quality of care.

If a health care organization is below standard, various sanctions may be applied, including revocation of license, law suits, and the withholding of governmental monies. In turn, these sanctions may lead to adverse publicity and difficulties in both attracting and holding staff and patients.

The *certification process* affects the health care provider in three major ways. First, it sanctions "appropriate" education and controls licensure of health care professionals. Second, it defines which tasks are appropriate for its members to perform. Finally, professional groups can determine continuing education and experience requirements for their members. As a result of increased training requirements and narrowed job definitions, providers find their labor costs increased considerably. Because specialists must be hired in the place of generalists, labor costs may be increased both by the higher wages paid to specialists and by the fact that more persons may have to be hired. One generalist could be shifted among jobs—there is not as much flexibility with specialists.

The cost and benefits of accreditation and certification are widely debated. Few would deny that in most instances standards of service are raised or maintained as a result of accreditation and certification. But there is concern as to whether or not (in specific cases) the resulting costs to the organization and thus ultimately to the consumer are worth the benefits.

Social and Religious Components

The social and religious components affect the delivery of health care and the health care administrator in many ways, from defining health, illness, and medical problems to defining appropriate types of remedies, care, and facilities. One of the most striking examples of the interaction of the social and religious components with the delivery of health care is the issue of abortion. Health service managers must give serious consideration to the effects of such sensitive issues upon the financial viability of the organization. Not only the revenue earned from offering abortion services should be considered. The potential loss of revenue in other service areas by those who object to abortion must also be taken into account.

The manager monitoring changing social and religious components within the external environment will find other types of constraints and resources emerging as well. As certain concerns come to the fore, the health care organization may find new demands on its already stretched resources. For instance, in addition to their traditional roles, health care organizations are being asked to monitor working environments for various types of pollution, such as radiation and other cancer-causing agents. Such services may be very costly, and management must see to it that costs of such services are covered.

Conversely, though, changing social concerns can also provide new sources of funds. For instance, various health care providers are beginning to be involved in nutrition programs for children, teens, or adults. Similarly, others are offering weight-loss classes and cooking classes for specific populations, such as heart attack victims.

Marketing Component

Closely related to the social and religious components is the marketing component. In fact, the marketing component can be viewed as a subset of the social component. All health care providers have at least one, and often two, major markets. The first is the consumer, usually called the client or patient in health care organizations. The second market is the source of funding, which may or may not be the same as the consumer. Each of these two markets can in turn be subdivided into segments whose characteristics can be fairly well defined.

Each segment of the consumer market has different characteristics, needs, wants, and desires which must be considered, and the health care provider should be well attuned to matching the services of the organization to those of the population it is trying to serve. For example, a health care provider serving an area that is undergoing population change should be aware of the services that the new population needs and wants. Just because services have "always" been provided does not mean that the population will continue to demand or even use them.

Health care providers which anticipate the changing market may find themselves at a competitive advantage. Once consumers go to Organization X for certain health services, they are likely to continue, all else being equal. The organization that wants consumers to change behavior patterns must develop new strategies. This may be done by manipulating any of the four basic factors of marketing: service, location, promotion, or price (Kotler, 1975).

It should be noted that there is considerable debate as to whether there is a direct link between the provider and the consumer in health services. Some contend that it is not the patient who makes the choice of providers; rather, it is the doctor who makes the choice on behalf of the patient. If this is the case in a particular instance, the provider should consider how best to reach the physician and how to reasonably meet his or her needs, wants, or desires regarding the working environment and patient care.

The second major market is the funding source, which may be either public or private. On the public side, the relationship between many providers and their public funding source is undergoing significant change. Various hospitals and community health organizations are finding that their funding sources are no longer "automatically" providing funds in response to "illustrative" cases of how well the organization is helping members of the community. Rather, funding sources are demanding cost-based statistics demonstrating the efficiency, effectiveness, or economy of the provider. With the proliferation of providers competing for the same pool of money, health care providers have to consider carefully how best to appeal to their traditional funding sources, as well as look to alternative and/or supplemental sources of funding where feasible.

Technological Component

For a considerable portion of health care, the technological component is becoming a significant factor. Rapid advances are being made in drugs and in other physical developments, such as CAT scanners, biomedicine, and computerized laboratory equipment. These changes will greatly affect both a health care organization's ability to provide services and its financial position. In providing services, the health care manager must assess both the cost and the benefits of such technological innovations and respond appropriately. Major medical breakthroughs can change the need for various medical services, and health care providers must be sure they are able to redirect their resources as needed.

Physical Component

The physical component is intertwined with the delivery of health care services. It both contributes to the need for various health care services and is affected by them.

Although humanity has always had to adjust to nature in its varied forms, the by-products of urbanization, industrialization, and technology have both contributed to a more healthy population and have brought about new health concerns.

A full discussion of the relationship between the physical component and the need for health care is beyond the scope of this book. Health care administrators of the future will, however, have to be more attuned to this factor than in the past. It is likely that the physical component interacting with the technological component will bring about many new health-related problems as well as remedies to other problems. Many of these will ultimately affect the resources of health care providers.

Organizational Component

In addition to the external environment, the very nature of the organization affects its ability to acquire and use financial resources. The organization's purpose, history, policies and procedures, management and staff, division of labor and organizational structure, professional relationships, and physical location are all important factors to consider in the planning for financial resources in terms of their effect on other resources.

For instance, in considering the initiation of a new service which will bring much needed funds into the organization, the manager must take into consideration a number of factors. For example, how will the board of directors react to the provision of this new service?

Imagine how different organizations would react to the initiation of abortion services even if they generate a considerable amount of new funds. Although some organizations would feel quite comfortable in making such a decision, others would consider it a gross violation of their purpose and history regardless of the financial implications.

Similar concerns must be addressed regarding management, staff, division of labor, and organizational structure. Not only do the financially related factors of hiring, promoting, or new facilities have to be considered in making organizational changes, but the effect on morale and turnover (which may result in lower productivity) has to be considered as well. Lower productivity eventually results in either decreased revenues and/or increased costs, both of which have to be factored into various management decisions.

PROGRAMMING

Once the environment has been assessed, the health service provider must identify its mission, goals, and objectives and determine how these are to be achieved. This process is called programming (Vraciu, 1979) and involves three interactive decisions: who is going to be served, what services will be offered, and how the offering of specific services will affect the financial viability of the organization.

Whom to Serve?

Answering the question "Who is going to be served?" has two facets: identifying the target population and identifying the target health problems. Although these two decisions are often considered simultaneously, there are various health care providers which have as their major focus one or the other: people, or health problems.

For instance, certain health care providers are concerned primarily with serving a specific population, such as women, the poor, migrants, children, the aged, athletes, and arthritics. Other health care organizations have as

110

their major focus health problems such as obesity, schizophrenia, gastro-
intestinal disorders, and blood disorders. For the most part, hospitals have
taken the latter approach, while community health care organizations vary
considerably in their orientation. In some cases, who is to be served is mandated by documents of incorporation, or funding source. For instance,
federally funded community mental health centers must serve all clients
regardless of income. In other instances, such as with for-profit hospitals,
there is a wide latitude of possible target populations.

Determining who is to be served must be based not only on humanitarian
concerns, but also on an assessment of the internal and external environments and economic considerations. To the extent that resources are no
problem, financial concerns play a reduced role in this determination. However, to the extent that resources are limited (and they usually are), the
effects of serving certain patients or clients rather than others must receive
close scrutiny as to their effects on the financial viability of the organization.

What Services to Offer?

The traditional approach to determining which services to offer is called the
incremental approach. Organizations operating in this mode usually continue
to offer the same services they offered in the past, but at an expanded or
more intensive level. This occurs largely because many health care providers
receive their funding from organizations that use incremental budgeting.
Under *incremental budgeting* each organization is given a certain percentage
increase or decrease each year. In turn, health care organizations under this
approach usually pass this same percentage increase to their various departments and subunits. To the extent that this pattern is followed, the
incremental approach tends to discourage innovation and change. The
organizational units soon realize that regardless of what services they propose to offer, they usually end up with a small increase to maintain or
moderately improve their present offerings.

Recently, a number of management techniques have come to the fore
which attempt to avoid the pitfalls of the incremental approach. Some of
the better known techniques are needs assessment, zero-based budgeting,
(Pyhrr, 1970) management by objective (Deegan, 1977), and modern marketing (Kotler, 1975). Each is based to one degree or another on two fundamental concepts: the responsive organization and organizational change.

Under the concept of the *responsive organization* (Kotler, 1975), each
health care organization assesses the current needs of its target population
and designs services to meet the more crucial of these needs. The *organizational change* aspect attempts to allow organizational units to bring to top
management their justifications for modifying service or service delivery so
that resource reallocation can occur. For instance, as a result of identifying
a high incidence of child abuse in their communities, certain health care

providers have reallocated their resources to treat either the abusers or the victims of such acts. Chapter 6 discusses organizational change in much greater detail.

A major advantage of these responsive approaches is that the setting of goals and objectives becomes more flexible in times of scarce resources. Rather than cutting back each program by a common percent, priority can be determined from among various alternative services. This concept is elaborated later in this chapter in our discussion of zero-based budgeting.

In addition to deciding *which* services to offer, the organization has to decide the quality and intensity of services. Decisions must be made concerning the excellence and the amount of service that will be given to various types of patients. Given unlimited resources, questions of quality and intensity of service would not be major factors. However, since resources *are* limited, the organization must resolve these questions. Every patient cannot be seen by the "best" practitioner, nor can each receive 24-hour care and the benefit of the latest technology. The health care organization must decide which level of care it intends to offer for each service and must identify the resources needed to provide these services.

Financial Viability

Integrated with the question of "whom to serve" and "what services to offer" is the question of financial viability. There are two aspects of a health care organization's financial viability: short-run cash flows and long-range survival. Questions concerning cash flow involve making sure that sufficient cash is available to meet current obligations such as payroll and credit. Long-range financial viability involves managing the organization so that it always has sufficient assets to provide needed services.

Of immediate concern to programming is the decision concerning the relationship between revenues and expenses. That is, any particular service must be judged not only in terms of its benefits to the community, but also in terms of its costs relative to the revenues it must generate.

Just as there is "no free lunch," health care providers can provide services only if funds are available. This is a complicated procedure involving juxtaposing the costs of a particular service, such as a pharmacy or cosmetic surgery, against (1) how it contributes to paying for itself and other services that may not pay for themselves but are deemed essential, and (2) how it contributes to future needs such as replacing equipment or building new facilities.

Tasks and Resources

The result of answering the questions of "whom to serve?" and "what services to offer?" in light of the financial viability of the organization is a specification of the tasks and activities to be undertaken by the organization in the time period in question. For instance, once a mental health center decides it will provide 24-hour year-round emergency care to approximately 1000 people, it must then decide how it will go about setting up and running such a service. It might decide, for instance, that in addition to procuring facilities and staff, it will also need to forge links with the police and other community social welfare groups. It might also consider the need to advertise its services through media and public-speaking engagements. These items comprise the tasks and activities necessary to provide 24-hour emergency care. The next step is to determine what resources are necessary to complete these tasks. This will involve an assessment of facilities and staff needs, as well as transportation, insurance, utilities, consultants, supplies, and other similar resources.

BUDGETING

Budgeting can be defined as the process by which an organization's plans are expressed in terms of dollars and cents—a quantitative expression of management's plans which is the end product of the planning process and which takes place in almost all health organizations (Herkimer, 1978).

Purposes of Budgeting*

One of the major purposes of budgeting is to force managers to *plan*. Second, as a by-product of the planning and budgeting process, it helps develop coordination and cooperation within the organization. Plans made by various departments have to be coordinated. For example, a laboratory or dietary department must know about changes in the surgical case mix if it is to prepare a budget for its services for the coming year. Third, within any particular department, budgeting can help staff members become aware of their role in the organization and bring to the fore the extent to which their jobs require resources. A fourth purpose of the budgeting process is communication. By documenting the plans for the coming year(s), a budget can help communicate the goals and objectives, the types and levels of services to be delivered, the resources needed, and the income generated for a particular program.

As well as communicating the information internally, the budget communicates information to external parties interested in the health organization. For instance, in for-profit health organizations, stockholders may be quite interested in the budget for the coming year. The board of directors,

---

*For a more detailed discussion of the purposes of budgeting, see Berman and Weeks (1979).

which represents the stockholders, is liable for reviewing the budget before it is passed for the coming year. Other external groups that may be interested in the budget include rate review commissions, planning agencies, labor unions, and state budget offices.

The final purpose of budgeting is cost awareness. By preparing a budget, members of the health care organization become aware of the resources they will consume, especially when budgets are compared to past budgets, and the effects of changing programs or new prices can be seen.

Who Budgets? Responsibility Accounting

There are essentially three general organizational approaches to budgeting: top down, bottom up, and participatory (Herkimer, 1978). In the *top-down* approach, top management of the health care organization determines what is to be accomplished the next year and does most of the budget preparation. There is little involvement by the rest of the staff. This approach has the advantages of being relatively quick and closely reflects the wishes of top management. On the other hand, it has the disadvantages of lack of involvement, coordination, and communication, which can be major benefits of the budget process. Top-down budgeting is most useful in smaller organizations where the top administrator is familiar with the total organization and there is little departmentalization. However, top-down budgeting is also seen in larger health care organizations.

An alternative to top-down budgeting is the *bottom-up* approach, in which each organizational unit independently identifies its goals, objectives, and resource needs. These separate assessments are then consolidated into overall organizational budgets. The bottom-up approach relies heavily on the knowledge and abilities of the subunit administrators, often called department heads. It has the advantage of having people prepare the budget who are most familiar with what the organization does on a day-to-day basis. However, it has the major disadvantages of having little overall coordination, and not having the overall goals and objectives of the parent organization taken into account by the subunits. The bottom-up approach is most useful in highly decentralized organizations.

The *participatory* approach is essentially a combination of the top-down and bottom-up approaches. This approach begins with top management setting forth the general parameters of the budgeting process, including the goals and objectives of the total organization for the coming year(s), expected sources of revenue, and forecasts of changes in patient load and case mix. With these general parameters in mind, the department heads develop their individual budgets. This approach has the advantage of involving management at all levels and optimizing departmental and organizational goals. Major disadvantages of this approach are that it may tend to stifle innovation because top administrators dominate the process, and it may be very time consuming.

Both the bottom-up and the participatory approach rely heavily on the concept of *responsibility accounting*. Responsibility accounting assumes that responsibility and accountability go hand in hand. Those who are ultimately accountable for various budgets should also be responsible for making the budget estimates. Therefore, when department heads submit budgets, it is their responsibility to defend the budgets and to be accountable for their implementation and achievement. To be fully practical, the responsibility approach must ensure that those who are accountable for budgets have available to them feedback about how they are progressing.

An important corollary of responsibility accounting is that persons are responsible only for costs over which they have control. For instance, if the head of a primary care unit must purchase pharmaceuticals from the hospital pharmacy and the prices of the pharmacy are raised 25%, the head of the primary care unit has no control over those costs. He or she should not be held responsible for the underestimate in the budget regarding drugs. Similarly, if there are unexpected increases in travel costs or utilities over which department heads have no control, they should be held responsible for these changes only to the extent that they should have reasonably been able to anticipate them.

Responsibility accounting is carried out through *responsibility centers*. A responsibility center is a unit of an organization headed by a person who is responsible for the conduct of certain activities. In a small organization in which there is only one department with an administrator and two staff members, the department is the only responsibility center. As an organization grows, the identification of various responsibilities and the linkage of responsibility centers becomes a major concern for financial management purposes.

There are two basic type of responsibility centers: cost centers and profit centers. *Cost centers* are the organizational units for which costs can be determined. Examples of cost centers include emergency clinics, radiology labs, and dietary units in hospitals. Examples of cost centers in health departments may include sanitation, immunization, and maternal and child health. A *profit center* has all the attributes of a cost center, but in addition it is responsible for producing revenue. A profit center not only incurs costs, but it is expected to earn a profit. Examples include emergency rooms, ambulatory care centers, pharmacies, and gift shops. Profit centers are often found in decentralized organizations such as those which have geographically dispersed clinics. A person responsible for a profit center must control costs and charge adequately so that a profit is earned.

THE BUDGET PROCESS

Thus far we have discussed the two initial steps of the planning process: assessing the environment and programming. As a result of these two activities, goals and objectives are set, tasks and activities are defined, and resources are identified. Thus budgets are ultimately based upon forecasts of resource needs. Once programming is complete, budget preparation can begin (Figure 4-3). The budget preparation process results in several types of budgets: the operating budget, the cash budget, the capital budget, and pro forma financial statements (American Hospital Association, 1971).

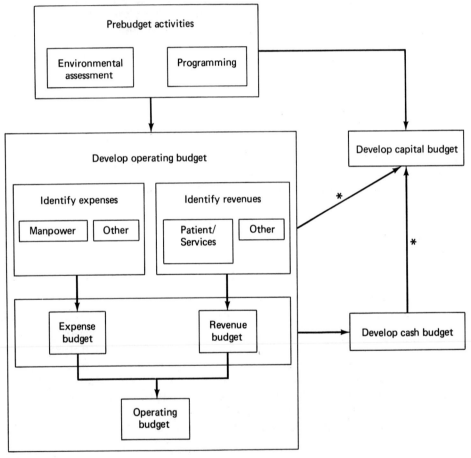

*From Long-Range Forecasts

Figure 4-3 Budget development sequence.

Types of Budgets

Operating Budget

The operating budget is actually composed of two budgets: the expense budget and the revenue budget. Theoretically, the expense budget is prepared first.

Expense Budget. The preparation of the expense budget is based on converting the resource needs identified in the planning process into dollar estimates. The first step in this process is to develop estimates of the cost of labor needed to provide services. Most health organizations have job descriptions and salary ranges for each position in the organization. With certain health care organizations, all staff is full-time and the development of the manpower cost estimate is relatively straightforward. However, with larger health care organizations, such as hospitals, HMOs, mental health centers, and various federal programs, there may be wide shifts in the number of clients seen on both a month-by-month basis and throughout each day. The task in such organizations is to develop a schedule of full- and part-time employees for the budget period, taking into account variations such as lower utilization during various months and at night and on weekends. Estimates must attempt to ensure that sufficient manpower is available to provide for regular needs, and to see that sufficient backup personnel are available in emergencies. An example of scheduling of nurses which takes such contingencies into account is given in Chapter 5. Once manpower requirements have been identified, salary expenses and disbursements can be identified.

The next step in developing the expense budget is to identify the non-labor costs for the coming year. This step is accomplished by identifying *direct* and *indirect expenses.* Direct expenses are those which are identifiable with specific services; indirect expenses cannot be traced to a specific service but are necessary for the facility to run. For instance, an inhalation therapy department might include as direct expenses the cost of oxygen and oxygen tents; a pharmacy might include the cost of pharmaceuticals; a lab might include the cost of chemical agents and disposable testing supplies; and dietary might include the cost of food and utensils.

Nonservice specific expenses, called indirect expenses, include general office supplies, administrative personnel, travel, utilities, membership dues, depreciation on buildings and equipment, insurance and bonding, mortgage interest or rent, and bad debts. These items comprise the general overhead of the facility. The manpower expenses together with the estimates of the other expenses are combined to make the expense budget (Table 4–2).

TABLE 4-2 *Expense Budget*

MGP

Expense budget, quarter ending December 31, 19xx

Salaries and benefits	$61,451
Cost of goods used	15,020
Laundry	300
Maintenance	600
Doubtful accounts	6,186
Day care	4,575
Rent	1,200
Depreciation	6,000
Telephone	405
Travel	520
	$96,257

Revenue Budget. The next step in developing the operational budget is to determine the revenues associated with the provision of services (Table 4-3). Projected service revenue is determined by multiplying the projected volume of service by the price charged for the service. The volume estimates are derived in the planning process when the amount of patients or clients using a service is projected.

There are essentially three ways in which prices may be determined. First, on the basis of rates allowable by a rate-setting commission or third party; second, on the basis of what the market will bear, that is, competitive rates; and third, on the basis of cost plus a reasonable profit. Whichever method is used, the actual cost of a service should be determined so that the amount of money earned or lost on each service is known.

After identifying service revenues, other revenues should be identified. Examples of other revenues include general donations, donations and grants for specific purposes, United Fund, investment revenues, nursing school revenues, revenues from television and telephone rental, cafeteria revenues, and funding from various tax levies in the form of budget appropriations from governmental units.

TABLE 4-3 *Revenue Budget*

MGP

Revenue budget, quarter ending December 31, 19xx

Staffing grant		$37,500
Patient revenues		
On account	$96,025	
Cash	20,435	$116,460
		$153,960

TABLE 4-4 *Cash Budget*

MGP

Budgeted statement of cash receipts and disbursements for the quarter ending December 31, 19xx

	Oct.	Nov.	Dec.	Total
Cash balance beginning	$ 1,000	$32,330	$ 9,004	$ 1,000
Cash receipts				
Collections from patients	7,260	36,620	32,328	76,208
Staffing grant	20,000	7,500	10,000	37,500
A. Total cash available before financing	28,260	76,450	51,332	
Cash disbursements:				
Supplies	1,925	4,025	3,638	9,588
Salaries and benefits	18,395	20,696	22,360	61,451
Laundry		100	100	200
Maintenance		200	200	400
Equipment purchase	23,500			23,500
Day care	1,575	1,650	1,350	4,575
Rent	400	400	400	1,200
Telephone	135	135	135	405
Travel		240	280	520
B. Total disbursements	45,930	27,446	28,463	$101,839
Cash balance before financing	(17,670)	49,004	22,869	
Minimum cash balance: 2500				
Financing				
Borrow from state	50,000			
Repayments		(40,000)	(10,000)	
Cash balance, ending	$32,330	$ 9,004	$12,869	

Cash Budget*

The next budget is the cash budget (Table 4-4). The cash budget, as opposed to the operating budget, looks at the flow of cash in and out of the organization. To clarify the difference between the cash budget and the operating budget, an understanding of the following two terms is essential: cash accounting and accrual accounting. On the *cash basis of accounting,* revenues are recognized when payments are received and expenses are recognized when they are paid. This is the way that most people keep their personal books, but it is not adequate for business. On the *accrual basis of accounting,* revenues are recognized when earned and expenses are recog-

---

*See the American Hospital Association, *Budgeting Procedures for Hospitals* (1971).

nized when incurred. Accrual accounting is recommended for all health care organizations. It has the advantages of matching revenues and expenses and more accurately reflects the use of resources in the organization. For instance, let us take an example of a small clinic that delivers $1500 worth of services and has $1000 worth of expenses.

In Table 4-5, examples 1, 2, and 3 illustrate revenues and expenses kept on a cash basis. In example 1, we assume that nobody paid cash for services; therefore, the revenues are $0. Similarly, we will assume that the organization will pay for its expenses next month. In example 1, the revenues are $0, the expenses are $0, and the net income is $0. This, of course, does not portray a very accurate picture of the financial results of the service delivery.

The second example, also on the cash basis, assumes that clients have yet to pay for their services, but the clinic did pay expenses of $1000. In this case it looks as if the clinic has a negative net income of $1000 even though it delivered $1500 worth of services. The third example assumes that two-thirds of the patients paid for their services in full, so the clinic recognized revenues of $1000. The clinic did not pay the $1000 in expenses. Therefore, net income was reported to be $1000.

It should be noted that in these three examples the recognition of revenue and expenses is dependent on (1) when the clients decide to pay for their services, and (2) management's discretion on when it pays for its expenses. This is a major reason why the accrual basis for accounting was developed.

Using the accrual basis of accounting shown in Table 4-5, the clinic recognizes that it delivered $1500 worth of services and, therefore, earned $1500 worth of revenue. Whether it collects the actual cash for earning that revenue is another question altogether and, of course, one for which management is held accountable. In earning the $1500 in revenue, $1000 worth of expenses were incurred and recognized. In other words, the accrual concept matches the use of organizational resources (expenses) and the benefits derived (revenues). Therefore, the clinic reports that it earned (not received) $1500 worth of revenue, incurred $1000 worth of expenses, and had a net income of $500.

Expense and revenue budgets, which are derived on the accrual basis of accounting, are not adequate to tell the organization what its cash flow will be. Although recognizing revenues and expenses are very important for stockholders and for determining costs, setting rates, and so on, they do not tell us about the cash flow in the organization. The cash flow, however, is very important on a day-to-day basis so that a health organization can meet its obligations to its creditors and employees. This is discussed further in Chapter 8. It should be noted at this point, however, that a cash budget helps the organization identify when it may need to borrow cash to meet its obligations and when it may have an excess of cash to invest.

TABLE 4-5 *Cash Versus Accrual Accounting*

A health clinic delivered services worth $1500, and it cost $1000 to deliver these services. What was the net income for the year?

	Cash Basis Accounting			Accrual Basis Accounting
Example:	1	2	3	
Revenues	$0[a]	$ 0[a]	$1000[a]	$1500[c]
Expenses	0[b]	1000[b]	0[b]	1000[d]
Net income	0	(1000)	1000	500

Conclusion: Only the accrual basis of accounting adequately matches expenses with revenues. The cash basis of accounting is dependent on cash flows, not service delivery and resource utilization.

[a]*Amount received from patients.*
[b]*Amount paid to creditors and employees.*
[c]*Amount of services delivered.*
[d]*Amount of resources used (expenses) to deliver $1500 worth of services.*

Capital Budget

Capital or fixed assets can be thought of as those which comprise the categories of plant, property, and equipment. These are items for which large amounts of money are often needed. Capital budgeting furnishes the organization with a systematic approach to determine which capital projects it wants to undertake, including replacement of existing fixed assets, and determining how and where it will obtain the money. A detailed discussion of capital budgeting is beyond the scope of this chapter.

Further Issues in Budgeting/Timing

Although we have discussed budgets as if they are for a single year, it is important for the administrator to look further than a year in advance. In fact, with the annual budgeting cycle in some institutions, the administrator does not even know the full budget picture a year in advance. One way to overcome such a disadvantage is to do multi-period budgeting: that is, to budget for at least three to five years in advance. Since things are more certain in the near run than the long run, the closer the budget is to the current time, the more detailed it should be. For instance, an administrator may want monthly budgeting for the current year, quarterly budgeting for the next two years, and annual budgeting for the next two or three years. By having multi-period budgets the administrator knows well in advance what the organization intends to do and how it intends to do it. The administrator also knows the organization's projected financial position (see Chapter 8), cash position, and results or operations several years in advance. If any major changes occur in the environment, hopefully there will be opportunities to adapt.

One useful approach to overcoming the nearsightedness of annual budgets is called the *continuous or rolling budget* (Herkimer, 1978). The continuous budget is like the periodic or annual budget in that it looks at the 12-month period. However, rather than developing the budget once a year, the budget is continually developed a full year in advance.

For instance, in January the budget projects a 12-month period from January to December. In February the budget is updated to include the subsequent January. In March, 12 months are projected to the next February, and so on. In this way information is provided at least a full year in advance.

Activity or Flexible Budgets*

Up to this point, budgets have been discussed as if they are static, as if they are developed for only one activity level. The problem with this approach is that forecasts in activity are not always accurate. What happens if the number of services delivered is somewhat higher or lower than forecasted? In these instances our budget may be misleading. To overcome such problems, some health providers use flexible budgets that make estimates based on different levels of activity.

Let us say that a provider has a free-standing laboratory which is estimated to deliver 10,000 tests and costs are estimated to be $40,000 (Table 4-6). Therefore, the cost is $4 a test ($40,000 ÷ 10,000). One assumption we might make is that within a reasonable range, our cost is $4 a test. Therefore, we could develop a budget for 12,000 tests and estimate that the total cost would be $48,000 (12,000 X $4). On the other hand, if we wanted to estimate for 8000 tests, expenses might be expected to be $32,000 (8000 X $4). Although this formulation makes sense intuitively, it is usually not accurate because all costs are not the same.

Returning to the 10,000-test level, costs were estimated to be $40,000. This $40,000 can be broken down into two components, fixed costs and variable costs (Cleaverly, 1978). *Fixed costs* are costs that remain the same in total regardless of the level at which we operate. For instance, whether we want one test or 10,000 tests, we will have to pay the same amount for our building each month. Other examples of fixed costs are maintenance and other overhead items, such as insurance. Let us assume that all fixed costs total $30,000.

---

*See Houser, "How to Build and Use a Flexible Budget" (1974).

TABLE 4-6 *A Flexible Budget*[a]

RVP Health Center

Flexible operating budget for January 198x

	Number of Immunizations		
	8,000	10,000	12,000
Variable costs			
Labor	$ 4,000	$ 5,000	$ 6,000
Supplies (syringes, cotton, serum, etc.)	1,600	2,000	2,400
Overhead	2,400	3,000	3,600
	8,000	10,000	12,000
Fixed costs			
Administrative	14,000	14,000	14,000
Rent, utilities, etc.	7,000	7,000	7,000
Maintenance	6,000	6,000	6,000
Other	3,000	3,000	3,000
	30,000	30,000	30,000
Total cost	$38,000	$40,000	$42,000

[a]*The flexible budget takes the fixed and variable components of cost into account. Note that regardless of the number of immunizations given, the fixed costs stay the same ($30,000) but change in their per unit cost ($3.75, $3.00, and $2.50). The variable costs remain the same per unit ($1.00) but change in total ($8,000, $10,000, $12,000) with the change in activity.*

Variable costs (Cleaverly, 1978) are costs that change in total as our volume changes, but stay the same per unit. For instance, the total cost of syringes, bandages, and supplies that we use will change depending on the number of patients. Assume that the variable costs are $10,000 to deliver 10,000 units of service. Therefore, our variable costs are $1 per unit. The total $4 per unit is made up of $3 unit fixed costs and $1 variable costs.

With this information, if we were to estimate what it costs to deliver 12,000 units, we would say that it costs $12,000 in variable costs ($1 per unit), but still only $30,000 in fixed costs. We therefore estimate that the cost is $42,000. (Note that this $42,000 is considerably lower than the $48,000 that we estimated before taking into account fixed costs and variable costs.) Also note that variable costs change in total with a change in volume (from $10,000 to $12,000) but remain the same per unit ($1). That is, the unit cost is $1 per unit at 8000, 10,000 or 12,000 units. Fixed costs act just the opposite. The fixed cost remains the same in total ($30,000) with changes in volume, but the cost per unit changes. Our fixed unit cost at 10,000 units was $3.00, but at 8000 units it is $3.75 and at 12,000 it is $2.50. You can see that flexible budgeting can be a very valuable tool. We will return to this when we discuss control.

Zero-Based Budgeting

The budgets we have discussed thus far are essentially incremental budgets. That is, we assume that the budget will be a certain percentage higher this year than last year. The disadvantages of this approach were discussed earlier in the chapter. An approach that has been developed to overcome these disadvantages is zero-based budgeting (ZBB) (Pyhrr, 1970). The basic idea behind zero-based budgeting is that no program is taken for granted. That is, just because it received funds in the past does not mean a program should again be funded or at least funded at the same level in the future. Each program or service should be justified each time it requests funds.

There are three key steps in zero-based budgeting: (1) preparing decision packages, (2) comparing the decision packages, and (3) allocating resources based on the priority of each decision package (Figure 4-4). A *decision package* is a description of one or more activities, services, or programs which are considered as a unit for funding purposes. Each decision package describes the activity, service, or units, and presents a short justification of its necessity. Finally, a request for funds is included describing what level of service can be performed at various levels of funding. For instance, the decision package for a particular service describes what could be done if the budget was funded as requested or raised or cut by 25% of the request. This is usually accompanied by a discussion of the impact of receiving various levels of funding. Of course, it takes considerable time and effort to prepare decision packages, but a number of health care providers around the country are beginning to implement zero-based budgeting programs.

Once decision packages are developed, the next step is to rank them in order of decreasing benefits to the organization. One way to do this is to first subdivide the decision packages into high, medium, and low categories and only review those which are at the highest priority level. If they are completely funded, the next level is then ranked.

The major advantage of zero-based budgeting is that it brings together in one planning process all the concepts that have been discussed in this chapter. That is, it forces administrators to plan to decide what resources are needed and to justify those resources. Although incremental budgeting was intended to do this, it is often nothing more than adding a given percentage of funds to already existing programs.

Pro Forma Financial Statements

The final step in budget preparation is to develop pro forma financial statements. There are three major financial statements: income statement, balance sheet, and statement of charges in financial position. These are discussed in detail in Chapter 11. Briefly, the income statement corresponds to the operating budget. The pro forma income statement projects the net

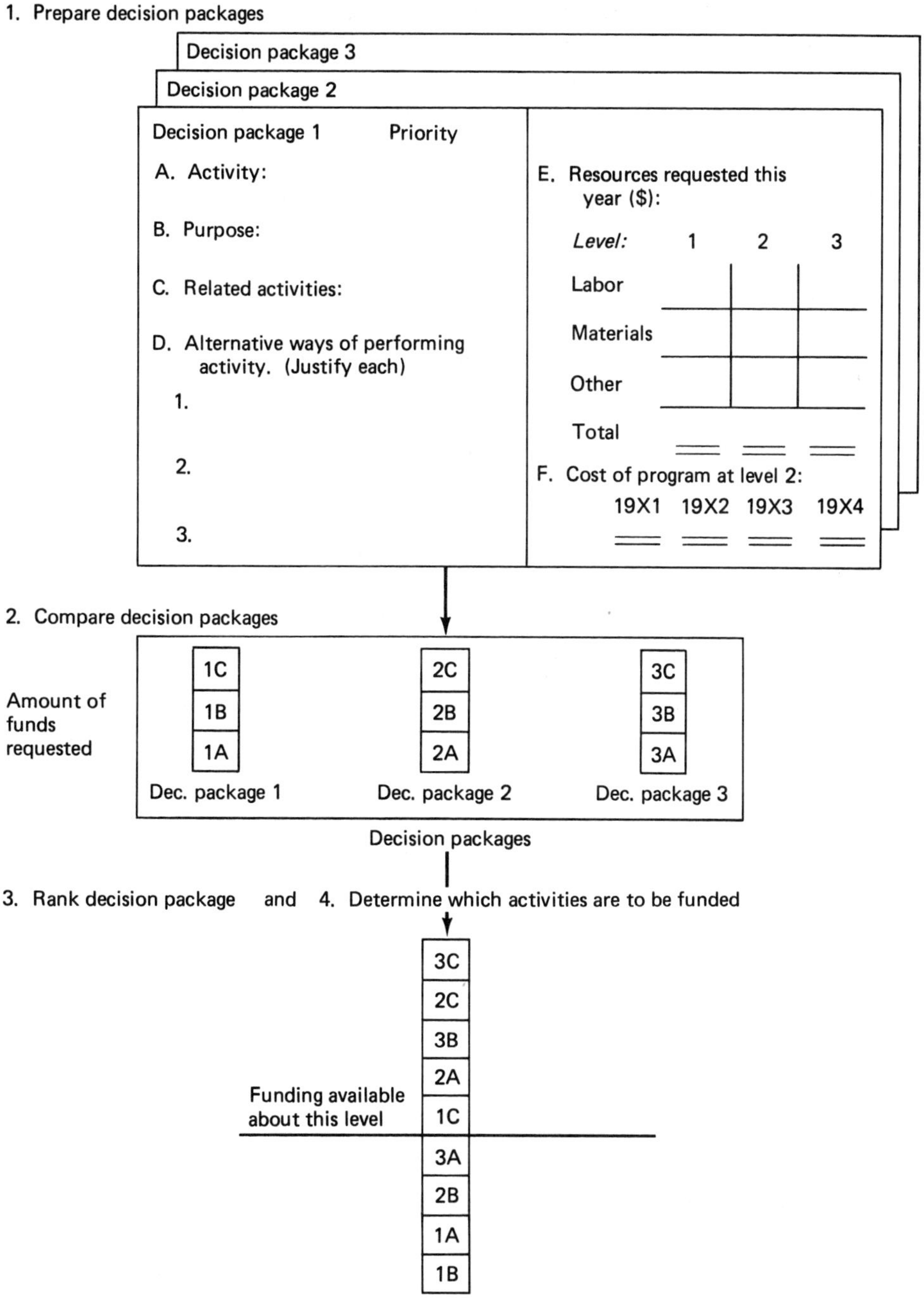
1. Prepare decision packages
Decision package 3
Decision package 2
Decision package 1
Priority
A. Activity:
B. Purpose:
C. Related activities:
D. Alternative ways of performing activity. (Justify each)
1.
2.
3.
E. Resources requested this year ($):
Level: 1 2 3
Labor
Materials
Other
Total
F. Cost of program at level 2:
19X1 19X2 19X3 19X4
2. Compare decision packages
Amount of funds requested
1C
1B
1A
2C
2B
2A
3C
3B
3A
Dec. package 1
Dec. package 2
Dec. package 3
Decision packages
3. Rank decision package and 4. Determine which activities are to be funded
3C
2C
3B
2A
1C
Funding available about this level
3A
2B
1A
1B

Figure 4-4 Basic steps in zero-based budgeting.

profit for the year if the budget is adopted. The pro forma balance sheet projects the assets and obligations of the organization at the end of the period if the budget is adopted. Finally, the statement of changes in financial position describes how changes in the financial position occurred.

CASE 1

The Budgeting Process: Conflicting Styles

Clearwater Hospital had 200 beds and a budget of approximately $10 million. It was a general medical hospital serving primarily federal beneficiaries. If there was one thing that Dr. McNamara, the director, prided himself on, it was that there were always funds available to run the hospital. His staff, though, was not quite so certain of this.

Jonas McNamara had been director of Clearwater Hospital for the last six years. He had been in the federal service for over 30 years and had been an administrator during the last 20 of these. He was approaching his fifty-fifth birthday and beginning to think of retiring.

One day over drinks, Mike Smothers and Tom Jacoby, chiefs of surgery and grounds, respectively, were discussing their plight as department heads at Clearwater Hospital. Their discussion began when they both complained about the inordinate amount of paperwork they had in relation to the forthcoming budgeting process. Dr. Smothers was especially concerned about his equipment requests for the coming fiscal year. The chief of surgery commented that this seemed to be such a futile effort, for he never knew what happened to his equipment requests once they left his office. In fact, he never did receive any feedback from the administrative officer in charge of fiscal affairs as to the disposition of his requests. This caused him considerable hardship in running his department because there never seemed to be sufficient equipment to provide services to patients at the level he felt was necessary.

Mr. Jacoby, on the other hand, revealed that he had no problems with the budget process. In fact, he was very pleased. Even though he always submitted his budget request late and with very few items, there always seemed to be more than enough money to carry out projects—even some that he did not request. For instance, just last year he was given an extra $300,000 to install a new underground watering system for the grounds. Last year he had received unrequested funds in the amount of $100,000 during the middle of summer for painting and renovating the director's home. In previous years he had received equipment to build a supply and carpentry shop as well as fill a number of staff positions he had not requested.

Dr. Smothers was so incensed with these facts that he immediately attempted to confront Dr. McNamara concerning the financial management of the hospital. Dr. Smothers was not only rebuffed, but told not to delve into areas that were not under his authority. Dr. Smothers submitted a letter to the director stating not only his concerns about the budgeting process in general, but as well, reminding the director about the number of promises of equipment he, McNamara, had made concerning the upgrading of the surgical department.

Having received no response to his letter, Dr. Smothers obtained another position and decided to resign in a very public manner. He not only sent letters of resignation to Dr. McNamara, but also sent letters to influential members of Congress.

Subsequently, an investigation was initiated which revealed, among other things, that the budgeting process took place in a rather unorthodox manner. First, all budget requests were aggregated into a single pool. Knowing that the hospital request would probably be cut back, Dr. McNamara inflated the budget figures before submitting them. Because of the federal budgeting policies at the time, he realized that once the money was allocated to the hospital, he had considerable discretion as to how it was spent. Wanting to have as much control over the budget as possible, he never informed his department heads how much money they actually received. Then, near the end of the fiscal year, he was able to decide how the money could best be spent. He usually put this money into facilities and grounds and other appearance-related items.

Within a year of Dr. Smother's resignation, Dr. McNamara was replaced by Mary Barbieto. Dr. Barbieto had graduated from the University of California with a joint M.D.-M.P.H. degree. This was her first assignment and she was hired largely because of her interpersonal skills. She set about redesigning the budget process to involve all department heads, fiscal personnel, and administrative staff.

The budget process under Dr. Barbieto began at the grass-roots level. Each department head was encouraged to meet with his or her staff to explore alternative programs. Dr. Barbieto made it known that her door was always open to anyone having any concerns about the budget process. All budget information would be shared and all department chiefs would have not only major input into the final budget, but would be kept informed of the budget process as it proceeded beyond their level.

Over time, to ensure that all essential input was available in the budgeting process, a number of forms appeared throughout the organization. By the end of the year, the budgeting process had been completely revised from that which existed under Dr. McNamara. As opposed to department heads spending approximately only one day developing their budgets, the budget process was designed to take place over a three-month period and was quite time consuming, involving many meetings, always ensuring that everyone had input into the process.

The new chief of surgery and the chief of medicine were meeting over drinks to discuss their burdens. Dr. Chandler, chief of surgery, indicated that he was relatively pleased with his new job. The major drawback was that although he had all the equipment he needed to go about designing a fine surgery department, he had to spend an inordinate amount of time in administrative tasks having to do with the means and forms connected with the budgeting process.

Discussion Questions

1. *Analyze the advantages and disadvantages of the budgeting process under Dr. McNamara.*

2. *Analyze the advantages and disadvantages of the budgeting process under Dr. Barbieto.*

3. *Compare and contrast the budgeting process under Dr. McNamara and under Dr. Barbieto. Discuss the relative advantages and disadvantages of each.*

4. *Which of the two styles of budgeting do you prefer? Why? If you are not comfortable with either style, what would you have done in Dr. Barbieto's case?*

CASE 2

The Budgeting Process: A Crisis Situation

Rodney Sneed walked into his office and sat down in his chair. Although there was a smile on his face, he had very mixed feelings about assuming the directorship of Alvondale Community Mental Health Center. On the one hand, he had achieved his goal of having his own agency within a year after having finished graduate studies in administration. On the other hand, this was really the first agency he had ever administered and he wanted to make sure that he impressed the board.

As he sat in his chair, he thought about the chain of events leading up to his present position. After graduating from college, he returned home to various jobs in the private sector, but knew that eventually he wanted to return and get a master's degree and work in local government. On completing his master's degree, he became an administrative intern with the county. In that position he performed quite well, impressing many superiors and other persons in the county. He was seen as being decisive, goal-oriented, efficient, and having a good knowledge of business principles.

As a result of the impressions he made, Mr. Sneed was asked to take over the community mental health center, which had been having a number of problems. Alvondale Community Mental Health Center had a budget deficit the last two years, and high staff turnover. Furthermore, there were allegations that it was not serving the community needs. In particular, the center was accused of having all the latest therapies, such as transactional analysis, behavior modification, and crisis intervention, which were seen as very trendy, but not relevant to serving the needs of the indigent, whom many members of the committee felt the mental health center should primarily be serving.

Mr. Sneed, of course, was concerned about accepting the position, as he did not have a background in mental health. However, it was his feeling that administration is administration and that a good administrator can work well in any organization. Later that day, Mr. Sneed sent out a memo to all staff saying that he would like to meet with each staff member and introduce himself. He completed this task within two weeks. His next major task was to develop the budget for the next year. He had some difficulties in doing this because (1) he was not completely familiar with the changes that were forthcoming in federal and state funding patterns, and (2) he was somewhat unclear as to the expectations of the community toward the Mental Health Center.

Given the problems that existed at the center, he thought it would be better not to involve all the staff in the budget process, for he felt their time was best utilized delivering services. Over the next several days he and one of the staff psychologists designed the budget for the coming year. Unfortunately, even trying to be as conservative as possible, there was a projected deficit of $100,000 in revenues to run the programs that Mr. Sneed and the staff psychologist set forth. He was now in quite a dilemma. Should he attempt to obtain more funds or cut back programs? If he decided on the latter alternative, which programs should he cut back? He really did not know which way to turn. Mr. Sneed had met his first major crisis.

Discussion Questions

1. *What are the advantages and disadvantages of the budget process undertaken by Mr. Sneed?*

2. *Was there any way that Mr. Sneed could have avoided the crisis he now finds himself in? If yes, what way? If no, why not?*

3. *What could you have done in Mr. Sneed's situation? What are the advantages and disadvantages of your approach compared to that undertaken by Mr. Sneed?*

FURTHER READING

AMERICAN HOSPITAL ASSOCIATION. *Budgeting Procedures for Hospitals.* Chicago: American Hospital Association, 1971.

AMERICAN HOSPITAL ASSOCIATION. *The Practice of Planning Health Care Institutions.* Chicago: American Hospital Association, 1973.

ANTHONY, R. N., and R. HERZLINGER. *Management Control in Non-Profit Organizations.* Homewood, Ill.: Richard D. Irwin, 1975.

BERMAN, H. J., and L. E. WEEKS. *The Financial Management of Hospitals*, 3rd ed. Ann Arbor, Mich.: Health Administration Press, 1976.

COOPER, P. D. *Health Care Marketing.* Germantown, Md.: Aspen Systems Corp., 1979.

DILLON, R. D. *Zero Based Budgeting for Health Care Institutions.* Germantown, Md.: Aspen Systems Corp., 1979.

HORNGREN, C. T. *Introduction to Management Accounting*, 4th ed. Englewood Cliffs, N.J.: Prentice-Hall, 1978, Chaps. 6–8.

SPEIGEL, A. D., and H. H. HYMAN. *Basic Health Planning Methods.* Germantown, Md.: Aspen Systems Corp., 1978.

5

Quantitative Planning

┌─────────────────────── OVERVIEW ───────────────────────┐

An important aspect of planning and design is the manner in
which basic resources are to be allocated. This in turn involves
considering numerous questions of size, such as number of beds
required, number of patients to be served, and so on. For example, in the management of hospitals: How many patients can we
expect to demand service? How large (how many beds, how many
examining rooms) should the facility be to meet demand effectively and efficiently? How many personnel should be hired?
How many days should the facility be open each week? This
chapter concentrates on the quantitative aspect of planning and
design and introduces not only a quantitative perspective, but
also some of the more typical and useful quantitative tools to aid
in planning.

└───┘

TYPES OF UNCERTAINTY

One of the most difficult aspects of planning is dealing with uncertainty.
Much of the value of quantitative techniques is in their ability to treat uncertainty in an objective, rational, and rigorous manner. This is not to say that
quantitative techniques *eliminate* uncertainty—there is no way to accomplish
that. These concepts and techniques are, however, useful for *containing* the
effects of uncertainty on the process of planning or, put another way, allow
us to plan even in the face of uncertainty.

There are two types of uncertainty. The first is uncertainty about what
will happen no matter what we (as an organization) do. In health services
delivery problems this type of uncertainty is illustrated in the question
"What will be the demand for a new outpatient clinic in five years?" Since a
clinic may have some influence on what demand will be by what services it
provides, a better question is: "What will demand be in five years if there are
adequate facilities to meet all demand?"

The second type of uncertainty is the uncertainty about what the consequences will be if we (the organization) take some action. For example, what
will be the average patient waiting time if a clinic provides exactly eight
examining rooms staffed by four physicians and six nurses, and is open five
days a week for ten hours a day? How many patients will be turned away?
How often will the eighth examining room be used? To approach this second
question, we must first have information about the first type of question:
What demand can we expect in the future?

It is useful to divide uncertainty into these two types because they are
sequential, and because two disciplines incorporating two areas of techniques
have been developed to deal with them: forecasting (for the first type) and
quantitative planning models (for the second).

We will treat each in turn, but first it is useful to review operations research as an approach, or as a framework for dealing with managerial problems. This framework will serve for both quantitative planning and quantitative decision making—the subject of Chapter 6.

THE OPERATIONS RESEARCH APPROACH

Consider a common problem faced by many health services managers: determining how many examining rooms to provide for 1986, or some other year in the future. Let us say that there are presently three examining rooms. These three rooms do not appear to be sufficient because patients have to wait for long periods of time, some patients leave without being seen, and no one knows how many people do not even come because they have heard about the overcrowded conditions. The manager's problem (actually, *part* of the problem) is determining the number of rooms to provide. What will happen if the clinic provides exactly four, five, six, or seven rooms? How long will patients wait under each alternative, and which one is "best"?

Operations research suggests that in order to solve this problem, the manager must "model" the problem, either in his mind, on paper, or perhaps in a computer. To model a problem is simply to abstract relevant aspects of the real-world problem into a conceptual model that can then be analyzed. This approach has been applied in various industrial organizations (Wagner, 1979; Hillier and Lieberman, 1974) and is receiving increased attention in health service organizations (Shuman et al., 1975). The process roughly follows that of Figure 5-1. The real world is separated from the conceptual

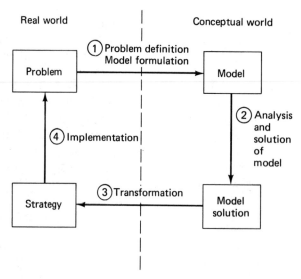

Figure 5-1 The modeling process.

world by a dashed line. The *problem,* of course, appears in the real world, and eventually it must be solved there. The modeling process calls for the problem to be carefully defined and then an *abstract model* of the real problem formulated in the conceptual world. This may be as simple as a mathematical equation, or as complex as a large computer program. For our example problems, we will first build simple mathematical models and then discuss more sophisticated and complex ones.

Once the model is formulated, the second step is to *analyze* the model in the conceptual world and to identify *model solutions.* This involves gathering data, making forecasts, taking measurements, and then determining which alternative seems best, as far as our model is concerned in the conceptual world. Usually, this analysis involves mathematics (and sometimes very complex mathematics), but common sense, rigorously applied, is extremely powerful and effective.

The solution we identify in the conceptual world (e.g., six examining rooms) must usually go through a process of *transformation* to meet the needs of the real-world problem. We call the end result of this transformation a real-world *strategy.* As the solution is transformed from the conceptual back to the real world, many considerations, such as timing, size of room, remodeling old space or building new, use of materials, and equipment, appear and must be addressed.

The last step of the process is the *implementation* of the real-world strategy, which is discussed further in the next section of chapters.

FORECASTING

Before the manager can resolve the problem of how many examining rooms should be provided, he must first have some idea of how many patients will demand service at the expanded clinic. There are more patients than can be easily handled now, but how many more? Will the number continue to increase (and by how much) each year into the future? This is an example of the first type of uncertainty described above, and we call this type of problem a *forecasting problem.*

There are two approaches to forecasting. The first is to use "expert" opinion about what will happen. In our clinic example, the manager might poll the several physicians who work in the clinic, the admitting clerk, and other "experts", and ask them how many patients they think will demand service in 1986. This might be done through individual interviews or a general meeting to "brainstorm" the question. The idea of a general meeting is that the group of experts will reach some consensus by the end of the meeting about how many patients the clinic could expect per day in 1986. More realistic than a single number of patients per day would be a *range* of patients —say "between 70 and 85."

A second method is to use the past behavior of patient demand for clinic service as an indication of future behavior. This method involves gathering data on the number of patient visits in the past, trying to establish some trend to that past behavior, and then trying to extend that trend to the future. Much of this method is quantitative in nature, and it is this method on which we will focus.

Forecasting can be divided into three types, based on the length of time into the future that the forecast must be made. We shall define the three types as:

- *Long term:* for a forecast of several years.
- *Intermediate term:* for a forecast of several months to a year.
- *Short term:* for a forecast of several hours to several days to several weeks.

In this chapter we are primarily interested in long-term forecasting, since most planning decisions require forecasts for more than a year. In Chapter 6 we discuss intermediate- and short-term forecasting with quantitative decision making.

AN ILLUSTRATION OF THE QUANTITATIVE APPROACH

To help illustrate the quantitative approach, consider the clinic manager's problem of determining the number of clinic examining rooms to provide, and the problem of how many patient visits can be expected in the future. An examination of clinic records from previous years has revealed the data presented in Table 5-1.

The technique that is most often applied to this type of forecasting problem is trend analysis. Trend analysis is the process of examining trends in the level of a phenomenon (in this case patient visits) over time. In long-term forecasting, the "over time" is usually by year, in intermediate-term by month, and in short-term by day or hour.

TABLE 5-1 *Average Weekly Examining Room Visits*

Year	Visits per Week
1976	240
1977	275
1978	279
1979	315
1980	325
1981	385

In all three cases, the method involves two important hypotheses:

1. There has been a recognizable trend in the behavior of the phenomenon in the past.
2. This trend will continue into the future.

The technique of trend analysis is applicable only to test the first assumption, and it is a powerful tool for establishing such a trend. The second assumption cannot be treated by trend analysis or by quantitative techniques in general, and is a problem for expert opinion and common sense.

In looking at the data in Table 5-1, the manager recognizes a trend in past behavior, which is that demand is growing. This is more easily seen and dealt with in graphical form as depicted in Figure 5-2.

Looking at the dots on the graph, the manager believes that there is a linear (or straight line) trend in the past data and draws a dashed line through the dots as shown in Figure 5-2. When this line is extended into the future, it seems to indicate that demand in 1986 will be 545 patients per week. This process—plotting the past data and drawing a line through them and on into the future—is forecasting by trend analysis in its simplest form. There are several pitfalls with this form.

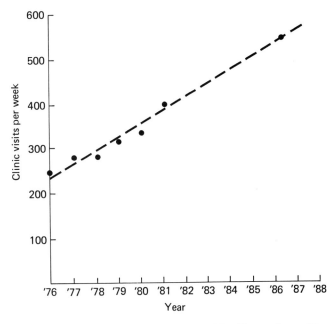

Figure 5-2 Average weekly examining room visits: Manager's trend line.

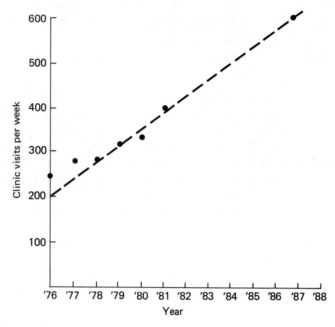

Figure 5-3   Average weekly examining room visits: Assistant's trend line.

First, when the manager's assistant draws the line, it seems to indicate that 1986 will have 600 visits (see Figure 5–3). Who is right? What is needed is some objective way to establish a "best fit" through the past data, and to use that line as the predictor. The method of least squares or linear regression is useful to address this issue, and it is discussed briefly below.

Second, the manager and his assistant tried only straight lines. Figure 5–4 shows a curved line through the dots that might explain past behavior as well as the straight lines, but it predicts a demand of 875 patients! We will address this issue after we look at the least-squares technique.

The linear regression technique for forecasting (one of several techniques under the general name of trend analysis) is a mathematical method of determining the line through the dots with the following quality: measuring the vertical distance between the dots and this line (Figure 5–5), squaring this distance, and summing up these squares; this line will have the smallest such sum of squared distances of all possible lines that can be drawn through the dots. The mathematics involved in determining this "best-fit" line by the least-squares method is beyond the scope of this book, but the analysis is easily performed on even the smallest computer and indeed on many hand calculators.

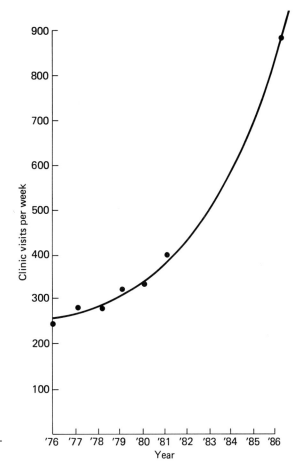

Figure 5-4 Average weekly examining room visits: Nonlinear trend line.

Once this line is determined, a tentative prediction can be made by extending it on the graph to 1986 (or any other year) as before. This must be a tentative prediction for at least two reasons: (1) we have tried only linear fits to the data, and (2) we still have no evidence that such a trend in the past will continue into the future.

The first of these reasons is addressed by trying to fit a nonlinear (curved) line to the past data. Now the mathematics is getting very sophisticated. There are computer programs that can "try" a wide variety of nonlinear trends to a set of data and compare the fits of several different nonlinear trends among themselves, and to linear fits. Using these comparisons together with knowledge about the past and common sense, the forecaster must pick the fit—linear or curve—with which he or she feels most comfortable.

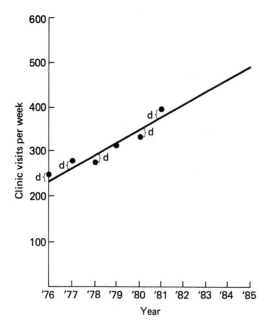

Figure 5-5 Average weekly examining room visits: Linear regression trend line.

The second reason to regard such a prediction as tentative is that the manager has yet to bring expert opinion (except his or her own) into the analysis. It is common sense and expert opinion alone that can address the question "Will the trend continue into the future?" This brings us back to our original comparison of the two methods: expert opinion and quantitative.

Both methods have advantages and disadvantages. The expert opinion method has the advantage of using insight and knowledge that no set of numbers can offer, but it also has the disadvantages of subjectivity, impression, personal bias, and other "human" qualities that limit its accuracy. On the other hand, although the quantitative method is precise, it lacks such human insight into what are usually very complex processes.

The best strategy is to combine the two methods when possible by (1) using experts to help identify which data are most useful and to make an initial prediction; (2) applying quantitative forecasting techniques to add additional insight and objectivity contained in past data; and (3) applying common sense and expert opinion to consider all evidence and to form a final prediction.

Assume that the manager follows this procedure and comes up with the estimates of Figure 5-6. These estimates of future demand are lower than the linear (dashed line) projection would suggest. This may be due to the

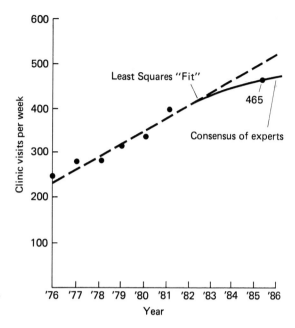

Figure 5-6 Average weekly examining room visits: Final projection.

strong consensus of the experts that some of the increase over the last several years can be attributed to a growth in popularity of the clinic, and that this growth will taper off in the future, leaving the increase to follow population growth rather than increasing popularity. These estimates, then, combine both quantitative and qualitative evidence.

This long-term growth of demand is only one type of trend that the manager must consider. There is a second type of behavior of demand for the clinic that can be seen from Figure 5-7. Notice not only the long-term growth over the years, but also the fact that demand fluctuates *within* years, being highest in the summer and lowest in the winter. Moreover, this fluctuation seems similar year after year. Such fluctuation is called "cyclical variation" and we consider it in Chapter 6.

SIMPLE QUANTITATIVE PLANNING MODELS

Once a forecast of demand is made, the second stage of the planning process is to determine the amount of resources (buildings, equipment, personnel) that the organization should provide to meet demand. The question of "how much" for our example involves not only how many examining rooms, but

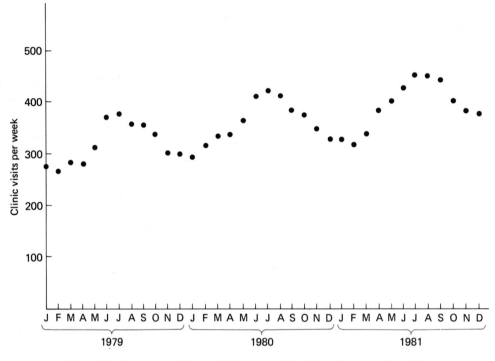

Figure 5-7 Average weekly examining room visits: Showing seasonal variation.

also how often the clinic should be open and for how long, how many physicians (and what type) should staff the clinic, what their schedules should be, and similar questions for other personnel. It also involves the size of waiting rooms, employee lounge areas, and so on. Initially, we consider (for the discussion of the planning process) the single question of how many examining rooms are needed. Our analysis will then be expanded by discussing how these other questions are addressed by quantitative planning models.

There are two important concepts to consider when converting forecasted demand to resources needed to meet demand: service time and utilization. *Service time* is the amount of time necessary to serve one unit of demand. For our example, the service time of interest is the amount of time it takes to treat the typical patient in a clinic. There are several simplifying assumptions we need to make with the concepts of "treat" and "typical" for our initial analysis. By "treat" we will begin by viewing the patient's time in the clinic (other than waiting time) as a single "service time," even though it will involve registration and perhaps some lab specimen taking, as well as examination, possibly treatment, and consultation with the physician. (Later we will break down this process into its several parts for a more sophisticated analysis.) This allows us to say that the typical patient "consumes" X number of minutes of examining room time per visit. Let us assume that we have carefully measured time spent at the clinic in a special study over several weeks, and have determined X to be 25 minutes.

The second concept, *utilization,* appears when we attempt to use the service time of 25 minutes per visit to convert demand to resources needed. From our forecast of demand (Figure 5-6) we have projected a weekly demand of 465 visits by 1986. If we assume that the clinic will be open six days a week, and demand is evenly spread out across the week, then the average daily demand will be 465 divided by 6 equals 77.5 visits. Since we have assumed that the typical patient needs 25 minutes, we then need 77.5 times 25 equals 1937.5 minutes of examining room time per day. Each examining room is available for 8 hours a day, or 8 times 60 equals 480 minutes. Our simplest estimate of how many examining rooms will be needed is 1937.5 divided by 480 equals 4 examining rooms.

There are several reasons why we may be unsatisfied with four examining rooms as our estimate of the number of rooms needed. First, the service time of 25 minutes per visit is too simplistic in two ways: (1) service represents a multi-stage process, involving registration, lab work, examination, consulting, and so on, and (2) the number of minutes per visit is not fixed, as some visits will take only a few minutes while others will take considerably longer than 25 minutes. Also, what if one day we have a nontypical mixture of service times with a preponderance of long ones? Another problem with the estimate occurs if we consider the possibility that on that same day, we have more than the average of 77.5 visits—say we have 95 on this day. Our estimate of four rooms will not adequately service this day, even if we keep all rooms busy all day.

This brings up a third problem: it is unreasonable to assume that the clinic can keep all examining rooms busy all day. We must assume that, even with patients waiting, there will be a utilization rate of something less than 100%. If there are slow spots in the day when the waiting line "dries up," there will be even lower utilization.

Utilization Model

To take into consideration all three of these variances: (1) service time, (2) daily demand, and (3) arrival patterns of patients and other room/equipment/physician scheduling problems that keep us from 100% utilization, we will use the following model, which is often called the *utilization model:*

$$\text{rooms needed} = \frac{\text{average daily demand} \times \text{average service time}}{\substack{\text{minutes per room} \times \text{target utilization} \\ \text{available per day}}}$$

This model differs from the "100% utilization" calculation only by the "target utilization" in the denominator. This is a factor used to represent the three variances discussed above in the simplest quantitative model we will consider. It is set to what is considered to be the "typical" utilization obtainable by this type of facility and it varies considerably by type of facility. For example, suppose we examine several clinics that are considered "well designed" in terms of size; that is, they seem to accommodate demand with little waiting by patients, and at the same time seem to keep rooms and personnel efficiently utilized. This assessment involves a value judgment of appropriateness, but such judgments can be made by experienced managers familiar with facility operations. The utilization of this "appropriate-sized" facility becomes the "target utilization rate" in our model. Let us assume it to be 80%, or 0.80, and our equation becomes

$$\text{rooms needed} = \frac{77.5 \times 25}{480 \times 0.80} = 5$$

The more general form of the utilization model, which can be used as a simple model for many facility size or staff (personnel) size problems, is

$$\begin{array}{l} \text{number of units} \\ \text{of resource needed} = \\ \text{per time period} \end{array} \frac{\begin{array}{l}\text{average number of} \qquad \text{minutes of resource} \\ \text{patients per time period} \times \text{needed per patient}\end{array}}{\begin{array}{l}\text{minutes of resource available} \times \text{target utilization} \\ \text{per unit per time period}\end{array}}$$

To illustrate this general model, consider two additional examples: nurse staffing and inpatient bed planning.

The nurse staffing planning problem involves the prediction of how many nurses are needed per shift to care for patients on a given nursing unit. To make the problem simple, we will consider the need for all skill classes of nursing personnel, instead of separately considering RNs, LPNs, and so on. The model for the nurse staffing planning problem is

$$\begin{array}{l}\text{number of nurses} \\ \text{needed for the day shift} =\end{array} \frac{\begin{array}{l}\text{average number of} \qquad \text{minutes of care needed} \\ \text{patients on day shift} \times \text{per patient per shift}\end{array}}{\begin{array}{l}\text{minutes per shift} \times \text{target utilization} \\ \text{each nurse works}\end{array}}$$

There are several forecasting and measurement problems involved in specifying the number for the terms in this model. First, the average number of patients on the unit is a common forecasting problem for hospitals, as it determines not only the need for nursing care, but also the need for most other hospital resources, including dietary, lab, and physical therapy, and it determines revenue. Let us assume that this number, called the average census on the unit, has been estimated at 35 patients for weekdays, and 25 for weekends. As with our clinic problem, this assumption carries with it the recognition that the actual census will be either higher or lower on any given day.

The second measurement problem is to determine the minutes of nursing care required per patient. Again, not all patients are the same, and even the same patient requires a different amount of care each day. Thus this number also represents the average over a range of time. Let us say that we have carefully observed nursing care on the unit for a study period of several weeks and have determined that the typical (or average) patient needs 60 minutes of nursing care per shift on the day shift.

In the denominator of our model, the first term is simply 8 hours times 60 minutes per hour equals 480 minutes. The second term, target utilization, can typically be set surprisingly high: 80 to 85%, even in the face of the consideration of variance discussed above. This is true for the nurse staffing model for several reasons. First, if the unit is running a census at near capacity on weekdays—say that there are 37 beds and that the average census is 35—the number of patients will not vary a great deal. Second, if the number of patients is large (as with our case of 35), the variance from different types of patients tends to "wash out" somewhat, with the high-care patients balancing the low-care patients. This would not be true with a small unit of, say, 10 patients. Third, nurses can adjust somewhat to peak demands, shifting their breaks or delaying certain nonessential tasks to nonpeak times, to take on peak inpatient care demand. Such adjustments, of course, should be counted on only to a limited extent, because too many can cause low morale and possibly questionable patient care. Let us assume that we choose 85% as our target utilization rate, a value judgment based on experience. For our example:

$$\frac{\text{number of nurses}}{\text{needed on weekends}} = \frac{25 \times 60}{480 \times 0.85} = 3.7$$

and

$$\frac{\text{number of nurses}}{\text{needed on weekdays}} = \frac{35 \times 60}{480 \times 0.85} = 5.2$$

We have considered the demand for all nursing personnel (RNs, LPNs, etc.) in this model. A more sophisticated model would include demand for each type of nurse, with some consideration to task substitution among skill classes. A further level of sophistication can be achieved by classifying patients by how much care they need (high, medium, and low), including separate "minutes of care needed per patient per shift" factors for each type of patient. Since approximately one-third of the total budget of the hospital is represented by nursing care cost, and since nursing care is such an important contribution to hospital care, a great deal of work has been devoted to developing sophisticated models for planning for nurse staffing needs.

A final example of the utilization model is in planning for inpatient bed needs. For this example, our model is

$$\text{beds needed} = \frac{\text{average daily census} \times 1}{1 \times \text{target utilization}}$$

The 1 in the numerator is for the service time: one patient needs one bed per day. The 1 in the denominator is the number of patients each bed can service each day. Average daily census is, in turn, usually broken down into the following:

$$\frac{\text{average daily}}{\text{census}} = \frac{\text{annual patient days}}{365} = \frac{\text{annual admissions} \times \text{average length of stay}}{365}$$

Combining these two models and leaving out the 1's gives

$$\text{beds needed} = \frac{\text{annual admissions} \times \text{average length of stay}}{365 \times \text{target utilization}}$$

For this example, the measurement problems are more straightforward than in previous examples, with the possible exception of annual admissions. With the increasing emphasis on regulation of the expansion of hospital beds, however, has come more systematic data gathering and planning for bed need, so that annual admissions for an area are often projected into the future by local health planning agencies. Thus the hospital has two sources of information about its annual admissions in the future: the local health planning agency and its own past data. It should use both to determine this crucial factor for bed planning. Let us assume that the hospital in our example has both projected annual admissions by trend analysis (similar to the example above for patient visits) and has used projections by the local health planning agency to arrive at a projection for 1990, the year for which it wants to plan. Let us assume that this number is 9000 admissions per year.

The second factor, average length of stay, deserves careful attention. The same two sources are available for this projection: past data at the hospital in question, and local (and also national) planning agencies. Trends in average length of stay for different types of patients have been carefully traced across the nation, and when this information is combined with past data at the hospital in question, an estimate for average length of stay can be made with which planners can be reasonably comfortable. Let us say that this has been done and that the estimate for average length of stay is 7.8 days for patients at the hospital in question.

The last factor, target utilization, has received close attention from health planning agencies, and usually shows up in health systems plans established by health planning agencies for their areas. Target utilization rates are best specified by service: 85 to 90% for medical and surgical beds, and 60 to 70% for emergency-type services such as intensive care units, obstetrics, and so on. To demonstrate this model, however, let us take an overall target utilization figure of 85% for our hospital, reflecting the predominance of medical and surgical beds. Our bed-need model then becomes

$$\text{beds needed} = \frac{9000 \times 7.8}{365 \times 0.85} = 226$$

Such an important (and expensive) resource as inpatient beds deserves maximum consideration by the planner with respect to both the sophistication of the model used, and in the projection of annual admissions, average length of stay, and target utilization. As you can easily demonstrate by using the example above, a small error in the average length of stay projection (say ½ day) changes the projection of bed needs significantly. The same is true for the other factors in the model.

Poisson Model

A final example of these simple resource planning models involves a slight variation for projecting bed needs. This model is useful for considering the fact that for some types of units (intensive care and obstetrics), a large unit can achieve a higher utilization than a small one. Consider an extreme example. A very small obstetrics unit, say 10 beds, can handle only one or two admissions a day without being overutilized, and must often turn patients away. If average daily admissions is 1.5 and average length of stay is 3, average utilization will be 45%, typical for small obstetric units. On the other hand, a large obstetrics unit, 30 to 40 beds, can maintain occupancies of up to 80% and above, due to a probability phenomenon sometimes referred to as the "law of large numbers," meaning that there is relatively less variance in the census of large units than in small units (relative to the average census).

A model using a fixed target utilization, then, cannot reflect this phenomenon. A variation model has been developed called the *Poisson model,* referring to a statistical term on which the model is based, the Poisson probability distribution. The statistical arguments supporting this model are beyond the scope of this book, but we will state the model and demonstrate it with examples. The model is

$$\text{beds needed} = \text{average daily census} + 2 \times \sqrt{\text{average daily census}}$$

or

$$\text{beds needed} = \frac{\text{admissions} \times \text{average length of stay}}{365}$$

$$+ 2 \times \sqrt{\frac{\text{admissions} \times \text{average length of stay}}{365}}$$

This model says that the number of beds needed will be the average daily census *plus* a factor to represent the variance in admissions and length of stay. This factor is two times the square root of average daily census and reflects statistical arguments about what sort of "buffer" in beds above the average daily census is needed to meet demand 95% of the time. (Incidentally, one may plan to meet demand 99% of the time by using a 3 instead of a 2 in this factor, and other percentages by adjusting this number. Of course, to meet demand 100% of the time would require a large number here, with a resulting utilization of very low magnitude.)

Let us take two examples to demonstrate the Poisson model: an obstetrics unit with an average daily census of 8 and one with an average daily census of 38. For the first:

$$\text{beds needed} = 8 + 2 \times \sqrt{8} = 13.7$$

For the second:

$$\text{beds needed} = 38 + 2 \times \sqrt{38} = 50.3$$

Now, for the first case, if we provide 14 beds and expect an average daily census of 8, we can expect a utilization of 8 divided by 14 equals 57%. For the second example, we expect a utilization of 38 divided by 50 equals 76%, demonstrating how this model reflects the phenomenon described above.

For some services, especially obstetrics and intensive care and other "emergency" services, the Poisson model is probably superior. For other services, the utilization model is probably superior. Thus for planning bed needs for an entire hospital, each service should be planned separately, using the most appropriate model (Griffith et al., 1976).

COMPLEX QUANTITATIVE PLANNING MODELS

The planning models discussed above have the advantage of being straightforward and of requiring measurements that are often obtainable from existing sources (e.g., average length of stay, annual admissions). They have the disadvantages, however, of relying on numerous simplifying assumptions for their application that have two significant effects on their contribution to the planning process.

First, their representation of the real-world problem (see Figure 5-1) is highly abstract and not as close a representation as more sophisticated models will allow. The implication of such representation is the possibility that solutions suggested by the models will not "fit" the real-world situation accurately, and incorrect decisions will be made. The second effect of the simplistic nature of these models is that they provide less information to the planning process than do more complex ones, as we shall see below.

The next stage of sophistication in quantitative planning models involves a rather large step in conceptual complexity, mathematical complexity, data gathering effort, analysis effort, and cost. It also often involves a considerable amount of computer expertise and time. Thus treatment of these models in this book will be at the introductory and survey level, with the goal set at attaining an appreciation of what these models offer, what effort is involved in undertaking an analysis using them, and a feeling for their limitations. Obtaining the skill to perform analyses using these models is not a goal of this book.

Recall the discussion of the service-time factor in the utilization model. A significant simplifying assumption was made that one service-time factor would represent all activities in the clinic: registration, history taking, examination, treatment, and so on. A second simplifying assumption was made that the *average* service time and the *average* daily arrivals would represent what were known to be variable, not fixed phenomena. Recall that the utilization factor was incorporated in an attempt to represent these compromises in modeling reality.

Queueing Model

A model that does not make these compromises is the queueing model or waiting-line model (the term "queue" is an English expression for a waiting line). These models have been applied in a number of health service organizations (Rising, 1977) and use the concept of how long patients must wait for services to attempt to measure the impact of providing alternative amounts of resources.

Figure 5-8 is a simplistic flow diagram of patients entering and being served in our clinic. The patient arrives and waits for the availability of the registrar (either receptionist or nurse or both). It is, of course, possible that the patient will wait for a zero amount of time to be registered. Then the patient is registered (with perhaps a history being taken, a blood pressure test, etc.), and assigned to a physician and to an examining room. The patient waits for an examining room and a physician, is placed in an examining room, is examined and treated, and then leaves the system.

This flow is simplistic in several ways. For example, it ignores the differ-

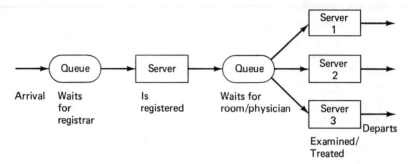

Figure 5-8 Queueing flow diagram.

ence between "first time" and returning patients, the role of x-ray and lab, and the fact that a patient may wait in the examining room for the physician. As we shall see below, there are several other "flows" not represented by Figure 5-8. We could incorporate some (but significantly not all) of these flows in a complex queueing model, but for our purpose of demonstrating the modeling method, we will keep to this simplistic representation.

There are several probabilistic (or variable) elements in this flow. The number of patient arrivals per hour varies considerably from hour to hour, both because of the time of day of arrival and because of the random nature of the arrival of patients to a clinic. The service time to register patients also varies, as does the service time to examine/treat patients. In the simple models of the preceding section, we represented these processes with average values. In queueing, these processes are represented by the distribution of the time to complete the process, or in the case of arrivals, the distribution of the number of arrivals per hour. For example, we could measure from past data the probability that for a randomly chosen hour there would be no arrivals, that there would be exactly one arrival, exactly two, three, and so on. Suppose that such a study had been done to measure these probabilities, with the results shown in Table 5-2.

Similarly, suppose that a study was performed to measure the probability that registration would take exactly 5 minutes, exactly 6 minutes, exactly 8 minutes, and so on, resulting in Table 5-3. If these distributions are similar in form to one of several theoretical distributions, a queueing model can be used to represent the patient flow process through the clinic as assumed in Figure 5-8. If these distributions are *not* similar to one of these theoretical distributions, the technique discussed below, *simulation,* must be used. There are statistical techniques to measure how similar these distributions are to the necessary theoretical ones, but these techniques are again beyond the scope of this text. Assume that a third study results in the distribution of the exam/treatment service time, as given in Table 5-4. Finally, assume that these distributions do indeed fit the form of a required theoretical one for using queueing models.

TABLE 5–2 *Distribution of Arrivals per Hour*

Number Arriving	Number of Times (hours) This Was Observed	Probability (column 2 ÷ 200)
0	2	0.01
1	9	0.05
2	21	0.11
3	33	0.17
4	38	0.18
5	35	0.17
6	26	0.13
7	17	0.08
8	10	0.05
9	5	0.03
10	2	0.01
11 or more	2	0.01
	200	1.00

Average number of arrivals per hour = 4.6

Given that we are willing to view the patient flow process as shown in Figure 5-8 (i.e., with the stated simplifying assumptions) and that the distributions are similar to certain queueing distributions, a queueing analysis can give us information on how long we can expect patients to wait at each of the queues of Figure 5-8 given that we provide alternative amounts of resources. Without presenting how this is done, Table 5-5 gives the type of information available from this type of analysis. It should be clear that this is considerably more information on which to make a planning decision than the simplistic models of the preceding section. Moreover, these queueing

TABLE 5–3 *Distribution of Service Time to Register*

Amount of Time to Register (minutes)	Number of Patients Observed Taking This Amount of Time	Probability (column 2 ÷ 100)
5 or less	9	0.09
6	15	0.15
7	20	0.20
8	20	0.20
9	16	0.16
10	10	0.10
11	6	0.06
12 or more	4	0.04
	100	1.00

Average service time to register = 8 minutes

TABLE 5-4 *Distribution of Service Time to Exam/Treat*

Time to Exam/Treat (minutes)	Number of Patients Observed Taking This Amount of Time	Probability (column 2 ÷ 200)
15 or less	11	0.06
20	12	0.06
25	18	0.08
30	23	0.12
35	26	0.13
40	26	0.13
45	24	0.12
50	19	0.10
55	15	0.08
60	13	0.06
65 or more	13	0.06
	200	1.00

Average service time to exam/treat = 36 minutes

models are closer representations to reality than are the simple ones, although they still encompass a great many simplifying assumptions.

There are many limitations of applying these models; many we have mentioned, but others are beyond the scope of this presentation. These limitations are especially severe in the health care delivery field, making queueing analysis a cut above the simple models, but still far short of accurate representations of the real-world process. We discuss the implications of the relative sophistication of planning models in the review section below.

Simulation Model

The most sophisticated—and accurate—technique for quantitative modeling is simulation. *Simulation* is an expansion of queueing and has received increased attention in the health services field (Valinsky, 1975; Kirkman-Liff, 1980). Simulation uses the basic idea of waiting-line analysis, but without the numerous limitations of the application of queueing. For example, a typical simulation analysis might represent the clinic flow as in Figure 5-9, incorporating many more of the important flows of the process. As in the queueing analysis, each part of the process that involves a service time would be represented by a distribution for that process similar to those shown in Tables 5-2 and 5-3, except that there would be separate distributions for all of these service-time processes. There would also be separate arrival distributions for each type of patient—first time and returning—and also a different distribution for morning versus afternoon, if activity is not similar across the day.

TABLE 5-5 *Output from Queueing Analysis*

Receptionist
Average time waiting = 12.7 minutes.
Average number of people in line waiting = 0.9 person.

Probability of having to wait more than 20 minutes = 0.20.
Probability of having to wait more than 30 minutes = 0.09.

Number of Exam Rooms/Physicians	Average Waiting Time (minutes)	Average Number Waiting
3	128	9.0
4	12	0.9
5	3	0.2

	Probability of Having to Wait More Than:			
	15 Minutes	30 Minutes	45 Minutes	60 Minutes
3	0.89	0.79	0.70	0.63
4	0.29	0.08	0.02	0.01
5	0.01	0.00	0.00	0.00

A special computer program would have to be written to simulate the flow of patients, as diagrammed in Figure 5-9. This program would then be run to simulate, for example, one year of clinic operation under each of several alternative arrangements of resources (e.g., four physicians versus three, five rooms versus four, two reception areas versus one, etc.). The computer would actually "create" patients one by one according to the arrival distributions, put them in line for registration, keeping track of when the registrar is free and putting the next patient into the registration process when the registrar is free, calculate from the service distribution how long this patient will take to register, check when the patient is finished registering, determine if an examining room is free, put the patient in the examining room, and so on. The program would keep track of how many patients waited where, and for how long, when examining rooms were busy or empty, when personnel were busy or not, and so on. It would even be possible to simulate personnel going on lunch breaks, physicians arriving late or on staggered schedules, and other factors. Of course, the more elements incorporated, the larger and more expensive the analysis.

Typical output from such a simulation analysis would yield the type of information shown in Table 5-6. Compared to the output from queueing—Table 5-5—output from this type of analysis gives substantially more information on which to make the decision of how many rooms, physicians, nurses, receptionists, and even waiting-room seats to provide.

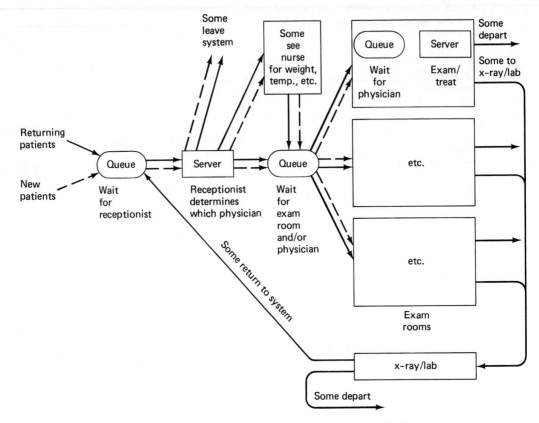

Figure 5-9 Flow diagram for simulation analysis.

MODEL APPLICATION

There are several points that should be kept in mind when considering these models as a whole and their relationship in the planning process. Both the simple and the complex models can be applied to each of the examples cited. Thus a problem does not automatically call for a specific type of model or a particular level of sophistication of analysis. The "number of examining rooms" problem for a clinic can legitimately be modeled by the simplest utilization model or by a very expensive simulation study. The decision of which model to apply rests on several considerations.

First, there is the question of whether a more sophisticated analysis will "pay for itself." The way an analysis pays for itself is by avoiding making incorrect decisions. Suppose, for example, that because of modeling inaccuracy, a simple model suggested one more obstetrics bed than would have been considered needed if the information from a more sophisticated model had

TABLE 5-6 *Output from Simulation Analysis*

RECEPTIONIST Both Returning and New Patients

Period	Average Waiting Time (minutes)	Probability of Waiting More Than:		Average Number Waiting
		10 Minutes	20 Minutes	
8 A.M.–10 A.M.	18	0.43	0.04	4.3
10 A.M.– 1 P.M.	13	0.33	0.01	1.6
1 P.M.– 4 P.M.	5	0.11	0.00	0.2

EXAM ROOMS/PHYSICIANS Return Patients: 8 A.M. – 10 A.M.

	Average Waiting Time (minutes)	Probability of Waiting More Than:				Average Number Waiting
		15 Minutes	30 Minutes	45 Minutes	60 Minutes	
Waiting Time to Obtain an Exam Room						
3 rooms	147	0.90	0.83	0.71	0.51	11.8
4 rooms	25	0.50	0.27	0.14	0.08	2.1
5 rooms	4	0.03	0.00	0.00	0.00	0.6
Waiting Time to See Physicians (once in an exam room)						
2 physicians	116	0.76	0.61	0.53	0.44	—
3 physicians	14	0.36	0.12	0.04	0.01	—
4 physicians	3	0.00	0.00	0.00	0.00	—

(and so on for new patients 8 A.M.–10 A.M., and for returning and new patients in the other two time slots)

been available. The marginal benefit of a more sophisticated model might thus be considered to be approximated by the cost of building and maintaining an unneeded obstetrics bed, perhaps $50,000 to $100,000. This determination of the possibility of making an incorrect decision is highly speculative, but must be kept in mind when considering what level of analysis is appropriate.

Another way an analysis pays for itself is in convincing decision makers that a proposal should be approved. The decision maker in this case could be the board of directors or a health planning agency with authority over such proposals for facilities expansion.

A second consideration, based on the first, is the type of resource being planned. Inpatient bed expansion involves a great deal of money and effort, and if too many or too few beds are provided, the consequences are considerable. Also, it takes a great deal of time to correct improper planning for this large a resource. Planning for the number of waiting-room chairs, to take an extreme example on the other end of the spectrum, involves little risk of serious consequences from faulty planning. Thus the type of resource being planned is a factor in considering the level of sophistication used.

Third, there are several practical considerations. There may not be time or money for anything but the simplest analysis. There may not be the talent (mathematical, computer, data gathering, etc.) available for an analysis as sophisticated as queueing or simulation. A very real consideration is the availability and quality of data to support an analysis. As can be gathered from even a brief description of the more sophisticated models, a great deal of high-quality data is necessary in these sophisticated analyses, which, even if available, is usually very expensive to obtain.

Finally, the decision maker to whom a proposal is presented must be receptive to whatever level of sophistication is represented by the analysis. It is easy to conceive of a proposal failing because the decision maker's tolerance for sophisticated mathematical analysis was overestimated. Considering all of these factors, the overwhelming argument in considering what level of analysis to perform is still the first: Will it pay for itself?

CASE

Planning for Additional Beds

For the past two years, your rural 100-bed general hospital has experienced higher and higher utilization, to the extent that patients now must wait several weeks to have general surgery, and several days for urgent admission. Some physicians are beginning to send some of their patients to hospitals some 60 miles away, requiring these patients to travel considerable distances and to stay in a hospital far from their family and home. Physicians, and other members of the community, are calling for an expansion of beds at your hospital. As administrator, you are faced with the decision of whether additional beds are needed, how many, and when to build them.

As a first step, you collect the following data on annual admissions to your hospital, average length of stay, number of beds, and average occupancy.

Year	Admissions	Average Length of Stay	Number of Beds	Average Occupancy
1971	2818	6.8	75	30
1972	2896	6.9	75	73
1973	3000	7.3	75	80
1974	3277	7.1	75	85
1975	3080	8.0	75	90
1976	3257	7.9	75	94
1977	3249	8.2	100	73
1978	3736	8.4	100	86
1979	3820	8.6	100	90
1980	3899	8.8	100	94

Your Service Area Population

The population or "community" that considers your hospital as their primary hospital, if not their only hospital, has grown substantially over the years. It was 22,410 people in 1980 and is predicted to be 28,500 people in 1985 by the census bureau.

The inpatient use rate in your service area for 1980 was 174 admissions per 1000 population. The local Health Systems Agency (HSA) has performed a special study of this community and predicts that this use rate will grow to 180 admissions per 1000 by 1985. Your hospital gets 90% of these admissions now. Moreover, your hospital gets 10% of its total patients from *outside* the service area. These two percentages have not changed over the years, and they are not expected to change in the near future.

The HSA has adopted a policy of trying to keep the number of beds in a community at or below the national standard of four beds per 1000 population. Also, the HSA uses an occupancy rate of 85% in its bed planning methodologies.

Required

Using as much information as possible, determine the number of beds that your hospital should build by 1985. Prepare graphs and tables that back up your decision. They should be clear and straightforward enough that they, together with a verbal presentation, can persuade the board of trustees of your hospital to approve the building of the beds.

FURTHER READING

CHURCHMAN, C. W. *The Systems Approach.* New York: Dell, 1968.

GRIFFITH, J. R. *Quantitative Techniques for Hospital Planning and Control.* Lexington, Mass.: D. C. Heath, 1972.

GRIFFITH, J. R., W. M. HANCOCK, and F. MUNSON. *Cost Control in Hospitals.* Ann Arbor, Mich.: Health Administration Press, 1976.

WAGNER, H. M. *Principles of Operations Research.* Englewood Cliffs, N.J.: Prentice-Hall, 1979.

WARNER, D. M., and D. C. HOLLOWAY. *Decision Making and Control for Health Administration.* Ann Arbor, Mich.: Health Administration Press, 1978.

PART

3

IMPLEMENTATION AND OPERATIONS

In the course of a study done by Earl Brooks on railroads, Brooks spent some time one afternoon observing and interviewing a man in a switching tower who was separating and recombining trains of freight cars. The electrical controls and relays were so worn that they failed to slow the cars properly. The violence with which they coupled led the researcher to inquire whether the cargo might not be seriously damaged. The switchman agreed that it might. "And shouldn't some of the equipment be replaced?" continued the researcher. The switchman agreed that it ought to be. "Then," said the researcher, "why don't you tell the regional office about it?"

The switchman's reply was oblique. "About how hot would you say it was in the tower?"

"It must be over a 100°" said the researcher looking at the afternoon sun beating in the west bank of the windows, "but what has that got to do with it?"

"I have been trying for six months to get a venetian blind for that window," said the switchman. "They told me that my job was to switch trains and they would make decisions about equipment. When they get around to that blind, I may get around to telling them about the relays and those braking controls." [Katz and Kahn, 1966]

Planning and design as future-oriented activities are important—yet managers must be aware of the implementation and operational aspects of the management process. The objective of this section is to consider various aspects of implementation and operations. Chapter 6 describes quantitative decision making. It considers the types of operational decisions made by health service managers and presents selected quantitative techniques to aid in the decision process.

Chapter 7 is concerned with the acquisition, protection, and use of financial assets to achieve organizational goals. The chapter discusses various types of assets and their implications for operations.

Chapter 8 centers on the actual implementation of new programs and technology. Implementation is considered one aspect of a change process and the chapter attempts to define different types of change and change strategies.

6

Quantitative Decision Making

Once the basic planning and design activities are completed, the health services manager is quickly immersed in many operational decisions involving quantitative logic and numbers. The objective of this chapter is to consider the types of operational decisions made by health services managers and to consider some of the techniques that are available for helping in the decision process.

TYPES OF DECISIONS

There are two general types of operational decisions: procedure decisions, which are very short-term planning decisions, and scheduling decisions.

Procedure decisions involve deciding on the best way to meet a certain operations objective. For example, should we hire four full-time nurses, or six part-time nurses whose full-time equivalent is four? Should we buy machine A or machine B? Should we buy a certain piece of equipment or lease it? Complicating these decisions is that old enemy of decision making—uncertainty.

Scheduling decisions do not involve *which* resources will be provided (which machine or which people), but how their availability will be *scheduled* over time. For example, how should the 28 nurses who comprise the staff of a nursing unit be scheduled (which days, which shifts) to meet their preference for weekends off, and so on, at the same time assuring that a minimum number of nurses are always on hand to care for patients? Another type of scheduling decision concerns how certain tasks should be sequenced so that they best "fall together" to complete some project. For example, when opening a new clinic, there may be 20 or 30 separate tasks to be performed: hiring nurses, implementing a promotional campaign, buying equipment, and so on. Some tasks cannot be started until others are completed, and some tasks are better started earlier than others, and so on. How to best sequence these tasks is the scheduling problem.

A third type of scheduling problem occurs when a consumable item (e.g., blood) is needed constantly, but must be ordered periodically in multiple units and stored for use. The decision involves when to order and how many items to order, and it has a special name: inventory problem.

Although both procedure and scheduling problems occur frequently and are of the "operations" or short-term variety, an important distinction between them is that although procedure problems are somewhat similar to one another, the same ones do not occur regularly. This is not true generally for scheduling problems, as essentially the same problem reoccurs every period. For example, nurses' schedules must be redone every four weeks, usually involving the same nurses and much the same parameters.

Ordering and storing blood is also a recurring decision. On the other hand, the decision to buy or lease a machine, or to buy machine A rather than machine B, is usually made only once for that machine or that type of machine.

Before we introduce these problems formally, we must first reintroduce two topics, the operations research approach and modeling, and we must update forecasting techniques to include intermediate- and short-term forecasting.

The Operations Research Approach Revisited

In Chapter 5 the operations research approach to planning decisions was presented as a process involving first building a model of the decision, and then analyzing this model for information and insight about the real-world decision (see Figure 5-1). The same approach is valid for the short-term procedure decisions described in the preceding section. The models that result from the analysis of short-term problems are different, however, and there are special classes of models for different types of procedure and scheduling decisions.

The important point is that no matter what type of model is built— planning, operations, or scheduling—the modeling (or operations research) *process* is similar. The process still calls for a conceptual model (usually mathematical in nature) to be constructed which describes important aspects of the real-world problem, serving as a special representation of the real-world problem or decision. This model is then analyzed using special quantitative techniques to reach a model *solution,* which in turn serves as information in deciding a real-world *strategy.* The model solution rarely serves as the strategy by itself, because the model from which it comes is only a representation of the real world. The solution must be carefully and wisely transformed into a real-world strategy in order to be implemented successfully.

Intermediate-Term Forecasting

The demand for health services often follows two trends simultaneously. The first is long-term growth (or decline), usually noticeable only by looking at several years' worth of data. This trend was the important one for the long-term planning decisions of Chapter 5, and it was this trend that was addressed by the techniques presented in Chapter 5.

The second trend is *cyclical;* that is, the behavior of demand repeats itself in cycles: annually, weekly, or daily, or some combination of the three. This phenomenon can be seen graphically in Figure 6-1, which shows clinic visits by month for the last three years, and in Figure 6-2, which shows clinic visits by day of the week for the last six weeks. Tables 6-1 and 6-2,

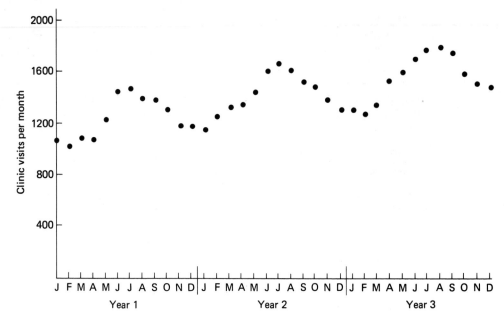

Figure 6-1 Clinic visits per month.

respectively, show the number of visits that are graphed in Figures 6–1 and 6–2.

Recall from Chapter 5 that there are two separate hypotheses that are important in all forecasting:

• There has been some measurable trend in the past.
• This trend will continue into the future.

The trend referred to in this case is the cyclical trend. To represent mathematically a cyclical trend of demand in the past, the technique of *cyclical*

TABLE 6-1 *Clinic Visits by Month, Monthly Means, and Indices*

Year	Jan.	Feb.	Mar.	Apr.	May	June	July	Aug.	Sept.	Oct.	Nov.	Dec.
1979	1100	1052	1116	1112	1244	1500	1532	1464	1452	1388	1224	1216
1980	1192	1276	1348	1368	1476	1616	1656	1624	1560	1524	1408	1304
1981	1308	1292	1352	1524	1600	1700	1804	1788	1772	1612	1564	1552
Monthly mean, M_i	1200	1207	1272	1271	1440	1605	1664	1625	1595	1508	1399	1257
Index, I_i	0.840	0.845	0.890	0.890	1.008	1.124	1.165	1.138	1.116	1.056	0.979	0.950

Grand mean 1428

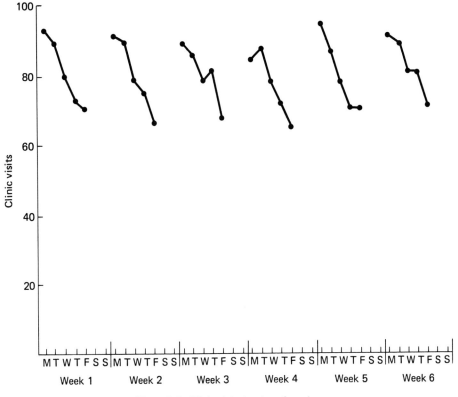

Figure 6-2 Clinic visits by day of week.

indices is useful. The technique is receiving increased attention as it relates to cost control in hospitals (Griffith et al., 1976).

To develop the notion of cyclical indices, consider the monthly demand data of Table 6-1. For each month we have three observations, one for each of the three years of data. The fourth row of Table 6-1 gives the average number of visits by month over the three years. When we take the average of these 12 numbers, we get the overall average monthly demand over the three years (end of row four). This latter figure is called the *grand*

TABLE 6-2 *Clinic Visits by Day of Week*

Week	Mon.	Tues.	Wed.	Thurs.	Fri.
1	93	89	78	71	67
2	91	89	77	75	64
3	87	85	80	83	64
4	83	87	77	71	63
5	94	85	78	71	71
6	89	87	80	80	72

mean (GM) and the means by month are called *monthly means.* Using M_1 for January, M_2 for February, and so on, we let M_i represent the generic monthly mean. When we assign i equals 1, it becomes January; and so on.

Also, let I_1 be the cyclical index for January, I_2 the index for February, and so on, and I_i the generic index. These I_i are calculated as follows:

$$I_i = \frac{M_i}{\text{GM}}$$

Therefore, the index is simply the ratio of the monthly mean to the grand mean. These ratios are displayed in the last row of Table 6-1. To interpret them, an index of 0.80 for a month means that demand for that month is 80% of the typical month (the grand mean), while an index of 1.21 means that demand is 21% higher than the typical month.

If all the indices are approximately 1.0, it means that there is essentially no cyclical trend, as the monthly means are not very different from the grand mean. A statistical test called the chi-square test can be used to statistically establish whether or not indices constitute a trend. This statistical test is beyond the scope of this text, but essentially it indicates how different the indices are from all being equal to 1.0.

Once indices are calculated and a trend has been established, either by statistics or judgment, we have an answer to our first hypothesis: there is some trend in the past. Unless we have reason to believe that this trend will not continue into the future, it might be useful to assume that it will. (What are some of the reasons that clinic visits would not continue to exhibit the cyclical trend of Figure 6-1?)

Since the indices measure only the *relative* difference between months, to use the indices to predict monthly demand in the future, we must first have an *absolute* prediction of the grand mean of demand in the future. We can obtain this from the long-range forecasting method discussed in Chapter 5. For example, suppose that it is 1981 and we want to predict monthly demand for 1982. From our long-range forecast shown in Figure 5-6, the demand in 1982 should be about 390 visits per week. Now 390 times 52 weeks equals 20,280 visits a year, or 20,280 divided by 12 equals 1692 visits per month for the typical or average month (the grand mean). To construct monthly forecasts, multiply this number times the individual indices. The results are displayed in Table 6-3.

Daily indices (to describe a possible cyclical trend in the behavior of demand by day of week) are calculated similarly and are used the same way.

Procedure Decisions

The most typical procedure decision involves choosing between two or more alternative ways to accomplish the same goal. In most cases, the objective

TABLE 6-3 *Prediction for Clinic Visits by Month for 1982*

	Jan.	Feb.	Mar.	Apr.	May	June	July	Aug.	Sept.	Oct.	Nov.	Dec.
Index	0.840	0.845	0.890	0.89	1.008	1.124	1.165	1.138	1.116	1.056	0.979	0.950
				... multiplied times 1692 as typical month in 1982 = ...								
Prediction for 1982	1421	1430	1506	1506	1706	1902	1971	1925	1888	1787	1656	1607

is to choose the alternative that accomplishes the goal at minimum cost. Consider the following procedure decision as an illustration.

Laboratory Utilization: An Illustration of Break-Even Analysis

Expansion plans for your clinic lead you to reexamine the arrangement your clinic uses for lab tests necessary for clinic patients. Currently, you use a nearby professional lab and pay an average of $20 a test. This saves you the expense of maintaining your own lab in the clinic and of related problems of quality control, maintenance of personnel in the lab, and so on. As the clinic grows, however, there may be a point where it becomes more cost efficient to develop your own lab in the clinic. The problem is: Should the clinic develop its own lab, and if so, when should it do it? Or should it continue to purchase lab services from outside the clinic?

This problem is typical of most procedure problems in that it involves a trade-off between fixed costs and variable costs, initially discussed in Chapter 4. *Fixed costs* are those costs that do not vary with the amount of output (lab tests in our example). Since we pay $20 a test, the outside lab alternative has no fixed costs. If we develop our own lab—the "inside lab" alternative—we would have very high fixed costs associated with building, equipment, and personnel. We must include personnel as fixed since we cannot hire and fire lab personnel as demand goes up and down, unless it fluctuates widely and we can predict such fluctuations well into the future. For our clinic, the monthly indices show that although there is monthly variation in demand, it is not such that we could expect to adjust the number of highly trained lab technicians to meet such fluctuations.

Whereas the inside lab alternative has large fixed costs, it has relatively low variable costs. *Variable costs* are those costs that vary with output, and in this case are expressed as dollars per lab test. These costs would essentially include supplies and other disposables. Let us assume that we perform a study to measure variable costs and determine that the variable cost per lab test is $3.

The fixed cost for the inside option is somewhat more difficult to measure, as it depends on the cost of the necessary rooms (including perhaps remodeling costs, etc.), equipment, and personnel. Let us assume that we do make this assessment and we determine that to do between 3000 and 5000 procedures a month would cost $50,000 a month in fixed costs, and to do between 5000 and 8000 tests a month would cost $70,000 a month in fixed costs.

Which alternative is less expensive, the outside or inside alternative? The two options can best be compared on a break-even graph such as that shown in Figure 6-3. This graph has dollars on the vertical axis and output (in tests per month) on the horizontal axis. The two lines show, respectively, the costs for the inside and outside alternatives as a function of output. For low output, the outside option is less expensive; for high output, the inside option is less expensive. The break-even point is that level of output below where the two lines cross, or where total costs (fixed plus variable) of the alternatives are equal. At this point we are indifferent about the two alternatives.

The answer to which alternative is less expensive comes down to the projected monthly demand. In the preceding section, we projected 1690

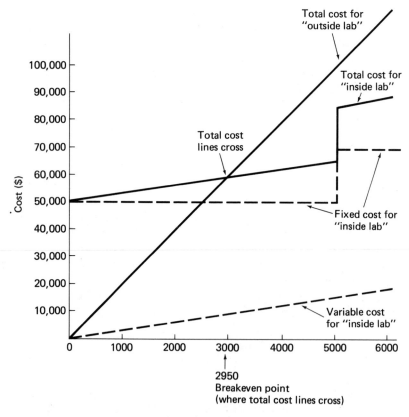

Figure 6-3 Break-even chart.

visits a month for 1982. Suppose we determine from past data that, on the average, each clinic visit generates 1.7 lab tests. Thus for 1982 we can expect 1690 times 1.7 equals 2873 tests.

For this level of output, the outside option remains less expensive, as can be seen from the graph, as the break-even point is about 2950. However, for 1985, when we expect approximately 465 visits a week, or 465 times 52 equals 24,180 a year, or 24,180 divided by 12 equals 2015 a month, we can expect 2015 times 1.7 equals 3426 lab tests per month. This puts us comfortably above the break-even mark of 2950, and makes the inside option more attractive.

Since it will take a year or so to organize the development of the lab as an inside option, we would probably be inclined on this evidence to consider beginning to plan for it immediately. There are, of course, a host of other reasons to choose inside versus outside, or vice versa. To name a few, there are changes in cost over time (we should try to predict these), quality control and personnel issues, and questions of turnaround, liability, and prestige. The economic analysis of the break-even model should be considered as only *one* of the factors in the decision.

There are numerous other examples for which break-even analysis is useful. The important element in all break-even analysis problems is the trade-off between the variable and fixed costs of the alternatives. The key to the analysis is to represent the fixed cost and the variable cost for each alternative as a function of the output, and then to compare the two on a break-even graph. The most difficult part of the analysis is the measurement of the fixed and variable costs involved, and the projection of these into the relevant future. A second consideration is the accuracy of the projection of the level of output into the relevant future.

We have used the break-even model to characterize a class of problems called procedure problems. There are other models that are applicable to procedure problems, and most are somewhat similar to the example presented above.

Scheduling Decisions

We now consider a different type of decision—scheduling. Scheduling decisions are distinct from procedure decisions in that the decision is not a choice among alternative machines or strategies, but how to schedule or arrange a *given* or previously established set of events to meet certain objectives. We consider two types of scheduling decisions: inventory decisions and task sequencing decisions.

Inventory Decisions

Consider the following problem. Your 180-bed nursing home keeps a full census of 180 patients. Each day, each patient consumes a certain item.

Your nursing home obtains this item from the supplier, who delivers the number you order to your storage facilities. It costs $40 to place an order with your supplier no matter how many items you order. This *ordering cost* does not include the price paid for the items, but includes only the cost of the "red tape" of placing the order.

Since it costs the same ($40) to order *any* amount, it seems to make sense always to order as many items as possible. However, it costs $0.01 per item per day to *store* the items (this includes costs of storage facilities, utilities, storage personnel, insurance, etc.). In addition, there is an *investment cost* of tying up cash with large amounts of this item in storage. Let us assume that you can earn 10% on idle cash by investing it in something else, so that you are forgoing a 10% return on whatever amount of investment you have tied up in inventory of this item. These *carrying costs* (storage and investment) seem to suggest that it is wise to keep the amount in inventory as small as possible. The problem is to balance these two conflicting costs—ordering and carrying costs—so that the total of these two costs is a minimum, and so that there is an ample supply of the item on hand to meet demand.

To find the minimum total cost, we build the following mathematical model:

$$\text{total cost} = \text{ordering cost} + \text{storage cost} + \text{investment cost}$$

Our model-building task continues by expressing each of the terms on the right-hand side as functions of a *decision variable,* or the variable over which we have control. In this case our decision variable is the number of items we order each time we place an order. (The amount ordered is called the *lot size,* and this model is called the lot-size model.)

Let Q be the number we order each time we place an order. How many times a year will we make an order if we order Q each time? We use 180 a day or $365 \times 180 = 65,700$ a year. Therefore, we must make $65,700/Q$ orders a year. Recall that each order costs $40 to place, so that we can rewrite our model as:

$$\text{annual total costs} = \$40 \times \frac{65,700}{Q} + \text{annual storage costs} + \text{annual investment costs}$$

(Note that we have picked annual costs as a basis. We could just as easily have picked monthly, weekly, or even daily costs as our basis.)

To express the last two terms as a function of Q, we must know the average number of items in storage over time. In Figure 6–4 the number of items on hand are plotted on the vertical axis and the horizontal axis is time. At time T_0 we receive a shipment of Q items. Since it makes sense

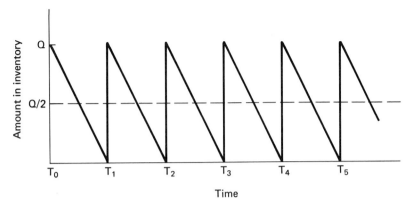

Figure 6-4 Amount in inventory over time.

to arrange for the reception of new items just as the inventory goes to zero, we have a total of Q items in inventory at T_0. Then we begin to use them up, so that at some time T_1, just as inventory goes to zero, we receive another Q items, and so on. (Since at this point we are assuming no uncertainty in our model, it would be easy to time the arrival of a new shipment to coincide with inventory going to zero. When there is uncertainty about how long it could take for the items to arrive once we order them, or uncertainty about using exactly 180 a day, the problem becomes more complicated.)

The average number of items in storage over time is $Q/2$, as seen from Figure 6-4. Now, if we assume that we incur storage cost on the *average* number in inventory, annual storage costs are going to be $\$3.65 \times Q/2$. (The $3.65 comes from multiplying the daily rate of $0.01 by 365 days a year.) Using the average ($Q/2$) implies that we can store other items in the place vacated by the use of this item. If this is not the case, we incur $\$3.65 \times Q$ in storage costs annually, since we must dedicate space for all Q items all year. If we assume the average is the correct amount, our model becomes

$$\text{annual total cost} = \$40 \times \frac{65{,}700}{Q} + \$3.65 \times \frac{Q}{2} + \text{annual investment cost}$$

The amount of cash tied up in inventory of this item is found by multiplying the price of the item times the average amount in inventory. Assume that the price for this item is $6. We then have on average $\$6 \times Q/2$ tied up in this item in inventory. Since the cost is the investment forgone by tying up cash in this item, our annual investment cost is $0.10 \times 6 \times Q/2$, where 0.10 is the investment rate assumed above.

Thus our complete model is:

$$\text{annual total cost} = \$40 \times \frac{65{,}700}{Q} + \$3.65 \times \frac{Q}{2} + \$6 \times 0.1 \times \frac{Q}{2}$$

Notice that we have expressed total cost as a function of our decision variable Q. This is an important step in mathematical modeling, as now we have total costs "under our control" by picking the correct value for Q.

Picking the optimal value for Q is called solving this model. By optimal, we mean that value of Q which minimizes total cost. There are two ways to find the optimal Q. The easiest way requires calculus, which is beyond the scope of this text. The other way is called the approximation method (or sometimes the trial-and-error method), and involves simple trial and error: picking a value for Q and substituting it into the model to calculate total cost, then picking another value of Q, and so on. By comparing the total cost associated with each Q, we can pick the Q that seems to have the lowest total cost, solving the model.

Table 6-4 calculates total cost for six different values of Q, to demonstrate the approximation method. Note that total cost first goes down, then back up, as a function of the size of Q. This is characteristic of most inventory problems. Figure 6-5 shows this relationship graphically, and shows that the curve is relatively flat around the optimal level of Q (i.e., the lowest portion of the total-cost curve). Thus the solution is somewhat insensitive to the exact level of Q as long as you choose one close to the optimal. Moreover, the curve rises faster to the left than to the right, meaning that it is better to err on the high side for Q than on the low side.

These phenomena are characteristic of many inventory problems, and therein lies an important point. By modeling inventory problems in general, insight can be gained about all inventory problems, with useful rules of thumb available even without gathering all the data necessary to solve the problem, as we did in the example above.

The model solution (from Table 6-4) is to order 1000 items each time. This model solution might have to be modified to meet real-world conditions, such as not being able to order on Sunday (or schedule an arrival on

TABLE 6-4 *Calculation of Optimal Q by Approximation Method*

Trail:	(1)	(2)	(3)	(4)	(5)	(6)
Q:	400	700	1000	1300	1600	1900
$\$40 \times 65{,}700/Q$	$6570	$3754	$2628	$2022	$1643	$1383
$\$3.65 \times Q/2$	730	1278	1825	2373	2920	3468
$\$6 \times 0.1 \times Q/2$	120	210	300	390	480	570
Total cost	$7420	$5242	$4753	$4785	$5043	$5421

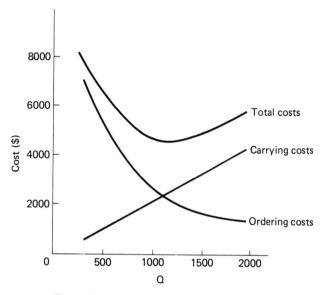

Figure 6-5 Inventory costs as a function of Q.

Sunday). Again, the model solution provides information and insight to the formulation of a real-world strategy rather than providing it directly.

As mentioned above, if we allow uncertainty into the model, the model becomes much more complex. It might be useful to consider the impact of the following types of uncertainty:

- Daily demand is not fixed at 180, but varies randomly between 160 and 200.

- Usually it takes five days to receive an order once it is placed, but it can come in as little as three days or take up to eight days. There are no deliveries on weekends.

- About 2 out of 100 of the items are found to be defective and must be returned unused.

All of these extensions to the basic lot-size inventory problem can be modeled and solved. A large body of inventory models have been developed over the years in industrial operations research and have been applied in various types of health service organizations (Cooperative Information Center, 1970, p. 82).

Task Sequencing Decisions

A second type of scheduling problem that is useful for demonstrating the quantitative approach to decision making occurs when a project can be divided into several tasks in such a way that, when the tasks are completed in a certain sequence, the project is completed. Consider the following problem.

You have been charged with designing the development of a new out-patient clinic (the "project"). You have identified the following tasks as components of the project (there would certainly be many more than this many tasks in a real clinic opening project, but these are sufficient for our purposes):

1. Find and lease *Space* for the clinic.
2. Hire lab and x-ray department *Chiefs*.
3. Purchase x-ray and lab *Equipment*.
4. *Remodel* the space.
5. *Install* equipment when it arrives.
6. Hire *Nurses* and other personnel.
7. *Train* personnel.
8. Design and implement a *Publicity* campaign.
9. Miscellaneous *Final* preparations.

The italicized words represent the tasks in the discussion and diagrams below. The problem concerns *when* each task should be initiated in order that the project be completed in the least amount of time. Clearly, not all of these tasks can begin at once, and some must follow others.

The first step in modeling this decision is to specify two things about each task: (1) how long (an estimate) it will take to complete the task, and (2) its sequence with respect to the other tasks, specified as which other tasks must precede the beginning of each task.

For our example, suppose that we establish the following:

Task	Time to Complete (weeks)	Predecessor Tasks
1. Space	14	—
2. Chiefs	16	—
3. Equipment	12	2
4. Remodel	6	1, 2
5. Install	2	3, 4
6. Nurses	5	—
7. Train	4	6
8. Publicity	11	—
9. Final	3	5, 7, 8

(Again, this sequencing is simplified from the real-world process, but suffices for our purpose of demonstrating the model.)

The next step in the modeling process is to build a PERT (program evaluation and review technique) network.* This network will be carefully constructed to graphically show the necessary sequencing of the tasks to make up the project. We first define an *event* as the end of one or more tasks and the beginning of one or more other tasks which must be preceded by the tasks that are ending.

The last event (we will denote events with circles) is the End event:

The tasks that terminate in the End event are those that precede no other tasks: only Final meets this criterion. We denote tasks as arrows:

Thus, when Final is completed, the project ends. Now, before Final can begin, three other tasks must be completed. This defines a new event as follows:

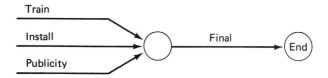

Continuing to work backward, we note that before we can Install the equipment, we must Purchase it, and we must also Remodel the space. This defines still another event, as follows:

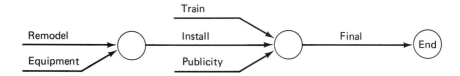

Proceeding in the same manner with all other tasks leads to the complete PERT network, as given in Figure 6-6. Note carefully how each task pre-

---

*For an extensive review of PERT and application in health programming, see Arnold et al. (1966).

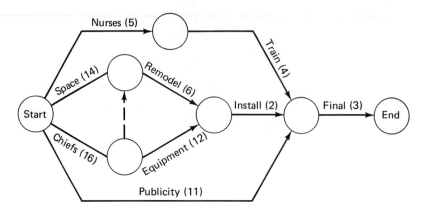

Figure 6-6 PERT network diagram.

cedes others as defined in the sequencing specified at the beginning of this section. Note also how the network begins with a single event—Start—from which all tasks that are not preceded by other tasks begin.

Figure 6-6 also includes a special task used for building the network, called a *dummy task,* represented by a dashed line. This dummy task is used to show that Space and Chiefs must precede Remodel, but only Chiefs must precede Equipment. Without the use of the dummy tasks, that section of the network would look as follows:

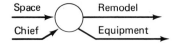

This would be incorrect, since it implies that Space must precede Equipment, which is not true in our example. The dummy task is instantaneous in that it does not take time to complete. It is used simply to show sequencing. The time to complete each task is shown in parentheses beside the task name on the PERT diagram.

Looking back to our general modeling process of Chapter 5, so far we have built our model of the real-world problem in the conceptual world. The next step is to solve the model. By solving, in this case, we want to identify when each task should begin so that the project can be completed in the shortest amount of time. To do this, we begin by specifying two things about each event:

- *Earliest starting time* (EST): the earliest time an event can happen, given that all preceding events happen at their earliest starting time.
- *Latest starting time* (LST): the latest time an event can happen without causing a delay in the completion of the project.

We first work through the network event by event to establish the EST as follows. Divide each event circle in half with a vertical line. On the left of this line we will note the EST, and on the right side the LST. Now, the EST of the event Start is 0:

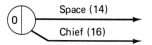

The EST of the event that terminates Chiefs is 16, as this is the earliest time that event can occur given that the Start event begins at time 0. Now, the event that terminates Space has an EST of 16 also, as it cannot happen until Chiefs is completed. (This is the function of the dummy task.) Thus we find the EST by taking the *longest* path to an event:

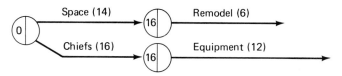

The event terminating Remodel and Equipment has an EST of 28. Why? The EST of the remaining events are shown on Figure 6-7. Thus the minimum completion time for the entire project is 33 weeks given that all tasks are started at their EST.

To get the LST of each event, we work backward from the last event, End. The LST of End must also be 33 weeks, as the definition of LST requires; that is, End must occur no later than week 33 in order not to delay the completion of the project.

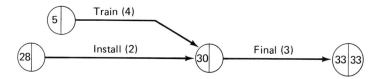

Consider the LST of the event from which Final begins. Since Final must end no later than week 33, and Final takes 3 weeks, it must begin no later than week 30 in order that the project not be delayed. Thus the LST of this event is week 30 (the same as its EST). Now consider the event from which Train begins. Since Train must end no later than week 30 and it takes 4 weeks, this event must occur no later than 30 – 4 = week 26. Using this logic, the LST of all events can be calculated as shown in Figure 6-8. Check these numbers carefully to see how they are determined for the different situations.

Now we have the EST and the LST of each event, and information on when tasks must be started and completed in order to keep the completion

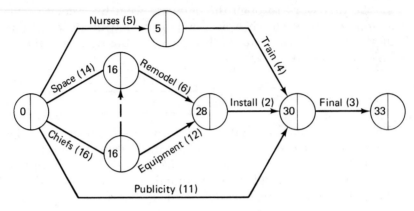

Figure 6-7 PERT network diagram showing ESTs.

time of the project at a minimum. Note that some of the events have their EST equal to their LST. This means that there is no slack time for the tasks that begin and end in these events. This path, the path along which tasks begin and end in events with EST = LST, is called the *critical path*. It is critical in that tasks along this path must be started as soon as possible to avoid delay of completion of the project.

Tasks that are not on the critical path have *slack time,* some amount of time that they can be delayed without delaying completion of the project. Slack time can be calculated as follows:

slack time = LST of the event that ends the task

minus the EST of the event that begins the task

minus the time to complete the task

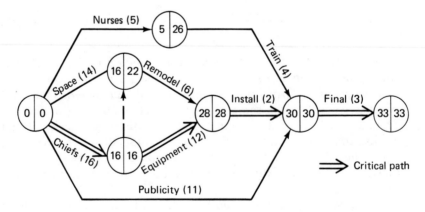

Figure 6-8 PERT network diagram showing ESTs and LSTs.

TABLE 6-5 *Slack Times for Tasks*

Task	Slack
Space	22 – 0 – 14 = 8
Chiefs	16 – 0 – 16 = 0
Equipment	28 – 16 – 12 = 0
Remodel	28 – 16 – 6 = 6
Install	30 – 28 – 2 = 0
Nurses	36 – 0 – 5 = 21
Train	30 – 5 – 4 = 21
Publicity	30 – 0 – 11 = 19
Final	33 – 30 – 3 = 0

For example, for the task Space:

$$\text{slack time} = 22 - 0 - 14 = 8$$

Slack times for other tasks are given in Table 6-5. As expected, the slack time is zero for all tasks on the critical path. There is an important concept to keep in mind when considering slack time. Slack time must often be associated with a *subpath* of tasks rather than with an individual task. For example, Table 6-5 lists both Nurses and Train as having a slack time of 21. In fact, the two tasks have a *total* of 21 weeks of slack, not 21 weeks each. Thus the 21 weeks of slack should be associated with the subpath made up of Nurses plus Train. Some subpaths have only one task, such as Publicity.

It is somewhat difficult to visualize the time relationships between tasks on a PERT diagram, as the lengths of the tasks are not drawn to scale. This is because the major objective of the PERT analysis is to analyze the *sequencing* of tasks. Once the PERT analysis is completed, a more useful representation for purposes of actually "blueprinting" a project is a *Gantt chart,* which is drawn to scale for time to complete tasks. A Gantt chart for our example is shown in Figure 6-9.

To construct a Gantt chart, begin from the last task and work backward, showing tasks in their LST position. (You could just as easily draw a Gantt chart in the EST position, or an inbetween position, depending on the individual needs of the blueprint.) First, draw in the tasks on the critical path. Then draw in the remaining tasks, using dashed lines to take up slack. Use vertical dashed lines to correspond to events. Once the chart has been drawn in its LST (or EST) position, the tasks with slack can be moved around within their slack to coordinate work load, and so on.

The arrows along the bottom of the Gantt chart indicate times when progress on the project can be reviewed. It may be necessary, at one of these reviews, to reanalyze the project using a new PERT network that begins at that date, and to redraw the Gantt chart for the remainder of the project. Thus PERT (and the Gantt chart) offers both a scheduling and a review function, as the name implies.

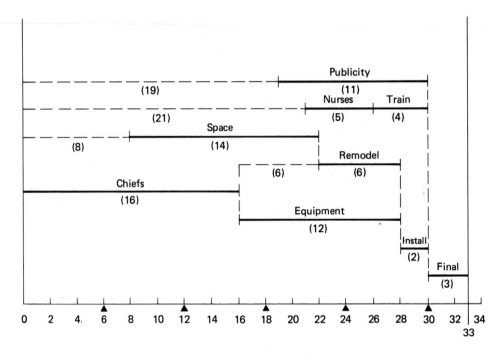

Figure 6-9 GANTT chart for PERT network.

So far we have considered the time to complete a task as fixed. In fact, most tasks can be completed sooner if more resources (usually money) are devoted to its completion. If the amount of money devoted to task completion is considered a decision variable, the analysis is called a *PERT/COST analysis.* In this case our objective is to complete the project in the most economically effective way (i.e., least amount of money).

To spend more money on speeding up the completion of a task, it must be worth something to complete the project as a whole sooner. Consider the following situation. Suppose that if the project could be completed in 32 weeks (instead of 33), it would be worth $2000 to us. If completed in 31 weeks, it would be worth $5000; if 30 weeks, $6000; and if 29 weeks, $7000.

Now, suppose that if we were willing to spend an extra $1000, we could reduce the time it would take to obtain Equipment by 1 week; if we spend $3000, by 2 weeks; and if we spend $8000, by 3 weeks. Should we spend extra money to speed up Equipment? How much extra money?

First, Equipment is on the critical path, so it makes sense to consider speeding it up. It is certainly worth spending $1000 to speed it up 1 week, because we "make" $2000 by having the project completed 1 week sooner. It is also worth spending $3000 for 2 weeks, because we "make" $5000. But it is not worth spending $8000, because we would only make $6000. Thus the optimal amount to spend is $3000 to speed Equipment (and completion of the project) by 2 weeks. A similar analysis could be used on all tasks where speeding is possible.

Two characteristics make large PERT/COST problems very difficult to analyze by hand, although it is easily done on widely available computer programs. First, after some point of reduction, a task on the critical path falls off the critical path and another task becomes critical (this happens to Equipment if it is reduced to less than 6 weeks). Second, there may be several ways to reduce the project by 1 week (or 2 weeks, etc.), and the least expensive way must be identified. Thus all but the smallest PERT/COST analyses must be done on a computer.

A final consideration is the ability of a PERT analysis to incorporate uncertainty. Suppose that the length of time to obtain Equipment is not fixed, but has probability 0.2 of taking 10 weeks, 0.3 of taking 11 weeks, 0.3 of taking 12 weeks, 0.1 of taking 13 weeks, and 0.1 of taking 14 weeks. Suppose also that all the other tasks have completion times described by their own probability distributions. This means that the time to complete the project will be uncertain, as well as all ESTs and LSTs. A PERT analysis can still be performed, but again the uncertainty requires a very complex computer program to allow analysis. The output of such an analysis specifies the probability that, given certain conditions (such that each task is begun at its EST), the probability of the project being completed in 31 weeks is 0.13, of being completed in 32 weeks is 0.41, and so on. By varying the conditions, the probability distribution of completion time of the project varies, giving an extremely useful insight into how sensitive project completion time is to how the separate tasks are undertaken.

CASE 1

Staffing Requirements for a CCU

The number of admissions by month to the CCU (cardiac care unit) of your hospital is displayed below for the past four years.

Year	Jan.	Feb.	Mar.	Apr.	May	June	July	Aug.	Sept.	Oct.	Nov.	Dec.
1977	93	101	84	71	69	74	86	83	83	89	101	90
1978	121	107	103	90	84	80	90	99	96	103	119	123
1979	143	120	110	117	103	100	97	106	117	124	130	138
1980	173	158	139	126	115	102	111	122	133	141	150	157

To plan the amount of staff needed on the CCU for next year (1981), it would be useful to know how many admissions, by month, to expect next year. From a previous analysis of CCU admissions by year, it has been estimated that there will be a total of 1800 admissions next year.

Required: Calculate cyclical indices. Does there seem to be a significant difference between months? If so, use the indices to prepare monthly estimates for 1981. If not, prepare monthly estimates using some other logic.

CASE 2

Inventory Decisions

The daily demand for a certain item used by all patients at your hospital is very stable and can be assumed constant at 200 units a day. It costs $50 to order any amount of the item (this ordering cost does not include the price per item, but includes the cost of making the order, communicating with the supplier, arranging payment, taking delivery, etc.). It costs $0.02 per item per day to store the items (this includes cost of warehousing, utilities, warehouse personnel, insurance, etc.). In addition, there is an investment cost of the cash tied up in inventory of 10% per year, with a price of $17 per item.

Required: Calculate the "optimal" number of items to order. Draw a graph showing how total inventory costs (on the vertical axis) vary with quantity ordered (on the horizontal axis).

CASE 3

Task Sequencing in a Training Program

The problem is to set up and conduct a training program for fieldworkers. The sequencing of tasks and the estimated times are as follows:

	Activities	Time Required	Predecessor Activities
A	Recruit fieldworkers	15	D
B	Write program materials	10	D
C	Select and invite trainers	5	D
D	Set out program objectives	3	—
E	Set up and reserve rooms, etc.	20	—
F	Assemble program notebook for participants	5	B
G	Arrange for field placement	5	A
H	Arrange for final placement	10	A
I	Present classroom training	10	A, C, E, F
J	Conduct field training	5	G, I
K	Prepare examination	3	B
L	Administer examination	1	J, K
M	Place trained fieldworkers	2	L, H

Required: Graphically construct the appropriate PERT network for this problem. Determine and label the critical path. Calculate the EST and LST and slack for each task.

FURTHER READING

CHURCHMAN, C. W. *The Systems Approach*, New York: Dell, 1968.

Cooperative Information Center, *Abstracts of Health Care Management Studies*, Ann Arbor, Mich.: Health Administration Press, 1965–present.

GRIFFITH, J. R. *Quantitative Techniques for Hospital Planning and Control.* Lexington, Mass.: D. C. Heath, 1972.

GRIFFITH, J. R., W. M. HANCOCK, and F. MUNSON. *Cost Control in Hospitals.* Ann Arbor, Mich.: Health Administration Press, 1976.

HILLIER, F. S., and G. J. LIEBERMAN. *Operations Research.* San Francisco: Holden-Day, 1974.

LEVIN, R. I., and C. A. KIRKPATRICK. *Quantitative Approaches to Management.* New York: McGraw-Hill, 1975.

SHUMAN, L. J., R. D. SPEAS, and J. P. YOUNG, eds. *Operations Research in Health Care: A Critical Analysis.* Baltimore, Md.: Johns Hopkins University Press, 1975.

WAGNER, H. M. *Principles of Operations Research.* Englewood Cliffs, N.J.: Prentice-Hall, 1979.

WARNER, D. M., and D. C. HOLLOWAY. *Decision Making and Control for Health Administration.* Ann Arbor, Mich.: Health Administration Press, 1978.

7

Financial Assets and Obligations

OVERVIEW

The implementation and operation phase of management is concerned primarily with the acquisition, protection, and utilization of the assets of the health organization in order to achieve specified goals and objectives as efficiently, effectively, and economically as possible within legal constraints. Accomplishing this involves a number of tasks, including ensuring the accuracy and reliability of accounting data, promoting the operating efficiency of the organization, and developing and encouraging adherence to prescribed managerial policy. Some of these items are discussed in more detail in Chapter 11. However, the objective of this chapter is to consider the management of the organization's assets and obligations.

ASSETS AND OBLIGATIONS

Assets are the resources of a health organization (Seawell, 1975). As presented in Figure 7-1, assets are used to provide services to clients and generate income or profits, which in turn are used to pay off obligations and provide more services. The assets of a health care organization originate from sources both outside and inside the organization. The top level of Figure 7-1 depicts the three major external sources of assets: public funds, such as those from federal, state, and local governments; private sources, such as creditors, stockholders, contributors, and foundations; and consumers. At this point we will focus on the cash that these sources provide, but it is important to

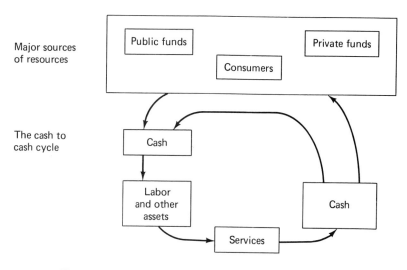

Figure 7-1 The flow of resources in and out of an organization.

realize that they provide credit as well as other resources to the organization. Initially, the cash received from these sources is used in large part to purchase other resources. For instance, cash may be used to purchase fixed assets, such as buildings and equipment, inventories, and labor, or overhead items, such as rent and insurance. In these cases, an asset internal to the organization, cash, is being exchanged for noncash assets such as buildings and labor. These noncash assets are then used to earn income by helping to provide services.

However, all income generated does not remain in the organization. In acquiring and using their assets, organizations assume certain obligations, such as payrolls, taxes, mortgages, accounts payable, and dividends to stockholders. This chapter focuses on the major assets and obligations of health care organizations and the interrelationship among them.

CATEGORIES OF ASSETS AND OBLIGATIONS

Part II of Figure 7-2 depicts the three major categories of assets and obligations of a health care organization. The first category is *working capital,* the second is *noncurrent assets and liabilities,* and the third is *residual equities.*

WORKING CAPITAL

Working capital refers to a health organization's current assets and current liabilities (Berman and Weeks, 1979). As shown in Figure 7-3, *current assets* include cash, marketable securities, accounts receivable, inventories, and prepaid items. *Current liabilities* are the current obligations of a provider to pay its creditors and employees. They include such items as wages payable, accounts payable, and the current portion of mortgages payable.

Current Versus Noncurrent
Assets and Liabilities

How do current assets and liabilities differ from those which are noncurrent? The first major difference is that *current* assets and liabilities are expected (to use the jargon of accounting) to be used up, converted, or extinguished within one year. On the other hand, *noncurrent* assets are expected to be used for periods longer than a year. Examples of noncurrent assets are buildings, x-ray machines, typewriters, and operating tables.

An administrator of a health care organization must ensure that there are sufficient assets to provide adequate levels of service, but not so many that assets are being wasted. For instance, there must be enough cash to pay employees and debts regularly, but not so much that cash is held idle and not

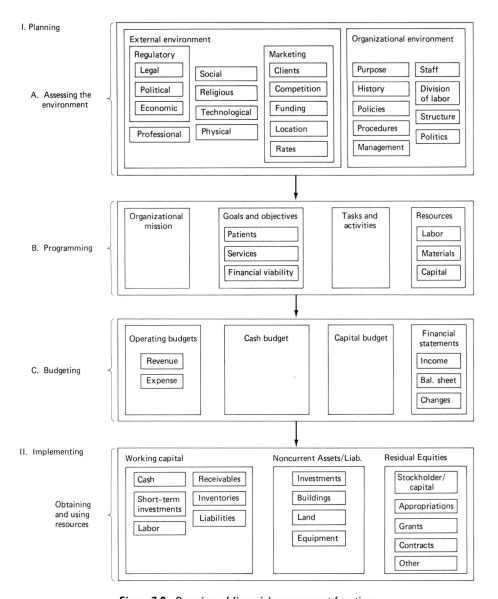

Figure 7-2 Overview of financial management functions.

invested in other assets such as marketable securities (i.e., certificates of deposit, Treasury bills, etc.) or supplies. Similarly, it is important to have sufficient supplies to meet everyday demands and certain levels of emergency, but if the supply inventories are too high, it costs the health care organization money both to store them and to pay for their purchase; the organization could be using the money for other purposes. The point is that the health care provider must manage the assets of the organization to ensure their optimal use (Aggarwal and Hahn, 1979).

Sources of cash

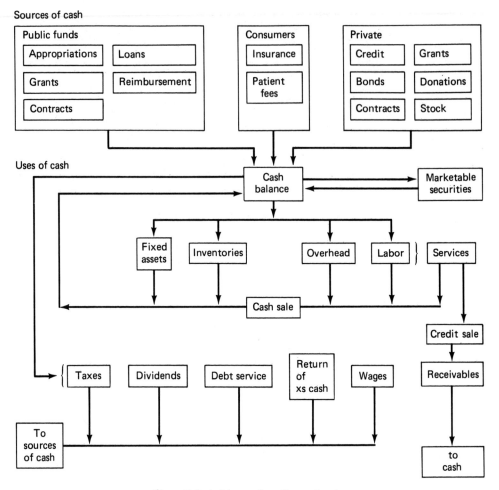

Figure 7-3 Inflows and outflows of cash.

Table 7-1 lists the assets and equities (obligations) of a health care organization. Notice that there is an order to the way both assets and equities are
listed. For instance, the current assets appear in the following order: cash,
marketable securities, accounts receivable, inventories, and prepaid items.
The basis for this order is called liquidity. *Liquidity* refers to the ability of
an organization to turn its assets into cash. Cash is the most liquid asset;
plant and equipment are the least liquid. Similarly, the liabilities are listed in
the usual order in which they must be paid. Listing the assets and equities
of an organization in terms of their liquidity is standard for all business of
organizations—this reflects the importance of cash in running a business.

TABLE 7-1   *The Categories of Assets and Equities*
of a Health Provider

Assets	Equities
Current assets	Current liabilities
Cash	Wages payable
Marketable securities	Trade accounts payable
Accounts receivable	Mortgage payable
Inventories (supplies)	
Prepaid items	
Noncurrent assets	Noncurrent liabilities
Investments	Mortgage payable
Plant	Bonds payable
Property	
Equipment	Stockholders' equity
	Common stock
	Retained earnings

Cash

Figure 7-3 illustrates the importance of cash by elaborating upon Figure 7-1. The cycle in Figure 7-3 begins with cash flowing into the organization from external sources. The importance of cash at this stage of the cycle is that it is used to purchase other assets and pay employees (labor). The labor and other assets are combined to supply services. As a result of receiving services, patients and third parties pay cash to settle their accounts. Money received from these sources can then be used to pay the government (taxes), creditors, employees, and stockholders.

If these steps are well managed, stockholders and creditors are more likely to invest in or provide loans to the provider when the organization needs cash. If a provider cannot easily turn to external sources of funding either on a short- or a long-term basis, the provider may find itself in financial trouble. By not having cash, it will not be able to purchase new assets or pay its employees. Without such assets and a sufficient complement of employees, it will not be able to provide various services at desired levels, so it will not be able to generate the cash it needs to operate. This will result in poor credit ratings, and creditors, funding bodies, and stockholders may well decide to invest elsewhere. This will place the organization in an even more distressing situation.

All organizations hope to avoid such a crisis. To do so requires an understanding of the sources and uses of cash by a health organization. We begin by discussing the three major sources of cash outside the organization: public funds, consumers, and private sources.

Public Funds. For many health care organizations, public funds are the major source of cash. Public funds come to the health care organization through five principal channels: appropriations, grants, contracts, loans, and reimbursement. Although many community health organizations receive their major source of funds through tax-based revenues in the form of appropriations or grants, others receive their funds from nongovernmental-appropriated donations such as the United Way. Regardless, each of these appropriation sources has a similar funding process, which is illustrated in Figure 7–4.

The process begins when the funding source issues guidelines to providers. These guidelines include the anticipated amount of money available and the priorities of the funding source for the coming year. Based on these guidelines, a budget request is submitted by a provider (such as a health department or county hospital) to the funding source or fiscal authority (such as a county board of commissioners). The funding source then develops a preliminary expense budget reflecting the amount of money it needs to cover its proposed activities (including funding the providers.) This process is analogous to that described in developing an expense budget in Chapter 4.

Once the funding agency has identified its expected expenses in detail, it develops a preliminary revenue budget, reflecting more specifically the amount of money it feels it can raise to cover the budget requests. If the revenues identified at least match the anticipated expenses, the providers' budgets are deemed to be appropriate both in amount and content, and the funding source's budget is approved by its fiscal authority, then the provider's budget is approved by the funding source. Once monies become available, they are allocated to the providers.

This is the basic process followed for appropriation-type funding. However, there are numerous variations in practice. For instance, some funding sources develop their anticipated revenue budgets in detail before they develop their preliminary expense budgets or even before they issue their budget guidelines. Similarly, in practice, as shown in Figure 7–4, the initial budget requests from providers are often not approved, and the providers are asked to either decrease the amount requested or perhaps modify the activities or programs they are proposing. One final point should be emphasized. Even though a budget has been approved, it does not mean that the provider is actually going to receive the money requested. This is because the funding source allocates its funds to the providers on the contingency that such funds will actually be available. Incidentally, in certain cases, funds are not only allocated but allotted. An *allocation* involves specifying that certain funds are designated for a specific provider or purpose. An *allotment* is a procedure by which only a portion of the funds are made available to the provider at any given time. For instance, if a health department requests

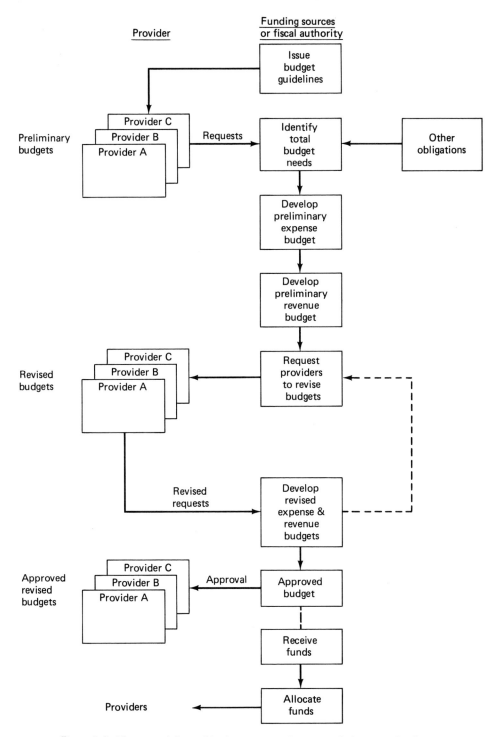

Figure 7-4 The general flow of budget requests for appropriations-type funding.

$10,000 for sanitation inspections throughout the year, the county may decide to allot the $10,000 in four quarterly $2500 payments. The purpose of allotting funds is to ensure that funds will not be spent prematurely.

In addition to budget appropriations, two other major public sources of cash are available to health organizations: grants and contracts. Both grants and contracts involve the funding agency supplying funds to a provider to accomplish certain outcomes. *Grants* are usually general in nature and do not have rigid or specific outcomes. For instance, grants have been made available to mental health centers for initially staffing their organizations as well as building some of their facilities; hospitals have been given grants for studying cancer-causing agents. *Contracts,* on the other hand, are more specific than grants. They usually specify an outcome to be accomplished or procedure to be followed. For example, the federal government may sign a contract with a voluntary health and welfare agency to provide 100 nutritional meals a month to senior citizens. The sanitary nature, nutritional quality, and quantity of the meals may be monitored closely, and the contractor paid accordingly.

A fourth possible source of cash from public funds is *loans.* In such an instance, a public agency may advance funds to an organization for a specific period of time with the stipulation that they be paid back at a certain rate of interest.

Reimbursement is a fifth way in which public funds are added to the cash balance on a health care provider. In reimbursement, an agency acts on behalf of an organization, client, or patient to reimburse the provider for all or some portion of the provider's cost or charges resulting from providing services. In such an arrangement the patient is called the *first party,* the provider the *second party,* and the agency acting on behalf of the client the *third party.* Although there are a number of different governmental reimbursement sources, the major ones at this point are Medicaid and Medicare. Medicare is federally administered; Medicaid is administered by the individual states.

Since their inception, Medicare and Medicaid reimbursement has become a—if not the—major source of funds for various health care providers. The rules and regulations involving Medicaid and Medicare reimbursement are voluminous, and many large health care providers, such as hospitals, have hired staff just to keep up with the latest regulations. Although a detailed discussion of Medicaid and Medicare reimbursement is beyond the scope of this book, it is important to know the extent to which each service offered is covered by reimbursement.

Providers have various tools available to them to maximize reimbursement, including providing highly reimbursed services rather than alternately lower reimbursed services, employing various cost-finding methods, and using various legal appeals (Frank, 1978; Hughes, 1972). These topics are beyond the scope of this book and are left for more advanced treatment.

Consumers. The term *consumers,* as used here, refers to the patients or clients of a health care provider who actually receive the health care services (Cooper, 1979). In their early development, many health care organizations, such as health departments, hospitals, and various clinics, received their funds mainly through appropriations from governmental and fundraising bodies. However, with increasingly rising costs and relatively restricted resources, many health care providers are now asked to turn to patients for amounts not covered by their funding sources.

The amount charged patients either by a for-profit or not-for-profit health provider should be an amount sufficient to cover expenses and to provide for future needs, such as new equipment, buildings, and land acquisitions. If the charges are too high, however, patients or clients may go elsewhere. On the other hand, if charges are too low, there may be an over-abundance of clients and/or a considerable amount of uncovered expenses.

There is an interesting relationship between governmental reimbursement, private insurance, and first-party (patient) payment (Dittman, 1976). As a wholesale purchaser of services, the government agrees to pay cost, or cost plus a certain percentage up to the amount charged the patient. However, the government only wants to pay for those "reasonable" costs which it feels are relevant to providing the services it is paying for. Conversely, it specifically does not want to pay for costs that are "unreasonable" or are not part of the services it is purchasing. This leads to a conflict between third parties and providers as to which charges can be included as "reasonable" for any particular service. At various times the government has not wanted to pay for depreciation, educational expenses, certain research expenses, or for such things as telephones or televisions in rooms. The government has felt that these are not an essential part of curative care. From a provider's point of view, however, these may be considered essential, and it is important that such expenses are paid by the third party. Although the government says that it pays cost, or cost plus a certain percent, it may be using a different definition of cost than that used by a provider. Therefore, providers may find themselves providing services for which the government will not pay the full amount, but not being allowed to charge the patient for the difference. In such cases, the provider must charge more to private pay patients to make up the deficit (Figure 7-5).

Insurance companies, as opposed to the government, will usually pay up to a certain fixed amount for various procedures. This amount is specified in the contract between the first party and the insurance company. As with governmental third parties, to the extent that insurance companies as third parties do not cover the full cost which the health care provider needs to operate, and to the extent that the health care provider cannot obtain funds to cover those costs from other sources, there is only one other place to recover their unreimbursed costs: self-paying patients. Figure 7-5 illustrates that to the extent that cost and a reasonably desired profit are not covered

Situation 1: The full cost of a service is $100. By agreement, the third party pays full cost for this service. In this case the third party and a self-pay patient would pay the same amount for the same service.

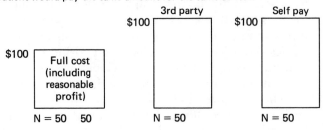

Situation 2: The full cost of a service is $100. By agreement, the third party does not pay full cost. In this case the self-pay patients pay even more than full cost to make up the amount not paid by the third party.

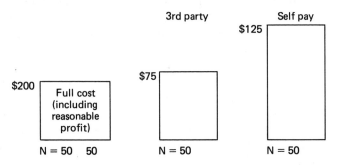

Note: In this instance the higher the proportion of third party reimbursed patients served by a provider, the higher the charges have to be. Self-pay patients make up the difference.

Figure 7-5 Relationship of third party and self-pay patients.

by other third parties, the self-paying patients will end up paying the difference. "Reasonable profit" means a profit that is sufficient to take care of future needs, such as plant, equipment, and pay raises, and to provide investors with a reasonable return on their investment if the provider is a for-profit organization.

Private Funds. Thus far two of the three major sources of funds flowing into the health care organization have been discussed. The first was public funds, which include appropriations, grants, contracts, loans, and reimbursements. The second is consumer funds, which include insurance and patient fees. The final source of cash that flows into an organization is called *private sources.* They include loans, trade credit, bonds, grants, contracts, donations, and stock. These are illustrated in Figure 7-3.

Credit: Credit takes two forms with health care providers (Van Horne, 1977). First is the type commonly thought of as a source of cash. It is a *loan* from various entities, including commercial banks, savings and loans, and various governmental agencies. In this instance, the health care provider receives cash which can be used for various purposes, and in return it promises to pay back the amount borrowed plus interest within a given time. There is a cardinal rule in borrowing which says that one should borrow short term for short-term needs and long term for long-term needs. This implies that for a short-term need such as meeting payroll or purchasing supplies, the health care organization should take out a short-term loan. A short-term loan may vary from a few days to a year. On the other hand, when monies are needed for long-term endeavors such as construction of a building, long-term funds such as bonds should be sought. The major reasons for this axiom are: (1) if one has only short-term needs, they should obligate themselves for only a short term to pay back the amount borrowed; that is, one should try to avoid paying for money beyond the time one gets the use of it; and (2) interest rates in the short run are more predictable than interest rates in the long run and tend to be lower. A major risk in taking any loan, however, is that one may not be able to meet an obligation when it is due.

In addition to loans as a major item of credit, there is another way in which health organizations are able to obtain credit from private funds: trade credit. *Trade credit* is the type of credit that merchants extend customers. With trade credit, the customer receives merchandise but does not have to pay for it until some later date. As opposed to a loan from the bank, in which there is an exchange of cash for a promise to pay it back with interest at a later date, with trade credit the provider receives merchandise in exchange for its promise to pay for the merchandise at a later date. In fact, then, the reason that trade credit is considered a source of cash is not because the health care provider is receiving additional funds, but rather because it is saving itself from an outflow of funds. This is illustrated in Figure 7–6.

In situation 1 (without credit) the health care provider has $500 in cash and no supplies and the creditor or merchant has no cash and $500 in supplies at retail. "At retail" is the amount the merchant charges "off-the-street" customers. After the transaction has taken place, the provider has $100 worth of supplies but $100 less cash, for it has given $100 to the creditor in exchange for the supplies. As a result of the cash transaction, each party has exactly the same amount of current assets as it had before the transaction. That is, the provider has $500 worth of current assets ($400 in cash and $100 in supplies) and the merchant has $100 worth of cash and $400 worth of supplies.

In situation 2 (with credit) the provider purchases $100 worth of supplies on credit, but the result is not the same. After purchasing the merchandise from the supplier, the provider has $600 worth of assets and the creditor has $500 worth of assets. That is, the provider has $500 in cash and $100 of supplies and the creditor has $400 in cash and $100 in accounts receivable. Accounts receivable represents the creditor's right to collect $100 from the

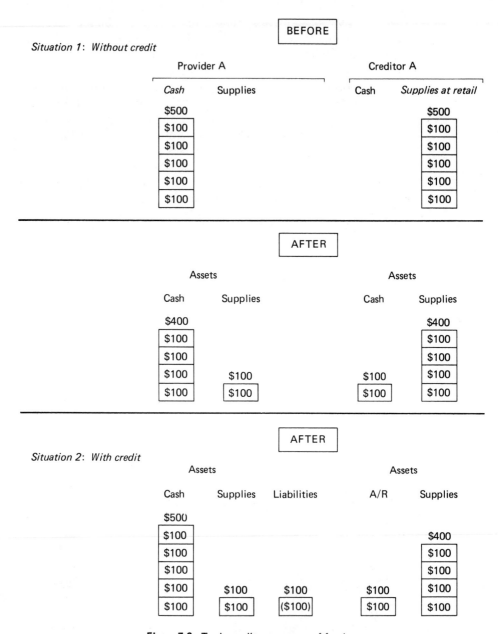

Figure 7-6 Trade credit as a source of funds.

provider. How did this happen? The provider has a $100 liability—the obligation to pay the creditor $100. This example illustrates that trade credit can be considered a source of cash because it allows the provider to have the use of cash it would not have if it paid for the merchandise upon receipt.

It is relatively easy to see why the provider likes to get credit. But why would a merchant want to give trade credit to a provider? The major reason is that extending credit will hopefully generate additional business.

Another source of funds, which is similar to trade credit, is the use of *discounts*. Rather than paying either full-wholesale or full-retail price, the creditor may offer providers a discount if they pay their bills within a certain time, or if they buy in bulk. The wise financial manager will attempt to take advantage of all these methods to the greatest extent possible. We now turn to a discussion of other sources of private funds.

Bonds: A bond is a long-term promissory note (Van Horne, 1977). In more detailed terms, a bond is a statement that the issuer (of the bond) will pay the holders of the bond periodic interest plus the face amount of the bond at a future date (Figure 7-7). A major reason why issuers of bonds like to use this form of financing is that it assures them of a certain amount of

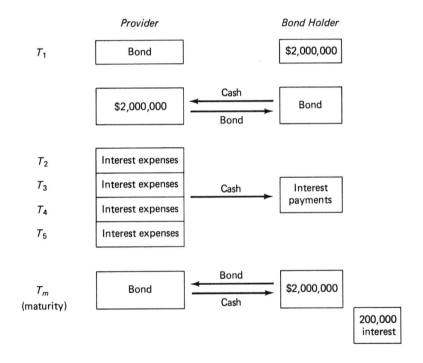

Note: At Time 1 (T_1) the provider issues a bond. The bondholders receive the bond and the provider receives the cash. Between the time when the bond is issued and it reaches maturity, the provider pays interest payments to the bondholders. When the bond matures (T_m), the provider pays the bondholders the face amount of the bond and receives the bond in return, thus ridding itself of its obligation to the bondholders.

Figure 7-7 Effects of issuing a bond.

funds when the bond is sold. For instance, a hospital may issue a $2,000,000 bond to improve its laboratory facilities. Upon selling the bond, the hospital receives $2,000,000 from the purchasers (bondholders) and issues the bond, which is a promise to pay: (1) $2,000,000 at a future date, usually a period longer than 10 years; and (2) a given amount of interest annually or semi-annually until the bond reaches maturity. Providers, as issuers of bonds, like this form of financing because they know exactly what interest they will have to pay in the future and the approximate amount of money they will receive upon selling (issuing) the bond.

Incidentally, because of fluctuating interest rates the provider may not receive exactly $2,000,000 upon issuing the bond. It may receive more (a premium) or less (a discount) depending on whether interest rates are, respectively, lower or higher than the amount stated on the bond.

The advantage to the provider of issuing bonds as opposed to stock is that the bondholders receive only the right to collect the principal, $2,000,000, at a future date (called maturity), and the annual or semiannual interest payments. The bondholders do not receive voting rights in the provider's company or rights to participate in dividends as do certain stockholders. A final advantage of issuing bonds as opposed to stock is that the interest payments are tax deductible.

With all these advantages, why might a provider turn to other forms of financing? There are two major reasons. The first is that if a provider does not have a good credit rating, it may have to pay an extremely high rate of interest to attract persons or companies to purchase its bonds. Second, the provider has no legal obligation to pay anything to stockholders, but there is an obligation to pay back both the principal and the interest to bondholders. If the provider cannot make these payments, it may be forced into bankruptcy or other litigation. Paying back the principal, of course, is no small matter. In the case of a hospital that issues $2,000,000 in bonds, it will have to pay back $2,000,000 at the end of 10 years to the holders of the bonds. This involves a large cash outlay that the hospital may not be able to accumulate. It is for these reasons that hospitals often turn to other forms of long-term financing, which include issuing common and preferred stock.

Equity financing: As just noted, by issuing bonds the provider assumes an obligation to pay creditors; issuing a bond is thus a form of *debt financing*. The issuing of stock incurs an obligation to the owners of the company and is referred to as *equity financing*. Equity in this case refers to the stockholders' interest in the provider. As noted in the preceding section (on issuing bonds) the purchasers of the bonds receive the right to certain interest payments throughout the life of the bond and a return of principal when the bond reaches maturity. When stockholders buy stock, they do not get these two advantages. This will be clearer as we discuss the two major types of stock: common stock and preferred stock.

Common stock may be a desirable method of financing for a health care organization because it does not obligate the provider to pay back either principal or interest (Van Horne, 1977). When stockholders purchase common stock they receive a piece of paper (called a stock certificate) which gives them the right to receive distributions of the net profits of the provider's corporation. From the provider's point of view, if no profit is made, no dividends have to be paid. For that matter, even if a profit is made, no dividends have to be paid. Although this sounds fine in theory, since common stockholders do not always receive dividends, they are less likely to invest in such a company because a major reason people buy common stock is to receive its dividends.

Besides the advantage of not having a definite obligation to make interest payments or to pay back the investment, equity financing has another major advantage: the provider can more easily borrow additional money from creditors. For instance, if instead of floating a bond for $2,000,000 as above, the company raised the money from stockholders, it might be easier for the company to borrow an additional $2,000,000. However, if it already has obligations to pay $2,000,000, creditors might be less likely to invest an additional $2,000,000 in the corporation.

As advantageous as these facts might seem, there are two major disadvantages to issuing common stock. First, dividends, unlike interest payments, are not tax deductible. Second, in issuing common stock, the provider is selling ownership interest in the company. As new common stockholders are brought into the corporation, they receive a right to vote in various matters of the corporation.

Although we will not discuss it in detail, there is one other type of stock that is often used: *preferred stock.* Preferred stock may have some of the characteristics of bonds and some of the characteristics of common stock. The holders of preferred stock, like the holders of bonds, are often entitled to receive their payments before the common stockholders. Second, to the extent that the corporation pays dividends, the preferred stockholders are usually entitled to a certain fixed percentage return. However, they may not be entitled to receive any excess earnings beyond the fixed percentage as do common stockholders. It should be noted that a not-for-profit corporation cannot issue stock. This makes sense, as stock dividends are a distribution of a corporation's profits.

Donations: The final source of funds for health care providers is *donations.* Although donations used to be the major source of funds for almost all health providers, this is no longer the case for many hospitals, health departments, mental health centers, and other federally financed organizations. On the other hand, numerous voluntary health and welfare organizations, such as those financed by the United Way, still rely heavily on donations.

Although many people think of donations in terms of cash gifts directly to health organizations, a large percentage of donations comes from United Way–type drives. If one looks at the roster of the United Way-type organizations, they would find many health-related organizations, including organizations devoted to arthritis, multiple sclerosis, heart disease, and so on. In these organizations, the budgeting process works much like that described earlier in this chapter under appropriations-type budgeting. A discussion of other sources of private funds, such as contributions, trusts, and gifts, is beyond the scope of this chapter.

Uses of Cash

The discussion above focused on the three major categories of outside sources of cash to a health care provider: public sources, consumers, and private sources. As noted earlier in the chapter, the cash received from these sources is then used to invest in other assets, which are used to earn interest or provide services or to pay off the obligation of the organization. The discussion continues with a focus on the other current assets of the organization which are used in or are a result of providing services. These are marketable securities, patient accounts receivable, and inventories.

Marketable Securities

When a health care provider has any short-term cash, it should invest that cash in a short-term investment (Schlag, 1976; Snelling, 1976). Besides banks, *marketable securities* are the main short-term investment for a health care provider. The most familiar marketable securities are certificates of deposit (CDs) and Treasury bills (T-bills). *Certificates of deposit* are receipts given by banks and saving and loans for money invested in special accounts for a specific period of time, usually over 90 days. They differ from regular accounts in which customers deposit their money and can essentially take it out at any time without penalty. Implicit in purchasing a CD is the idea that customers intend to leave their money in the account for the full period specified. Since it is important for the bank to know this, the bank pays higher interest to customers who purchase CDs as opposed to those who deposit their money in regular accounts. Although customers can turn in their CDs early and receive the money they deposited, usually they will be penalized for doing so—even to the extent of receiving no interest.

Treasury bills are obligation notes issued by the federal government and backed in full by the government (Berman and Weeks, 1979).

How does a provider decide among its different investment alternatives? It should weigh three factors: return, risk, and liquidity. *Return* refers to the interest or yield from an investment. *Risk* refers to the safety of the investment. For instance, an investment in a government-backed Treasury bill is far safer than an investment in most new, poorly financed small businesses (over half of which fail in their first year). Liquidity, as noted earlier in this chapter, refers to the ability to convert an item into cash. Unfortunately, these three factors tend to work against each other. For instance, the safer an investment, usually the lower its yield. Since this is the case, a health care organization should set forth its investment policies beforehand to identify how conservative or risk taking it will be. Of course, such policies should be reviewed periodically to reflect changing circumstances—such as changing interest rates or new needs for money by the provider.

Accounts Receivable

Accounts receivable is the name given to the monies owed to the provider usually for services rendered to patients (Seawell, 1975). Accounts receivable exist because health providers offer credit to their patients. The process is almost exactly the opposite of that discussed earlier in this chapter, where the provider was offered credit by merchants. In the case of accounts receivable, rather than a merchant supplying credit to a provider, the provider is granting credit to its customers—the patients. As with the merchant, health care organizations extend credit to patients with the hope of attracting more patients than if they charged cash for all services. However, extending credit has a major disadvantage—not all patients pay their bills.

To ensure an optimal balance between the amount of credit extended, increased consumer demand, and the possibility of not receiving payment, the health care provider must establish detailed credit and collection policies. *Credit policies* should identify patients' eligibility for services, focusing mainly on their ability to pay (Stamps et al., 1978; Assunta, 1970). *Collection policies,* on the other hand, are applicable once credit has been granted and service has been rendered (Smejda, 1978). Collection policies focus on how the health care provider goes about collecting unpaid bills. The major concern is to see that collection efforts do not result in ill will or unnecessary hardship on patients, but do ensure prompt receipt of cash by the provider. Figure 7-8 shows the place of credit and collection policies in the whole patient accounts receivable system.

Beginning at the upper left-hand corner, credit policies are established. When the patient applies for service, a credit review is completed. Many health care organizations find it advantageous to screen the patient's credit before the patient arrives for service. In this way the valuable time of patients is not wasted filling out forms when they arrive for service. It has been found that much of the information about patients can be collected over the phone before the patient arrives.

After credit has been approved and the patient admitted, services are delivered and charges are determined. Charges are based upon the services that the patient receives and may be a result of hourly computation or standard rates or a combination of the two. These charges are entered on the patient's

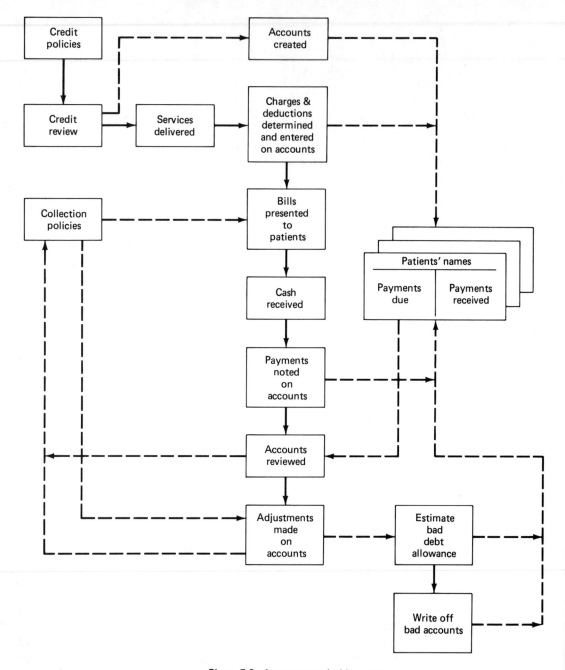

Figure 7-8 Accounts receivables system.

account, which was created after the credit check was completed. Notice that not only are the full charges noted on the account, but the deduction from charges is also noted. The reason for this is that various patients receive discounts (Seawell, 1975). *Charity discounts* are discounts given to persons who are not financially able to pay their full bill. Some charity accounts are mandated by law; others are instituted as part of the policy of the organization. For instance, since by law federally funded mental health centers must treat all clients regardless of their ability to pay, patients are charged on a sliding scale that reflects this fact. Therefore, a person with a large income and few obligations may be billed the full amount of charges; a person with a low income, numerous obligations, and a large family to support may receive a 90%+ discount.

A second type of deduction from charges is called a *courtesy discount.* Various health organizations offer discounts to their employees and various members of the community, such as clergy, teachers, or other health professionals. Such discounts are also deducted from full charges. The final type of discount is called a *contractual adjustment.* The contractual adjustment discount reflects the fact [as discussed earlier (Figure 7-5)] that various third parties, such as Medicare and Medicaid, do not pay full charges. In the case of each of these three types of discounts, the full charges should be entered into the account and then the deductions from charges should be noted. How this process is handled greatly affects the reported financial results of the health care provider.

Continuing with Figure 7-8, after charges have been entered on a patient's account, a bill is presented to the patient in person, by mail, or by some other means, according to the collection policies of the provider. As payment is received from the patient (or a third party) it is noted on the patient's account (or in an account established directly for the third party). The account is reviewed periodically to see if any amount remains to be paid. If so, the patient (or the third party) is then sent another bill, according to the established collection policies.

Periodically, the health care organization reviews its accounts in an attempt to identify and *write off* bad accounts. That is, it determines that certain accounts will never be collected. If the probability is very high, providers will decide not to carry them any longer and remove such accounts from their books. Hopefully, this will be a small percentage of their accounts. Incidentally, the amount of accounts written off can be a very good indicator of the efficacy of the credit and collection policies of the health care organization.

The final step in adjusting accounts is to estimate the amount of the accounts currently on the books that will be written off in the future. A discussion of the procedure is beyond the scope of this book.

In larger health care organizations, with literally thousands of patients receiving multiple services from all parts of the organization, it should be apparent that keeping track of all services, medicines, and so on, delivered to a particular patient can be quite an intricate job. As the importance of running an efficient organization increases, more and more health care providers are beginning to focus upon increasing the accuracy of their cost-determination and billing systems. It is not that they have necessarily been negligent, but rather that they have not been as precise as they could be or for various reasons their methods of determining charges do not fulfill the requirement of various government agencies and third parties. It can be expected that future activities in this area will increasingly focus upon uniform accounting and reporting among health care providers for the cost of goods and services delivered to patients.

Inventories

The fourth major class of current assets is inventories. The term *inventories* is a generic term referring to the various medical and office supplies that a health care organization expects to use up in its day-to-day operations within one year (Seawell, 1975). Examples of medical supplies include drugs, syringes, disposable thermometers, and tongue depressors. Business supplies include typing paper, computer cards, paper clips, pens, and pencils.

Inventory control is often a major concern in the financial management of health care facilities. It is important to have enough supplies on hand to meet everyday needs and certain emergencies, but a provider does not want too much money tied up in excess inventory (Bates, 1979).

As shown in Figure 7-9, the cost of inventory includes not only the amount of money paid for it, but also the costs to order, transport, store, account for, and distribute it. These costs may be considerable, and an increasing number of health care organizations are hiring people to attempt to cut costs in each of these areas.

For instance, a good purchasing agent can identify reliable suppliers and be concerned with negotiating the best terms for the provider (Boergadine, 1979). In a recent case, just before the price of silver was expected to double, a hospital purchased the remaining inventory of an x-ray maker who was going out of business. It is felt that this one purchase saved the hospital over $50,000 in one year.

Once goods are on hand, they must be stored safely and monitored for three main reasons. First, some goods are perishable and must be kept in appropriate storage environments or providers will lose their investment from deterioration of the supplies. Second, to prevent unauthorized usage, the provider must make sure that only those who are authorized have access to the goods, and then only in amounts that are appropriate. This process is part of internal control and is discussed further in Chapter 11. Finally, the goods must be monitored in order to assign the costs of goods to the patient when they are used.

A large health care organization may use hundreds of thousands of dollars of inventory a year. With this much involved, it should be easy to see why inventory control is so important (Aldurf, 1980; Henning, 1980).

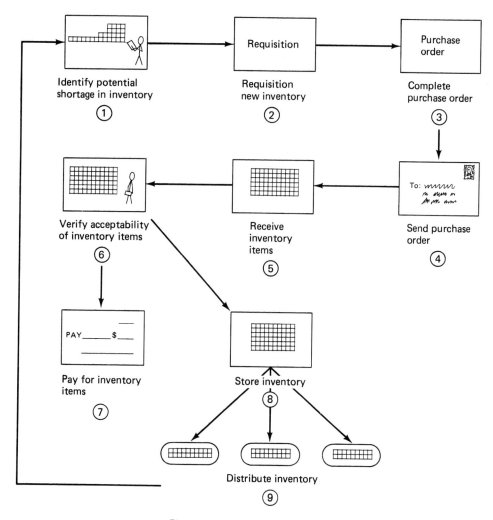

Figure 7-9 Inventory acquisition.

Labor

Thus far this chapter has discussed four of the six working capital items: cash, short-term investments, receivables, and inventories (see Figure 7-2). The next item appearing under working capital is *Labor*. Labor is considered in a different way from the other four current assets and therefore does not appear in the list of assets of an organization (see Table 7-1). Traditionally, labor is treated as an expense but is thought of as an asset. Technically, a resource must be owned by an organization to be considered one of its assets. Since employees are not owned, but rather are paid for their labor, they are not listed as an asset for financial accounting purposes. It is included in our list of working capital items though, to emphasize its importance as a resource of health care organizations. As labor is discussed in Chapter 4 under developing the expense budget, and receives considerable attention in Chapters 5, 9, 11, and 12, it will not be discussed further here.

Current Liabilities

The final category of working capital is *current liabilities*. Current liabilities are liabilities that must be paid within one year. They are usually incurred by the organization in the course of its business. For instance, Table 7-1 lists three categories of liabilities: wages payable, trade accounts payable, and mortgages payable. *Wages payable* are the obligations that an employer has to pay its employees for work they have already done. *Trade accounts payable* are the obligations the health care provider incurs, as discussed earlier in this chapter. *Mortgages payable* appear both as a current and a noncurrent liability. A mortgage can be thought of as the long-term obligation incurred when one buys some equipment, land, or a building. Only that portion due during the current year is listed as a current liability.

Thus, although not commonly thought of as such, liabilities necessarily result in the course of providing services, and are an important component in managing a health care organization's working capital. As opposed to being avoided, incurring liabilities allows the organization to purchase and use assets, while delaying payment for them.

NONCURRENT ASSETS AND LIABILITIES

Fixed Assets

There are two major categories of noncurrent assets: investments; and plant, property, and equipment (Seawell, 1975). The items in this last category are often called *fixed assets* and are fundamental to health care organizations providing service. That is, they give the organization the *capacity* to provide service. The current assets then convert this capacity into service. Thus both current and fixed assets are essential before service can be provided (see Table 7-1). As plant (buildings), property, and equipment usually require a considerable cash outlay, both initially and over time, considerable consideration should be given to the acquisition, protection, and disposition of fixed assets. In acquiring fixed assets, health care administrators must be concerned not only with the cost of the assets, but also the terms, the quality, and the new benefit of a new fixed asset to the organization. Although purchasing a new piece of equipment may seem advantageous on its face, it may not be. Numerous quantitative techniques have been developed to decide among competing alternatives, including capital budgeting, lease–buy, and keep–sell techniques. A discussion of these techniques is beyond the scope of this chapter.

The protection of assets has two major facets, physical protection and maintenance. *Physical protection* is discussed under the topic of *internal control* in Chapter 11. *Maintenance,* as its name implies, refers to the upkeep of facilities and equipment once they are purchased. In this regard the health care administration has several major concerns. First, it must keep the fixed assets in working condition so that they are available when needed. Second, it must keep the fixed assets in working condition so they do not wear out unnecessarily or prematurely; third, it must keep the fixed assets in acceptable condition so that they meet accreditation standards (see Chapter 4). Maintaining buildings and equipment in health care facilities can be extremely costly. The health care administrator must consider the costs in light of the benefits of various levels of upkeep.

Finally, the disposition of fixed assets involves concerns similar to those discussed under their acquisition.

Noncurrent Investments

Noncurrent investments are investments that providers intend to hold over a year. Just as in the earlier discussion of sources of cash, when other companies purchased a provider's bonds or stocks, a provider has purchased the stocks or bonds of other companies (Figure 7-7). The purpose of these investments is to help earn money for the provider and involves the same consideration as those discussed under marketable securities.

Noncurrent Liabilities

Noncurrent liabilities are obligations to other than owners which are expected to last over a year. For the most part, these obligations are incurred in order to purchase fixed assets. For instance, mortgages payable are incurred to pay for the purchase of buildings from their owners. On the other hand, bonds payable may be incurred to finance major equipment purchases or to provide capital for providers constructing their own buildings. In either case, the provider undertakes a long-term obligation it intends to liquidate at some future date longer than a year. The relative advantages and disadvantages of noncurrent liabilities compared to selling stock are discussed earlier in this chapter under "sources of cash."

RESIDUAL EQUITIES

Residual equities refers to the claim on the assets of the organization by those who own a company (if it is a for-profit organization) or by supplying its funds through appropriations, grants, contracts, and so on (if it is not-for-profit). In for-profit corporations, residual equity is called *stockholders' equity*. In not-for-profit organizations the residual equities are classified under the term *fund balance*.

CASE

Operating Concerns: The Royster Health Initiative

Miller Johnovich became director of Royster Health Initiative upon his graduation from a health administration program. He found the situation to be most interesting and challenging. The previous director had left before Mr. Johnovich assumed his position and, essentially, he found that he had to start his organizations from scratch. Not only were the books considerably behind, but he had major problems in locating physicians to spend two years in this rural community. However, because of a considerable amount of hard work and some excellent consultation, Mr. Johnovich was able to turn around the rural health initiative in short order.

With the challenge of the position at Royster Health Initiative behind him, and for reasons relating to family concerns, he readily decided to accept another directorship when it was offered to him. This position was with Vernal Rural Health Initiative, located approximately two hours from Royster by automobile. In discussing the position with Vernal Staff and board members, he was most impressed with the operation.

After two weeks on the job, he returned to his old graduate program to do some library research and to stop by and talk to one of his professors. In the conversation Mr. Johnovich revealed that he really had not realized what he had gotten into. Over the past four months, the previous director had just "not shown up." Therefore, his staff was used to doing essentially what they wanted to do. Furthermore, he was losing two physicians and had no way of knowing what the new administration in Washington was going to do in terms of funding rural health initiatives.

It was his feeling that the community definitely needed medical services, but how best to provide such services was still problematic. He knew that he had to reduce costs. One attractive approach to reducing costs was to enter into purchasing arrangements with other health initiatives. Second, he thought of sharing resources with surrounding health initiatives or clinics. Since each rural health initiative had a business manager, it was possible to pool their resources and have one run all three organizations. He also found out that he was getting a new computer that would be used for a number of purposes—all of which were not yet fully conceptualized.

Mr. Johnovich noted further problems. For example, the previous director had kept a balance of $40,000 in a checking account so that it could be used whenever needed. It was of some concern to Mr. Johnovich whether this was the best way to invest these funds. He was also concerned about the large amount of inventory that was kept on site. The previous administrator felt that it was extremely important in keeping physicians happy to have an abundance of medical supplies. Therefore, the initiative had over a year's supply of some items on hand.

Mr. Johnovich noted that not everything was bad—the organization did have a good credit standing because it always paid its bills on time. In fact, as soon as it received its bills, they were paid. The problem he noted was not that Vernal did not pay its bills promptly, but rather that Vernal did not do a good job of collecting the money that it was owed. The organization was extremely lax in charging its patients, allowing them to pay whatever they could, whenever they could. A third note of concern to Mr. Johnovich was how the Rural Health Initiative could finance a new wing on its building; however, he was unsure of the advantages and disadvantages of various methods of funding. He did not want to work under federal constraints, but did not know what alternatives were available to him. He was thinking of dropping the federal status of Vernal and seeking ownership by members of the community. Finally, Mr. Johnovich believed there would be a cash shortfall in the next year due to the receivables policy. He wondered what sources of funds he could seek to carry him through the next year.

Discussion Questions

1. *Discuss the advantages and disadvantages of the shared service arrangements Miller Johnovich was proposing. What other shared service arrangements might he consider?*

2. *Would you continue the policy of keeping $40,000 in the bank? What alternative should be considered?*

3. *Evaluate the current policy of keeping a large inventory on hand. What would you suggest? Discuss the advantages and disadvantages of the alternative you propose.*

4. *Are you in agreement with Vernal's payment policies? Discuss the reasons behind your answer.*

5. *Criticize Vernal's credit and collection policies. What alternatives would you suggest?*

6. *Discuss the advantages and disadvantages of equity and debt financing.*

7. *What alternatives might be available to Vernal to overcome its projected cash shortfall?*

FURTHER READING

AMMER, D. S. *Purchasing and Materials Management for Health Care Institutions.* Lexington, Mass.: Lexington Books, 1975.

BERMAN, H., and L. WEEKS. *The Financial Management of Hospitals,* 4th ed. Ann Arbor, Mich.: Health Administration Press, 1979.

FRANK, C. W. *Patient Account Management Techniques.* Chicago: Hospital Financial Management Association, 1976.

FRANK, C. W. *Maximizing Hospital Cash Resources.* Germantown, Md.: Aspen Systems Corp., 1978.

FRANK, C. W. *Managing the Patient Account.* Chicago: Hospital Financial Management Association, 1979.

VAN HORNE, J. C. *Fundamentals of Financial Management,* 3rd ed. Englewood Cliffs, N.J.: Prentice-Hall, 1977.

8

Implementation and Organizational Change

OVERVIEW

Planning and the subsequent operational activities result in the development of new programs, organizational designs, and a host of other proposed activities that need to be successfully implemented in the organization. Implementation is really one aspect of a larger ongoing process of organizational change in which the critical management issue is to assure that programs, structures, and technologies, once planned and designed, are made operational within the organization and accepted by organizational personnel. The objective of this chapter is to identify different types of change and change strategies. Emphasis is given to relating the specific strategies to the types of changes being proposed together with considering some of the unique problems facing certain types of changes in health service organizations.

TYPES OF CHANGE

In a single day an administrator may be involved in the implementation of a new piece of equipment, a home care program, and a screening program for hypertension. To classify an almost endless array of activities, consider the means–ends classification scheme in Table 8-1. Any change involves some modification of both ends and means and it is important that administrators have a framework by which to order a vast array of apparently random events.

Change may or may not involve a modification of organizational ends or goals, as indicated in the right-hand column of Table 8-1. The means by which an organization accomplishes its goals may or may not be modified, as indicated in the left-hand column of the table. The resulting three possibilities are designated technical change (a change in means but not in ends), adjustive change (a change in ends but not in means), and adaptive change (a change in both means and ends). What are the characteristics of these three types of changes, and what is their significance for health service organizations?

Technical change may vary in its cost and impact on the organization. For example, the decision of a hospital to replace a four-test blood analyzer with a twelve-test blood analyzer may represent little cost beyond the replacement price, and it may have little impact on the overall organization. On the other hand, a decision by a hospital to install a cobalt machine or to devote a major portion of its resources to a cardiac care unit will have substantial impact on the hospital financially. Moreover, such a decision will affect many of the hospital functions because the cobalt machine or the cardiac care unit will place a demand on available resources. Neverthe-

TABLE 8-1   *Types of Organizational Change*

Types	Means	Ends
Technical	Change	No change
Adjustment	No change	Change
Adaptive	Change	Change

SOURCE: Kaluzny and Veney (1977).

less, both of these changes will remain, at base, technical changes, because they are changes primarily in the *means* by which the normal and usual activities of the hospital are carried out. They do not represent changes in the basic goals of the organization.

Adjustive change represents change in organizational goals but no change in the essential means. The provision of nontherapeutic abortions and the movement of a hospital toward becoming an area's major provider of primary care are examples of adjustive change. In both situations, the technology (i.e., the organizational means) is already available within the organization. However, the organizational goals must be focused. Thus change involves the decision to apply the available technology to provide a service not provided in the past.

Adaptive change is the most extreme form of change. In adaptation, a change occurs not only in the means the organization uses to reach its end, but also in the ends themselves. Adaptation occurs infrequently, but when it does it involves a basic modification in overall organizational direction and reflects changes and means by which the organization accomplishes these modified ends. A classic but rarely observed example of such a change is that of a community hospital providing preventive health care services for the total community. Community hospitals, despite the name, have traditionally provided acute or chronic treatment services to individuals entering the hospital through the emergency room or the admitting office. Hospitals are generally not concerned with disease or disability unless it is brought to their attention from the outside. A shift to preventive health services on a broad community base requires the hospital not only to change a major goal—that is, to move from treatment of illness to the prevention of illness—but it also requires the hospital to change its means. Prevention requires the addition of people skilled in community outreach, case finding, social work, family medicine, and prevention, or it requires redefining the roles of existing personnel within the organization.

STAGES AND CHARACTERISTICS OF THE CHANGE PROCESS

Whether technical, adjustive, or adaptive, change is a process involving a number of different stages. Figure 8-1 describes the basic stages in the process.

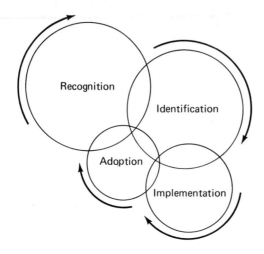

Figure 8-1 Stages of the change process.

The first stage is the *recognition* of a problem by organizational participants who perceive a gap between what the organization is currently doing and what it should or could be doing. The second phase occurs when decision makers *identify* a possible course of action to narrow the gap between action and desired performance. The third stage involves the actual *implementation* of this action within an organization. The final stage, *adoption,* is the acceptance of the implemented change by relevant actors within the organization.

A number of points about the process require special attention:

First, the stimulus for change occurs when there is a perceived discrepancy between how the organization is performing versus how relevant actors think the organization should be performing. This discrepancy creates a performance gap, which when made visible to appropriate individuals within the organization, provides a stimulus to initiate corrective action (Downs, 1967). The performance gap becomes a driving force for organizational change and implementation.

Second, the particular type of change has a set of attributes or characteristics that influence the various stages of the change process. While understanding of the specific attributes is embryonic, these attributes include such things as complexity, the compatibility with existing activities, the cost, and the overall effectiveness of what is proposed. Moreover, it is important to distinguish between what Downs and Mohr (1976) term the primary and secondary attributes of the proposed change. *Primary attributes* are those characteristics of the proposed change that exist without reference to the specific adopting organization. For example, a financially well endowed hospital and an organization with no endowment might describe a particular type of change in the same way. *Secondary attributes,* on the other hand, are those characteristics of the change which are highly inter-

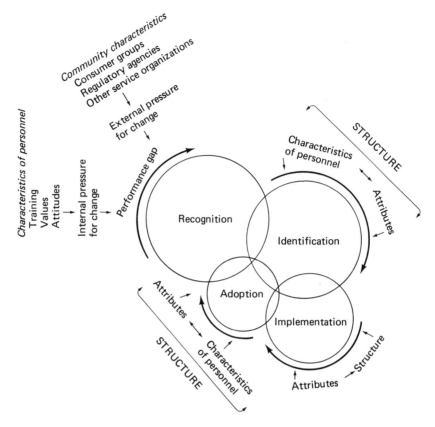

Figure 8-2 Factors influencing change process.

related with particular characteristics of the implementing organization. Thus the financially well endowed hospital might classify a particular type of change as relatively inexpensive, whereas the organization with no endowment may classify the same change as prohibitively expensive.

Third, stages of the change process are influenced by a variety of factors.* Figure 8-2 suggests some of the factors that may facilitate or impede change in the various stages. As suggested by Figure 8-2, recognition (the initial stage of the change process) is affected by both internal and external pressures for change. External pressures for change are a function of the changing needs and demands of the environment. These pressures may be generated by consumer groups, regulatory agencies, or other service organizations in the community.

Internal pressures for change are the results of individual characteristics,

---

*For review of factors associated with various stages of the change process, see Zaltman et al., 1973; Hage, 1980; and Greer, 1977.

such as level of training, values toward change, and the cosmopolitan out-look of organizational personnel. For example, highly trained personnel who keep abreast of latest developments in their respective fields will have higher expectations of what their organization should be doing. This can result in a performance gap and recognition for change.

Identification, that is, where decision makers select a possible course of action to resolve a recognized problem, is affected by characteristics of personnel, selected characteristics of the organization, and secondary attri-butes of the change. Of particular importance are the information networks available within the overall organizational design configuration. One study (Kimberly, 1978) specifically examines the role of information networks on innovations and suggests that many, but not all, information networks facilitate the change process. For example, the amount of physician travel to professional meetings and the percentage of physicians holding joint appointments in medical schools were found to be unrelated to innovation. However, the level of research activity and the amount of resources allo-cated to bring outside speakers in as well as sending physicians out were good predictors of the amount of technological change occurring within the organization.

At the implementation stage, the design characteristics of the organiza-tion and their interaction with attributes of the proposed change are much more important. Here the degree of horizontal and vertical differentiation, availability of slack resources, and integrating mechanisms are important characteristics in determining whether a particular program or set of new activities moves from the identification to the implementation stage. More-over, these characteristics appear to interact with attributes of the proposed change and thereby affect the rate of implementation. For example, organi-zations that already are structurally differentiated, and formally committed to a particular area are more likely to implement programs and technology in that area than are organizations that are not. In essence, the change takes on the characteristic of a technological change rather than an adaptive/adjustive change, and it is therefore more compatible with the existing structure.

Adoption represents the final stage of the change process and it is im-portant to emphasize that implementation of the change is not tantamount to ultimate acceptance by organizational personnel. The extent to which adoption occurs is contingent on the basic design features of the organiza-tion, the previous stages, and selected sociodemographic and personality characteristics of those involved in the adoption process.

Adoption itself involves degrees of attitudinal and behavioral change which vary along a continuum from compliance to internalization (Kelman, 1958). Compliance relates to behavioral change which occurs because the individual, seeking a reward or avoiding punishment, complies with the change. This level of adoption is associated with implementation in the absence of any recognition of a problem or identification of the change as the appropriate action to resolve the problem.

The ultimate in adoption, however, is internalization. This process occurs when individuals perceive an action as relevant and credible, and they incorporate this action within their own set of values. Internalization is most likely when the change has progressed through the stages of recognition, identification, and implementation. The challenge to managers is to achieve internalization.

Moreover, in health service organizations, many changes involve autonomous actors who have a secondary choice as to whether the new program or technology is to be used after it is implemented by the organization (Rogers and Shoemaker, 1971). For example, the adoption of a home care program requires (1) implementation (i.e., the service is available within the organization) and (2) patient referrals to the program by physicians once the program is available. Many programs are implemented but later terminated because of lack of patient referrals by physicians.

Fourth, the change process and the implementation of the various types of programs and activities are not totally random. There appears to be a predictable order which administrators need to follow as they attempt to implement programs (Kaluzny et al., 1971). For example, in the implementation of various types of health service programs such as family planning, social work, chronic disease screening, and rehabilitation services, data reveal a predictable pattern in hospitals. Rehabilitation services are usually the first to be provided. Organizations then implement mental health services, medical social work services, family planning services, and home health services in that order. Armed with this information, administrators might consider the overall sequence of implementation rather than simply implementing programs without providing the appropriate groundwork for subsequent implementation. In many cases the administrator might first think about organizational redesign programs to provide the proper milieu for the implementation of various programmatic innovations which would have significant impact on both the means and the goals of the organization.

TECHNIQUES AFFECTING THE CHANGE PROCESS

Techniques affecting the change process are limited only by the imagination of the manager and the relevant actors involved in the process. Some of the techniques may be executed by the manager or in some situations by a third party or agency. In any case, the administrator should be familiar with the approach and its application. We have limited our discussion to those approaches that are likely or have been used in a health services setting.

To provide some order to the various approaches, we have borrowed the classification scheme developed by Zaltman and Duncan (1977). Under this scheme, four basic strategies are identified: reeducation strategies, persuasion strategies, facilitative strategies, and coercive strategies (power). While we feel that the scheme is useful, it is also important to note the difficulty of classifying approaches. As a result, assignment is sometimes arbitrary.

Reeducation Strategies

Reeducation strategies refer to the unbiased presentation of fact. The approach focuses on individuals within the organization and assumes that personnel within health service organizations are rational, capable of discerning facts, and able to adjust their behavior accordingly. The approach does not, a priori, state a particular course of action for the organization but serves as a potential source for generating discussion concerning the discrepancy between what the organization is doing and what it should be doing.

Continuing Education

The accelerating rate of technological as well as programmatic changes facing health service organizations has placed increasing emphasis on continuing education as an approach to affect the change process. The underlying assumption is that if personnel are well trained and are kept current in the latest developments in their respective fields, they will be more likely to recognize problems within the organization, identify solutions, and ultimately enhance the performance of the institution. This belief is well developed among nursing and medical personnel who pursue an extensive program of continuing education.

Although it is difficult to generalize among various occupational groups, evaluation of continuing education for physicians has shown no consistent association between participation in continuing education programs and the quality of performance (Palmer and Reilly, 1979). The one exception is continuing education programs that are designed around feedback. Here studies suggest an improvement in physician performance, at least in the short run (Brown and Uhl, 1970).

Several reasons may be cited for the limited effect. First, individuals tend to self-select for participation in continuing education efforts. That is, better trained persons tend to participate, whereas less qualified individuals tend to avoid such activities, leaving the overall organizational performance unchanged. Second, the acquisition of new information provides no explicit contrast with what the individual or organization is currently doing, and therefore does not provide stimulus for problem recognition and corrective action.

Survey Feedback

The approach provides a mechanism for systematically gathering data about the operations of the organization. The underlying premise is that one cannot impinge directly on organizational processes (Bowers and Franklin, 1977). Instead, one must work with specific individuals and be able to help these individuals change behaviors that create ineffective processes within the organization. The approach gives individuals an opportunity to understand basic organizational problems and to begin to resolve them.

Figure 8-3 provides an outline of the basic sequence of activities involved in the survey feedback approach. The basic idea is to begin the change process by collecting data on the operations of the organization from

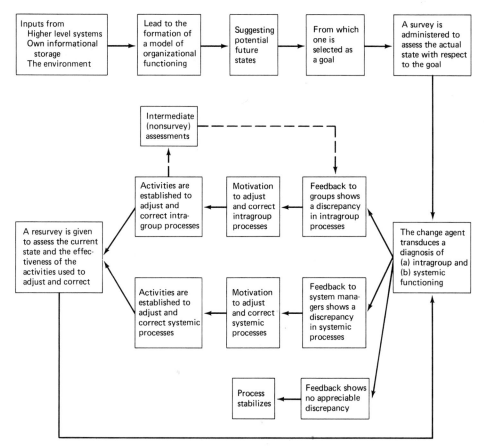

Figure 8-3 Survey-guided development. [D. G. Bowers and J. L. Franklin, "Survey-Guided Development: Using Human Resources Measurement in Organizational Change." *Journal of Contemporary Business* (Summer 1972), 43-55.]

detailed questionnaires administered to organizational personnel. The results are fed back in tabular form, usually to groups of personnel who are given an opportunity to explore its meaning and arrive at some corrective action. Data are again collected and reassessed to determine the effect of the corrective action.

The major function of the feedback process is to develop a discrepancy between what the organization is doing versus what the organization should be doing, and make this discrepancy visible to participants within the organization. Feedback affects behavior in two ways (Nadler, 1977). First, it generates energy and motivates individuals to initiate corrective action. That is, it provides information inconsistent with the perceptions or beliefs of individuals or groups within the organization. For example, the medical staff of a local community hospital may feel that the staff is providing the highest-quality care to its patients. Yet when data are collected on a number of indicators reflecting overall quality of care (e.g., postoperative infection rate), it is found that a significant number of patients have postoperative infection rates or lengths of stay that are considered excessive for selected conditions.

Second, feedback directs behavior where motivation already exists. That is, given the existence of the discrepancy, feedback provides the basis for plans or programs to resolve the discrepancy. Where such plans or programs are not available, the feedback data trigger a search activity to develop plans or programs which at subsequent times may become predetermined plans of action to resolve a discrepancy. For example, returning to the case of postoperative infection rates, the feedback data may provide the basis for problem recognition as well as point to the solution—implementation of an educational program or some other type of program to increase the quality of care provided.

Whether the feedback will actually generate energy or direct behavior is largely contingent on identifying factors affecting the ultimate direction of behavior change. Three factors seem particularly important: the characteristics of the feedback data, the characteristics of the feedback process, and the characteristics of the group or individual task performed. As described by Nadler (1977):

> The first factor, feedback data, must be specific enough to get activity, goal setting, or search behavior going in the right direction. The data should include some evaluative content—comparisons to standards or past performance. The more accurate the data, the more likely it is to bring about change in desired directions.
>
> The second factor, the process of using feedback data, contains two important issues. The group process and the behavior of leaders (or other powerful individuals) should emphasize participation in using the data, use in a nonpunitive manner, and goal-setting activity. In addition, for feedback to serve

as an external motivator, valued rewards must be seen as contingent upon the feedback data. At the same time, connecting rewards to feedback data without developing a constructive and nonpunitive approach for using the feedback can cause defensive behavior.

The third factor is the nature and difficulty of the tasks being performed by the group or individuals. If the level of performance needed to obtain favorable feedback and/or rewards is unattainable, change in the desired direction may not occur. Similarly, tasks which are not challenging or meaningful (in the absence of external rewards) may be poor targets for motivation by feedback. In group situations, the greater the interdependence, the more emphasis that should be put on group feedback and group-level processes to work on feedback. [P. 80]

The feedback approach has been used in initiating and guiding change affecting the total organization as well as dealing with change in specific groups within the organization. One study (Bowers, 1973) has attempted to compare the effectiveness of survey feedback with other change strategies such as process consultation and sensitivity training in initiating and guiding change within the organization. The study involved 14,000 respondents in 123 business organizations and revealed that survey feedback had the most significant impact on organizational functioning. Data were gathered on basic design variables initially outlined in Likert's model of organizations.

Persuasion Strategies

Persuasion strategies attempt to bring about change through bias in structuring and presenting the message. Here the focus is on selling an idea based on substantive facts or on totally false information and/or manipulation of the individual. These approaches, like the reeducation methods, are most appropriate at the early stages, that is, the recognition and identification stages, or in the final acceptance stages of the change process. At the early stages of implementation, persuasion strategies provide a mechanism for increasing expectations of what can be accomplished through a particular change, thereby initiating the innovation process. Moreover, by presenting an advocacy position for a particular activity, persuasion strategies provide identification of a solution to the recognized problems as well as assuring its ultimate acceptance.

Most persuasion approaches focus on attitudes of individuals. The objective is to persuade without creating resistance or reaction to the content of the persuasion. Below is a list of various persuasion techniques derived from our understanding of fundamental behavior patterns (Smith and Kaluzny, 1975).

Successive Approximation

Individual attitudes about new programs, equipment, or activities vary along a continuum. An individual may be very positive about certain aspects and have negative feelings toward other aspects. For example, physicians in a hospital may feel quite positive about the educational implications of a quality assurance program. On the other hand, they may feel quite negative about other aspects, such as the amount of paperwork and the possibility of having to sanction one of their colleagues.

The approach of successive approximation develops a scale reflecting the range of attitudes about the particular program. The objective is to change those attitudes with which the individual disagrees only mildly. With each minimal change there is a change in the individual's overall attitude, thus leading to further change. Obviously, this approach involves a gradual process, and is not suitable for inducing sudden change on major issues.

Analogy

Using an example unrelated to the context of the attitude problem toward which persuasion is directed but getting the individual to commit himself to the logic of the example involved can prove quite useful. Such an unrelated discussion has the advantage of not touching on sensitive issues.

This approach is based on the general finding that individuals seem to have a need to perceive of themselves as consistent. If individuals accept the logic of an unrelated context, and the inconsistency with the arguments they use in another context are exposed, they will experience a certain amount of tension and in turn will try to reduce the tension by changing their attitudes. For example, many health professionals are very skeptical about the use of management science techniques in hospitals and other health service organizations, yet are impressed with the efficiency of industrial organizations. In attempting to persuade these individuals to use management science techniques in certain areas of hospital activities, the job of persuasion can be made easier by pointing out to the individual that operations research methods are used in industrial settings. Since the individual is impressed by the efficiency of industrial organizations, the obvious discrepancy between the individual's two attitudes should result in a change. Although it is hoped that the attitude changes toward supporting operations research in health service organizations, the individual may simply change his or her attitude toward the efficiency of industrial organizations. This possibility is always one of the limitations and unanticipated consequences of some persuasion approaches.

Social Pressures

Groups exert a great deal of pressure toward conformity. In a classic experiment it has been demonstrated that if naive subjects are immersed in a group of confederates who will judge the length of a line incorrectly, more than a third of the subjects will conform to those judgments. Many of the remaining subjects will experience a good deal of confusion (Asch, 1952).

This finding can be applied directly to many group situations in health services. In fact, manipulation by peer pressure is undoubtedly used at an intuitive level by many managers dealing with committees and hospital boards.

The New Wing

The hospital board has been called together to make a decision on two alternative designs for a new wing. The administrator, as a result of his own personal "edifice complex," would prefer to see the construction of a modern glass structure. The most influential board member, however, prefers the more conservative design that looks like the bank he represents. The administrator seats the board members so that they can't see each other's faces but the administrator has a clear view of each of them. He then proceeds with a discussion of the options, complete with flip charts and slides. He makes his pitch for the glass-walled facility and scans his audience for signs of approval and disapproval. The bank representative frowns, but another member leans forward with interest and nods his head slightly. He turns to this board member and asks his opinion of the option. The board member indicates that he likes it, and the adminstrator asks him why. (This helps to obtain full commitment from the individual and also allows the administrator to scan the group for signs of approval from the other members.) Some of the things the board members say are likely to trigger signs of approval from other members, and their opinions will then be sought. The most influential resistant member will, of course, be left to last. By this time he should be feeling sufficient pressure to revise his opinions somewhat about the modern structure. (More rigid authoritarian individuals tend to have a low tolerance for ambiguity, and seem to be more susceptible to such pressures.) The seating arrangements have prevented the more ingratiating members of the board from giving initial support to the banker. The administrator will have his glass edifice. [Smith and Kaluzny, 1975, pp. 317-318]

Complying with Small Request

Persuasion may also be achieved by first obtaining an agreement on a small and apparently reasonable request. Once such a request is met, the individual is likely to comply with more dramatic or greater requests for behavior changes. The approach is similar to successive approximation; however, it is not based on the development of an attitude scale and deals more directly with individual behavior.

This approach is often used in interviewing. The interviewer begins by obtaining fairly innocuous information and then proceeds to request more revealing data.

There are many opportunities for the use of this strategy in health service organizations. The approach is further enhanced by the development of credibility over time. For example, a university program may be interested in developing an outreach program with a number of hospitals. Cooperation with the hospitals might be facilitated by limiting initial requests to information easily accessible within the organization. After this initial commitment is obtained, more sensitive information such as fees for different procedures, access to medical records, and so forth could be requested in subsequent years. As agreement is reached on each of these issues and there is a further establishment of credibility by the university program, the likelihood of encountering resistance to other requests will diminish.

Distraction

Social psychological experiments have shown that persuasion often works best when the subjects are not forewarned of the persuasion attempt and when there are sufficient distractions built into the design to prevent the marshaling of a counterargument. Thus effective persuasion design should, at the very least, start with some kind of distraction. In fact, even a causal observation of most meetings where persuasion is to take place reveals a beginning with some unrelated conversation or activity. This is a part of our social norms and provides a convenient pattern of interaction. Most distractions need not be elaborate. Discussions of sports or the latest joke are perhaps the most traditional distractions. As many individuals may be impatient with these topics, the creative persuaders will probably look for other kinds of distractions to incorporate into the persuasion design.

Curiosity

It is well known that most people exhibit curiosity. As described below, individuals can capitalize on this human tendency to achieve their own purposes.

Salesman: Let's see, I've got some of the more standard stuff in the bottom of this case. (The salesman carefully lifts out a small shiny gadget and places it ever so slowly on the side of the desk and then returns to rummage in the bottom of his case.)

Pathologist: Hey, what's that thing?

Salesman: Oh, that's the new ____. I don't think you'd have any interest in it. Only the big teaching hospitals in the city are using it.

Pathologist: Oh yeah, why not?

Salesman: Oh, I doubt that you do many of those kinds of tests in a hospital like this.

Pathologist: That's not true! We do some of those.

Salesman: Well, it's pretty expensive, and Anderson [the administrator] would probably put up a big fuss about purchasing it.

Pathologist: That idiot! What the hell does he know? I'll make the medical decisions in this department. Show me how it works!

[Smith and Kaluzny, 1975 p. 321]

Obviously, the skillful use of curiosity takes advantage of both sensitive professional pride and traditional medical/administrative antagonism. The salesman has maneuvered the pathologist into believing that the hospital needs the new gadget. If the salesman tried to push his sale directly, the pathologist probably would have told him that the item was too expensive and they would have little use for it. Instead, the hospital will probably purchase a new piece of equipment, one with limited use.

Facilitative Strategies

Facilitative strategies are those interventions that make the implementation of a specific change easier. The use of facilitative strategies assumes that organizations (1) already recognize the problem, (2) agree on a remedial action, (3) are open to external assistance, and (4) are willing to engage in self-help efforts.

Many of the organizational development methodologies are appropriate facilitative strategies. These include such activities as sensitivity training, process consultation, and team building approaches. Each of these methods provides a mechanism through which organizational members are able to gain additional insight into themselves or relevant work groups, enhancing the overall change process.

Process Consultation

One way to facilitate the change process is to gain a better understanding of the personal, interpersonal, and group processes within the organization. Process consultation is a method by which an outside consultant helps the client, usually the manager, to perceive, understand, and act upon process events confronting the individual. Consultation focuses on five areas of organizational activities: communications, role and function of group members, the way groups solve problems and make decisions, development and growth of group norms, and the use of leadership and authority.

Under this approach the process consultant provides insight to the client on various events going on around him or her. Various remedial solutions can therefore be developed to enhance the overall workings of the organization and to facilitate the overall change process. Although the approach has been widely accepted and used in industrial settings, there are few documented cases of process consultation within health service organizations. A specific application of process consultation to groups in the form of team building has been applied to health organizations as described below.

Team Building

Health service organizations are composed of many different working groups or teams involved with providing health and managerial services. Yet all too often these teams are engulfed in conflict, confusion, and ambiguity, which inhibit the overall effectiveness of the group and its ability to effectively participate in various stages of the change process. As viewed by one observer (Weiss et al., 1974):

> It is naive to bring together a highly diverse group of people and expect that, by calling them a team, they will in fact behave as a team. It is ironic indeed to realize that a football team spends 40 hours a week practicing team work for the two hours on Sunday afternoon when their team work really counts. Teams and organizations seldom spend two hours per year practicing when their ability to function as a team counts 40 hours per week. [p. 56]

Team building represents an approach to enhance the overall performance of the work group and the ability to facilitate and effectively participate in the change process. The approach is much like process consultation, but the primary emphasis is on providing insight to the group rather than to any individual client. Attention is given to assessing critical variables known to be important to the group's operation, and feeding this information back to the group to permit it to develop plans for resolving identified problems.

The approach has been used to enhance the performance of health care teams composed of physicians, nurses, and social workers in a community health center (Rubin and Beckhard, 1972). The approach focused on seven selected characteristics known to be important to the functioning of the group: goals of the group, internal and external role definitions, decision-making patterns, communication patterns, leadership style, and group norms. Data were collected through the use of questionnaires and interviews on each of these characteristics, with feedback provided to the respective health teams. Based on this information the groups attempted to diagnose specific problems as well as to develop corrective actions. Several short-term changes were observed:

- Greater work productivity, particularly with respect to team conference meetings.
- Increased clarity of role expectations plus mechanism for negotiating changes in role behavior as they were needed.
- Greater flexibility in decision making.
- More widely shared influence and participation among all team members.

Funds

The simple availability of funds provides an important facilitating mechanism. Fund availability provides the slack necessary to avoid making hard decisions. This places less strain on the basic structural features of the organization.

Although funds will obviously facilitate the implementation of various changes, the simple availability of dollars does not facilitate the development of a performance gap or the assurance that the implemented change will be accepted by relevant personnel. In fact, the use of funds as a sole intervention method can be dysfunctional to the overall change process. For example, funds may facilitate implementation, but if implementation is not based on a perceived need, it is likely that the implemented programs will not be ultimately accepted by personnel within the organization.

Power Strategies

Power strategies involve the use of sanctions and/or coercion to obtain implementation and subsequent compliance. The success of such a strategy is contingent on the degree to which the organization depends on the individual or organization that is imposing the strategy. The availability of alternatives to achieve organizational goals decreases the effectiveness of the power strategy.

Power strategies are particularly useful when the organization or relevant unit fails to perceive a performance gap and thereby fails to initiate the overall change process. The obvious limitation of this approach is that although power strategies can guarantee implementation, they do not assure acceptance by relevant actors within the organization.

In health service organizations this approach is best illustrated by standards imposed by external agents. Illustrations are presented below.

Affirmative Action

Racial and sexual discrimination is a pervasive problem affecting many organizations. Affirmative action represents a power strategy for organizational change (Neely, 1978). Initiated by the federal government, affirmative action requires organizations to go beyond a neutral "nondiscriminatory" and "merit hiring" policy and establish a goal-setting program with measurement and evaluation criteria for all employment practices, including, but not limited to, recruiting, hiring, transfer, promotion, training, compensation, benefits, layoffs, and terminations (U.S. EEOC, 1974).

The approach has two distinguishing characteristics. First, it designates the process by which compliance is to be achieved. Organizations are required to go through a series of steps. First, the organization must identify the number and percentage of minorities and female employees in the organization in each division, office, and major job classification. The purpose of this step is to determine areas of underutilization or concentration in a particular job category more than would be expected by the presence of minorities or women in the relevant labor market.

A second step involves the establishment of goals and time tables to achieve "representation of each group identified as 'underutilized' in each major job classification in reasonable relation to the overall labor force participation of such groups" (U.S. EEOC, 1974, p. 26). The difference between the number of minorities and women currently employed and the number that should be employed determines the goal for proper representation in job categories and in the total organization.

The final step involves the identification of causes of underutilization. These include (1) the recruitment process and personnel procedures; (2) selection standards and procedures; (3) upward mobility systems: assignments, job progressions, transfers, promotions, seniority, training; (4) wage and salary structure; (5) benefits and conditions of employment; (6) layoff, recall, termination, discrimination, action discharge; and (7) union contract provisions affecting areas (U.S. EEOC, 1974, p. 28).

A second distinguishing characteristic is that failure to comply with the process results in the threat of legal action. This legal action is the responsibility of several agencies, including the Equal Employment Opportunity Commission and the Office of Civil Rights. During 1979 the Office of Civil Rights trained more than 700 investigators to assure monitoring and compliance among health and human service program activities (Washington Report, 1980).

Accreditation by the Joint Commission on Accreditation of Hospitals

The purpose of the JCAH is:

1. To establish standards for the operation of hospitals and other health-related facilities and services.

2. To conduct survey and accreditation programs that will encourage members of the health professions, hospitals, and other health-related facilities and services voluntarily:
   a. To promote high quality of care in all aspects in order to give patients the optimal benefits that medical science has to offer.
   b. To apply certain basic principles of physical plant safety and maintenance, and of organization and administration of function for efficient care of the patient.
   c. To maintain the essential services in the facilities through coordinated effort of the organized staffs and the governing bodies of the facilities.

3. To recognize compliance with standards by issuance of certificates of accreditation.

4. To conduct programs of education and research, and publish the results thereof, which will further the other purposes of the corporation, and to accept grants, gifts, bequests, and devices in support of the corporation.

5. To assume such other responsibilities and to conduct such other activities as are compatible with the operation of such standard-setting, survey, and accreditation programs.

Since 1970, the Commission has participated in an extensive review of hospital standards. The review culminated with the implementation of a number of new or substantially revised standards in 1980 which affect the governing board, ambulatory care services, management and administrative services, quality assurance, and utilization review activities. Quality assurance standards are the most far reaching in terms of their implications. The standards require that hospitals demonstrate a consistent endeavor to deliver patient care that is optimal within available resources and consistent with achievable goals. The major component in the application of this principle is the operation of a quality assurance program.

The ability of the Joint Commission to force compliance to standards was greatly enhanced with the passage of the 1965 Public Law 89–97 (Medicare). Written into this legislation was the provision that hospitals participating in the Medicare program were to comply with the standards of the Joint Commission. These standards and conditions of participation for hospitals were subsequently promulgated and published by the Social Security Administration. Thus hospitals in compliance with the Joint Commission standards are automatically deemed to be in compliance with the federal Medicare conditions of participation and are therefore eligible for participation in Medicare reimbursement. Since participation in Medicare is an important mechanism for reimbursement, the standards and the Joint Commission have a great deal of power for achieving compliance.

Combined Strategies

The ultimate selection of strategies and specific approaches within each strategy are contingent upon (1) the type of change involved, and (2) the particular stage of the overall change process. Table 8-2 outlines the relationship of the types of strategies to the types of changes.

As seen from the table, there is a close relationship between the type of strategy and the type of change being proposed. Technological changes that require a change in means but not in ends are most compatible with reeducation and persuasion strategies. The greater the extent to which change will require a change in ends and, in the case of adaption, a change in both means and ends, the more likely that power strategies and appropriate facilitative approaches are required. In essence, the latter changes require a basic realteration of the organizational structure, thereby requiring greater external pressures.

The application of multiple strategies also requires consideration of the different stages in the implementation process. As reflected in Table 8-3, it is particularly important to emphasize the idea of sequence as well as the difference in target groups involved at the particular stage of the process. Failure to consider sequence and the appropriate target group may be counterproductive to the use of change strategies. For example, at the recognition and identification stages, change strategies must be targeted at individuals rather than at the larger organization. Recognition and identification are cognitive activities that can be accomplished only by individuals, whereas implementation involves the basic structure of the organization. Moreover, to achieve implementation without first achieving recognition and identification fails to provide the basis to sustain the change over time.

Consider the combined effects of power, facilitative, and reeducation strategies in the implementation of some quality assurance activity. Power strategies could provide the basis for recruiting full-time directors of medical education to meet accreditation guidelines. The recruitment of new faculty within the organization would affect horizontal lines of communication and challenge the existing power structure within the organization (Hage, 1974). The reallocation of power may place individuals knowledgeable or at least more sensitive to the performance problem of the organization in a position to initiate corrective action. It is unlikely, however, that without

TABLE 8-2 *Types of Change and Change Strategies*

Types of Change	Change Strategy			
	Reeducation	Persuasion	Facilitative	Power
Adaptative	Yes	Yes	Yes	Yes
Adjustive	Yes	Yes	Yes	
Technical	Yes	Yes		

SOURCE: Kaluzny and Veney (1977).

TABLE 8-3 *Combined Strategies by Stage and Target Groups*

Stage	Target Groups	Strategy
Recognition	Individuals ◄───────	Reeducation Persuasion
Identification	Individuals ◄───────	Reeducation Persuasion Power
Implementation	Organization ◄───────	Facilitation Power
Adoption Compliance[a] Internalization[b]	Individuals/groups ◄───────	Reeducation Persuasion Facilitation

[a]*Occurrence of implementation but no recognition/identification.*
[b]*Occurrence of implementation, identification, and recognition.*

facilitation strategies such as supplemental funds, the particular quality assurance activity would be implemented within the organization. But to assure the acceptance of participating physicians within the hospital, neither facilitative nor power strategies are sufficient. Here attention must be given to basic reeducation efforts to increase the probability that the new quality assurance activities will be accepted by professional personnel.

IMPLEMENTING ADAPTIVE AND ADJUSTIVE CHANGES

Health service organizations are increasingly faced with the need to reassess their overall objectives and design to ensure their ability to provide appropriate quality care. As part of this assessment, organizations have attempted to use various types of facilitative strategies (e.g., team building and process consultation) to assure appropriate adaptive and adjustive change. Although these efforts have been well developed and applied in many industrial settings, their application has encountered unanticipated difficulty in health service organizations. This difficulty centers around four factors (Rubin et al., 1974):

1. *The nature of the task:* The provision of health services is characterized by its vague and ambiguous task, making it difficult to set meaningful and measurable goals. This difficulty is further confounded by the fact that health service organizations deal with serious issues of life and death.
   Both characteristics have significant implications for the imple-

mentation of adaptive and adjustive changes. First, these changes are perceived as having a direct effect on the individuals involved in the delivery of care. This alters the way in which individuals function in the delivery of health care and affects the quality of care itself. A second limitation is that health service organizations are predisposed to assess the efficacy of the proposed change. Most adaptive and adjustive changes have not been made before and there is no clinical or empirical evidence to support the efficacy of these approaches.

2. *The nature of internal resources—the people:* A critical factor affecting the success of adaptive and adjustive changes is the personnel within the organization and their orientation to change interventions. First, physicians operate from the general assumption that one should first do no harm. Any act that implies risk taking or the use of unproven methods may result in peer criticism or legal risk. Adaptive and adjustive changes are usually viewed as taking unnecessary risks or as the least conservative approach to remedy a situation.

   A second factor is the nature of the medical model in the doctor-patient relationship. The medical model is contradictory to the normal organizational development approach involved in most adaptive change. The medical model is characterized by fairly active intervention on the part of the physician. The patient presents a problem and it is expected that the physician will diagnose and resolve the problem. In contrast, the organizational development consultants operate from a different perspective. They attempt to work out problems in full consultation with the major actors within the organization. The failure of the organizational development specialist to meet the expectations of the medical model undermines the credibility of the organizational specialist as perceived by many health professionals in the organization.

3. *The organization's structure—power and control:* The distribution of power within an organization makes it very difficult to map critical influence points. In developing an adaptive or adjustive change, one would normally focus on the prime actors in the organization. However, much of the power may be held by individuals not appearing on the organizational chart. For example, physicians not involved in earlier consultation efforts to initiate an adaptive or adjustive change may later very easily veto the change.

   Another limitation is the fact that many health care organizations have little experience with collaborative problem solving and joint decision making. The dominant actors are trained primarily to make decisions in a largely authoritative manner. This makes it difficult for them to adapt to the more consultative approaches characterizing planned change efforts.

4. *The wider environment:* A final factor making adaptive and adjustive changes very difficult is the environment impinging upon the health service agencies. Particular emphasis needs to be given to the funding patterns, which contribute greatly to the uncertainty of the task. Money is often allocated according to criteria that have little relevance to delivery of health services. It is difficult to develop an adaptive or adjustive change to enhance the operations of the organization unless relevant actors see such changes as assuring external funding.

CASE 1

Using Survey Feedback in a Short-Term General Hospital

Federal Hospital is a 200-bed public health service general medical and surgical facility serving federal beneficiaries, located in a major metropolitan area. Administratively, it is composed of a director, associate director, and three assistant directors (one each for clinical services, hospital services, and ambulatory services) and a full complement of medical and surgical departments. The hospital has a staff of approximately 400 and a large outpatient service. It is affiliated with the local medical school and, although federally supported, has maintained positive relationships with local and state government as well as the nongovernmental sectors of the health care community. The hospital is a desirable employer because salaries in most personnel categories are significantly higher than those in other health institutions in the area.

Despite these favorable salary conditions, there has been a growing amount of dissatisfaction among professional and nonprofessional personnel. For example, physician members of the staff (full-time employees) have complained that they were not being supported by management; they were unable to communicate with management; and they were often the subject of harassment, either directly or indirectly, by the hospital director.

As a federal hospital, management had access to a recently established managerial consulting team. This team conducts intensive diagnostic studies, and although it does not make recommendations, it provides information to local management to plan activities to improve the operations of the hospital. Several of the assistant directors felt that the team could provide an important resource to the identification and eventual resolution of various operating problems. The director initially opposed the idea but was ultimately convinced that there was sufficient grounds for such an effort and proceeded to invite the team to conduct its diagnostic survey. It was understood that information generated from this survey would not be shared outside the participating facility.

When the team arrived, the director and his associates, together with the personnel officer, met with the team for instructions and the setting of ground rules. The team leader described the purposes of the visit and the procedures for gathering information and reporting. He reiterated that this visitation was the result of a purely voluntary request and informed the administrative staff that the work load would be divided among the three team members and a fourth team member, the associate director of the hospital. The director had selected this individual to serve as a team member in response to a request by the team leader.

The associate director would provide logistical support as well as function as a full team member. Tentative dates were set for the reporting, and the team leader stressed that all reporting would be oral and that there would be no written documentation, thereby assuring greater confidentiality. The director informed the team that it would have his staff's fullest cooperation.

To initiate the process, the team requested that all employees complete a standardized questionnaire. The questionnaire was composed of 50 statements describing the workings of the hospital. For each statement the employee was to check one of five possible responses, indicating the extent to which this condition *actually* occurred. For example, one statement was: "To what extent are decisions made at those levels where the most adequate and accurate information are available?" For this statement, each employee was to indicate the extent to which this condition was true: to a very little extent, to a little extent, to some extent, to a great extent, and to a very great extent. The employee was also requested to check another set of responses for the same statement, indicating the extent to which this condition *should* occur.

The survey was followed by interviews with a subsample of respondents. Respondents were selected on a sampling basis according to the size of the department. In smaller departments all members of the department were interviewed, and in larger departments (e.g., nursing) a sample of personnel were interviewed. The associate director was assigned departments for which he had no direct authority and thus could be more impartial and objective.

Prior to the interviews, employees were informed of the interview procedure, assured of anonymity, and requested to cooperate. Employees discussed the forthcoming process and were generally supportive and interested in cooperating. The hospital personnel office provided employee data and scheduled all appointments.

Each afternoon, after eight hours of interviews, the team met in the associate director's office to discuss either administrative problems or general tendencies that had been elicited during the interview process. The individual team members were encouraged to keep notes of each interview while preserving the anonymity of the interviewees. The team members retained identification of departments, so that in the reporting process departmental problems could be identified as well as positive findings that would be beneficial to the administration.

At the conclusion of the interview process, the team met for two full days preparing its report. The team discussed its manner of presentation and agreed that individual team members would report on the departments which they had surveyed, as well as present a summary report. It was agreed that only indisputable findings would be presented and no recommendations made, since the purpose of the team was to provide information rather than make recommendations.

During the summary preparation it was noted that all evidence pointed toward a highly autocratic administration, focused on the director, with little or no delegation, and that communication was a major problem area. Interviews revealed that the associates were hindered in their performance by the autocratic nature of the director, who refused input and revealed little to his associates of his intentions and desires. It was obvious that he was seen at all levels as a major problem.

At the department-head level the difficulties that existed between the director and his associates became even more evident. Specific comments regarding traits of the director were discarded, and the team recognized that its report would be extremely sensitive. Thus considerable effort was made to generalize the problems that were identified and to refrain from any accusatory statements regarding the director. The team felt that employees were unusually cooperative and trusting, and felt that they had been properly advised as to the nature and content, as well as the purposes, of the survey. A large number of employees reported their satisfaction with the procedure and the fact that it was their first, and perhaps their only, opportunity to provide frank input and evaluation. To a great many of these employees the process seemed to have almost a therapeutic effect. There was also considerable interest in the survey results.

In recognition of the earlier agreement between the administration and the team, all employees were informed that they would receive feedback through administrative channels by a mechanism yet to be determined but which would be decided when the team met with the administration to provide its report. The employees were uniformly pleased and filled with a sense of expectation concerning the final report.

As the summary report was being prepared, the associate director emphasized to the team members that the director was unpredictable and was likely to challenge the report if he perceived it as a personal attack. Further efforts were made to avoid this likelihood, although the results of the survey were quite clear in pointing to the director as a major problem to the effective operation of the hospital.

On the day that the team was to begin its presentation to the director and his associates, the team leader first met with the director individually to discuss the report and to provide some insights into what might take place. This had been agreed to earlier to resolve any last-minute problems as well as to allow the director to develop insight into problem areas that had been identified. The meeting lasted approximately an hour, and at its conclusion the team and administration gathered in a conference room.

At the beginning of this meeting, the team reminded all present that this had been a voluntary effort and that it had been especially satisfying in view of the cooperation of the director and his staff, as well as the frankness and openness of the employees interviewed. He also reminded the director that he would be responsible for further dissemination of the information presented, either with or without the participation of the team. The director assured the team leader that subsequent to the summary sessions, his associates would meet with their respective department heads, present the information, and later share the information with all hospital employees.

The discussion began with an overview of findings by the team leader. Within twenty minutes the director became defensive and expressed dissatisfaction with the process, the team members, and the results. Although his associates remained quiet during this period, one suddenly spoke in defiance of the director, challenging him to remain quiet and listen to the presentation. He then delivered a scathing attack on the director, in which he claimed that the summary was a verification of what all had known—specifically that the director was responsible for all the problems in the hospital. Following this intense attack a loud and dramatic exchange occurred between these two individuals, at the conclusion of which the director stood, ordered the team to cease the report, to gather its materials, and to leave the hospital immediately. He advised his associates that there would be no further discussion of the survey, there would be no report to the employees, and there would be no explanation of the lack of a report. The team prepared to leave the hospital. The director dictated a memorandum to all employees in which he informed them that the survey process had failed and that there would be no further information regarding that process. Six months later the director and his associate, who were in such severe conflict, both retired and were replaced.

Discussion Questions

1. *What would be your response to the charges raised by the director at the time of the summary meeting?*

2. *How successful was the team in creating a performance gap? What other data collection and feedback approaches might have been considered?*

3. *Evaluate the role of the hospital director and his associates. What action might have been taken to prevent the collapse of the development program? Where does the program go from here?*

CASE 2

An Application from a Doctor of Osteopathy for Medical Staff Privileges*

A doctor of osteopathy applied for staff privileges at a Fort Worth hospital after she had been practicing medicine for three years in the specialty of family practice in a nearby rural town. She was also a member of three other hospital staffs.

She attended a local college, where she received her undergraduate degree, and graduated from the Texas College of Osteopathic Medicine. She is licensed in the state of Texas and had a one-year rotating internship in an osteopathic hospital in the adjoining city of Dallas.

The hospitals where she had privileges were queried and all responded favorably. Additionally, three physicians on the medical staff of this hospital attested to the applicant's knowledge, training, and experience. The privileges she requested were for admitting privileges with immediate referral to a specialist, and for assisting in surgery on her own patients. She did not request any surgical privileges on a primary basis, nor did she request any special procedure privileges.

Two days after receipt of the application, she requested temporary privileges to

---

*Adapted from Harris (1979a).

assist in surgery. The request was considered by both the chief of staff and by the vice-chief of surgery. They both felt that there was no urgency in giving temporary privileges and preferred to process the application in the usual manner.

The first step in the process for appointment of new physicians is for the appropriate clinical section to review the pertinent data on the application. The medicine policy committee reviewed the application and recommended to the credentials committee the physician's appointment to the provisional medical staff. The committee stipulated the privileges as the applicant requested, "admitting privileges for referral to a specialist and surgical assistance on her own patients."

The credentials committee then recommended to the executive committee that a provisional medical staff appointment be granted with privileges as delineated by the medicine policy committee.

The executive committee reviewed all information and subsequently upheld the recommendation that admitting privileges in medicine be granted, but that surgical assistance on her own patients be denied. In addition, the members concurred that referral to a specialist within 24 hours of admission was unrealistic, and therefore this constraint was removed. During the meeting, the administration informed all that even though there were four practicing doctors of osteopathy on the staff, this applicant was the first who did not have postgraduate allopathic training.

The recommendation was made and carried without dissenting votes that the applicant be recommended to the board of trustees for appointment to the provisional staff. A subcommittee of the board (the professional activities committee) recommended that this physician, together with other candidates, be granted staff membership. It is interesting to note the composition of this board committee:

Chairman:	Board member, who is an attorney
Physician:	Active practice and a board member
Chief of staff:	Board member
Physician:	Chairman of Utilization Review Committee
Administration:	Two board members
Representative of nursing:	A sister of the religious order

When the motion from the professional activities committee was made at the board meeting to approve the appointment of this physician, it drew immediate discussion. One board member reported past conversations with colleagues and friends which led him to believe that the city would soon be saturated with osteopathic physicians, and that this trend would drive away medical doctors planning to practice in this and other hospitals. His argument was quickly supported by another trustee, who announced that the dean of the Texas College of Osteopathic Medicine is on the board of directors of the county hospital. It was also discussed that it was rumored (and feared) that the county hospital may lose or choose to disengage itself from Southwestern Medical School in Dallas and offer its facilities to the Texas College of Osteopathic Medicine. Further, the same trustee relayed a conversation he had with a respected surgeon (chief of surgery at another hospital) while at a local country club. This surgeon indicated that the M.D. community was concerned about the increasing number of graduating osteopaths and their effect upon the quality of medical care in the community.

Again, it was brought out that there were four doctors of osteopathy already on the staff, but that each had completed an approved M.D. postgraduate training program, whereas the present applicant had not. The board elected to table the motion and suggested that the discussion be continued at a joint conference meeting. The board desired clarification on two questions before making a decision. They were: (1) specific delineation of privileges as to limitations, and (2) implications for the future in the context of precedents." They also indicated that they had no intention of negating the recommendations of the executive committee, only that several members of the board of trustees desired further deliberation with the medical staff prior to any action on this particular applicant.

The joint conference committee met and discussion centered on the problem of setting a precedent for future applications from osteopaths and how best to determine and document the training and experience of osteopathic physicians. Concern was expressed about the future effect that the Texas College of Osteopathic Medicine would have on the practice of medicine in Fort Worth, and more specifically on the quality of membership within the medical staff of the hospital.

With respect to the doctor's application, there seemed to the committee to be three alternatives:

1. Rejection.
2. Acceptance with limited privileges as she had requested (that of admission for referral to a consultant and privileges to assist at surgery on her own patients).
3. Acceptance as previously recommended by the executive committee (admitting privileges in medicine only).

The committee unanimously voted to reject the application, for two reasons: membership in the district osteopathic society made her ineligible for professional membership in the Tarrant County Medical Society, and by precedent, the hospital is not accepting applications from osteopathic physicians who do not have formal training in an AMA-approved allopathic internship or residency.

The committee felt that before any action was taken on the recommendation, a joint meeting should be held with voting members of the executive committee, board members, administration, and legal counsel. In light of the questions raised with this applicant, discussion was held to determine whether or not a statement should be included under membership qualification regarding the requirement that applicants complete an AMA-approved internship or residency program.

The hospital's attorney advised the group that the two reasons given by the joint conference committee for rejecting the application were unacceptable. The first reason was invalid because membership in a local osteopathic society does not disqualify a person from being eligible for local medical society membership. Even it if was a valid reason, counsel said it would not "hold water legally." The second reason for denial centered around the lack of an AMA-approved internship or residency.

The attorney reemphasized that membership in any organization, whether AMA, medical society, or other, could not be used as a criterion for acceptance to or rejection from a medical staff, and that the same principle applied to training programs. Objection to the training program would have to be based on something other than the organization sponsoring it.

Counsel proposed three alternatives in regard to the applicant and the future practice of other osteopathic physicians:

1. Reject the application of the applicant because she is not M.D.trained.

2. Approve the applicant and have an "open door" policy to any and all osteopathic physicians of good standing.

3. Amend the medical staff bylaws to include a statement requiring an approved internship or residency training program for any future applicant. An exception should be made with the present applicant and stringent restrictions placed on her practice.

Since the responsibility of the medical staff and board of trustees is to assure quality care, all applicants must be screened and determined to be appropriately qualified. Since this particular applicant did not complete an M.D. internship or residency program, the medical staff was unable to judge her qualifications for membership to the staff as they had with the previous D.O.s who were accepted. It was the consensus of the group that the application be rejected because the applicant had not completed a formally approved training program that could be properly evaluated. The board subsequently upheld the decision to reject the appointment. Also, the recommendation was made that the medical staff bylaws be revised to define applicant qualifications more precisely, to include, at the minimum, one year of American or Canadian postgraduate training in an institution employing an M.D. faculty.

The physician applicant was notified of the board's decision not to appoint her to the medical staff. She chose not to exercise her right of appeal.

Discussion Questions

1. *What type of change is being proposed?*

2. *What accounted for the apparent reversal of the change process?*

3. *Illustrate the use of various reeducation, persuasive, facilitative, and power strategies appropriate to various stages of the change process.*

FURTHER READING

CHASE, G. "Implementing A Human Service Program: How Hard Will It Be?" *Public Policy* 27(4) (Fall 1979):385-435.

GREER, A. L. "Advances in the Study of Diffusion and Innovation in Health Care Organizations." *Milbank Memorial Fund Quarterly, Health and Society*, 55 (Fall 1977):505-532.

The Journal of Applied Behavioral Sciences, 14(3) (July-Aug.-Sept. 1978). Special Issue: "Towards Healthier Medical Systems: Can We Learn from Experience?"

RUSSELL, L. B. *Technology in Hospitals: Medical Advance and Their Diffusion.* Washington, D.C.: The Brookings Institution, 1979.

TICHY, N. M. *Organizational Design for Public Health Care: The Case of the Dr. Martin Luther King Health Center.* New York: Praeger, 1977.

WIELAND, G., ed. *Improving Health Care Management: Organization Development and Organization Change.* Ann Arbor, Mich.: Health Administration Press, 1980.

PART

CONTROL
AND
EVALUATION

Imagine a group of elderly men sitting around the fire discussing the glories of the past and the hopes for the future. During the conversation one gentleman comments: "I've not been born to greatness—nor have I achieved greatness—but I am still waiting to have it thrust upon me"—Adapted from the *New Yorker*, November 1980.

So it is with the management process. Planning and design as well as operations and implementation have come and gone—and there is always the eternal hope that if all else fails, control is still possible. The objective of this section is to consider control and evaluation as the last phase of the management process. Plans are created/implemented and are now operational. Control and evaluation is concerned with whether or not the organization is meeting its planned activities and, if not, why not.

Chapter 9 defines the concept of control and emphasizes the control of human resources. Attention is given to various control strategies appropriate to health service organizations. Chapter 10 presents a more quantitative approach to control. It describes a control framework and the issues relevant to data measurement and analysis. Chapter 11, which deals with financial control, focuses on the protection of the organization's assets and the reliability of its accounting records.

Chapter 12 considers the legal aspects of control. Emphasis is given to recognizing the types of legal problems which management faces as well as an understanding of how the law operates to assist in management decisions. An underlying premise is that a basic understanding of the law will enhance all aspects of the managerial process.

239

9

Controlling Human Resources

Managers at various levels within the organization are constantly confronted with "people-type" problems. Essentially, these problems center on the issues of motivating individuals to make contributions to the organization and assuring that behavioral contributions are in the desired direction. Motivational and behavioral problems are extremely difficult because they involve individuals each with a set of values, needs, and perceptions which may or may not be congruent with the overall organizaional values and activities. To confound the situation further, all individuals are members of various types of formal and informal groups within the organization, and many individuals are members of professional groups external to the organization, each with its own function, orientation, and dynamic. The objective of this chapter is to explore the concept of control as it relates to individual and group activities within organizations.

COMMON MISCONCEPTIONS

Most people accept the idea of control, yet they have rather simplistic views about control and how it operates in organizations. For example, control is often thought to reside in a particular position or result from the development and execution of a formal set of rules. Individuals work long and hard to achieve positions or to establish a set of rules only to find they have little effect on the overall operations of the organization. We tend to underestimate the potential of the individual in exercising control and overestimate the control that positions and rules have in the operations of organizations. Below is a list of some other common misconceptions.

Control is hierarchically linked to structure: Imagine a chief executive officer sitting at his or her desk, which has an elaborate panel of dials, gauges, buttons, and levers. Although the panel gives the image of control, a quick look behind the panel indicates that only a few of the dials, gauges, buttons, and levers are connected to anything. Although the position gives the image of control, it is necessary to look elsewhere to get an accurate picture of control within the organization.

First, control is quite diffuse and involves many relationships beyond those designated in the formal hierarchy of the organization. This situation is best illustrated by the role that physicians play within the hospital and their relationships with various types of organizational personnel. As described by Freidson (1970):

> Unlike the foreman, who is caught in "the middle" between his legitimate superiors and subordinates, the nurse is caught between two superiors,

administrative and medical. The latter, however, is not your bureaucratic superior: that is to say, while the floor nurse is subject to the orders of her superior, who is her official superior in the hospital hierarchy, she is also subject to the orders of physician involved in the care of her patients by virtue of his superior knowledge and responsibility. Similarly, justifying his demand by reference to the well being of his patient, the physician can and does give "orders" to other hospital personnel even though he is not bureaucratically defined as superior. In this way the functioning of the hospitals seems to be disruptive and broken, lacking the clear, linear authority upon which Weber predicts efficiency and reliability in organizational performance.

The situation is further complicated by physicians' abilities to intervene and justify their actions on the basis of a "medical emergency" (Freidson, 1970). Although there is no doubt that these actions are often legitimate, they are all-too-frequent occurrences, suggesting that they provide an opportunity for physicians to label ambiguous events as emergencies to gain additional resources which they consider necessary. Thus, even though an organization may have a well-developed set of rules and regulations, they can be abrogated by a physician's declaration of a "medical emergency."

Second, a great deal of control is often lodged in what David Mechanic (1962) has termed the "lower participants" of the organization. Lower participants are health attendants, secretaries, and other workers widely spread throughout the organization, who, over time, obtain and maintain access to persons, information, the physical plant, or equipment. The control of lower participants is enhanced when they develop special knowledge about the organization that higher participants do not have because of lack of interest or lack of tenure in the organization.

The amount of control is enhanced further by the development of coalitions among lower participants. These coalitions provide the mechanism for accomplishing relatively mundane, yet time-consuming tasks. For example, a secretary may know the person responsible for assigning parking stickers. Such an acquaintance may give her the ability to handle informally certain needs that would be extremely time-consuming and difficult to handle formally. Her ability to handle services informally makes higher-ranking participants and professionals dependent upon her, thereby increasing her ability to bargain on issues important to her.

Finally, managers tend to overestimate the amount of control exerted by various groups in the organization. In a study of hospitals in New York State (Kaluzny and Veney, 1972) it was found that hospital administrators consistently overestimated the amount of control exerted by physicians, trustees, and department heads on a range of issues. For example, administrators claimed that department heads, physicians, and trustees had more influence in decisions involving the allocation of total hospital income, adoption and implementation of new hospital-wide programs and services, development of formal affiliation with other organizations, appointment of medical staff, and long-range planning than physicians, trustees, and department heads themselves believed they had. This type of misperception can create a void in the decision-making activities of the organization, resulting in missed opportunities to provide managerial leadership.

Control is unidirectional: A second misconception is that control, when exercised, is unidirectional. That is, managers are viewed (or view themselves) as persons who initiate actions for others and whose interaction ends once these directions are issued (Campbell et al., 1970). In reality, the execution of control is a reciprocal action in which the responses made by individuals to the control attempts represent stimuli for the manager which cannot be ignored. Control efforts must be viewed as a constantly unfolding process involving "debits and credits." That is, individuals complying with various control efforts or assisting in the development of control activities develop credits with colleagues in the organization which may be drawn upon at a later date to accomplish some favor or accommodate some deviant or idiosyncratic behavior.

Control is finite: Individuals often see an increase in control by one party accompanied by a corresponding decrease in control by some other parties. In effect, they view control as a "zero-sum" game in which there is a finite amount of control and that, by increasing control of one party, there is a corresponding decrease in control of the other.

A different view of control is presented by Arnold Tannenbaum and associates (1968). Here control is viewed as an infinite quantity in which the total amount of control within an organization may grow and managers and various types of personnel may enhance their power jointly. The approach also emphasizes the distribution of control among groups within an organization and between different types of organizations. For example, in a comparative study of community- and university-based clinics there was a substantial difference in the distribution of control among various types of personnel over diagnosis and treatment decisions and over decisions involving clinic policy (Nathanson and Becker, 1972). The total level of control over clinic policy and over diagnosis and treatment was higher and more equally distributed in the community-based clinics. Paramedical personnel, such as nurses and social workers, in comparison to clinic physicians are attributed relatively more influence over policy issues in community clinics. There is little variation among university- and community-based clinics in the amount of control ascribed to clinic physicians over diagnosis and treatment or over policies.

Control is management: An underlying assumption of many control efforts is that there already exists an understanding of the cause-and-effect relationship of the area in question. This assumption is implicit in many control strategies, such as management by objectives, planning, programming, and budgeting as well as various types of management information systems. The role of management is to use these various strategies to produce or present some stipulated outcome.

Although there are many areas in which the assumption is valid, the universal application of this approach is limited, particularly in the area of human resources, where there is little understanding of the cause-and-effect relationship. The use of control techniques and the dependency on these techniques by management, eliminates the organization's risk-taking ability and the opportunity for management to discover creative solutions to many of the critical problems involving human resources (Landau and Stout, 1979).

Consider the story of Edward Teller (1963) and imagine its extension to the health services field, where the technology is less developed and requires greater management risk.

> One word about my impression of effective management. . . . We [at the Lawrence Radiation Laboratory] were told to go ahead on a program and were given a charter to do something new which required major advancements in science and technology. We tried and we failed. Then we tried again and we failed again. At that time any *reasonable* management would have shut us down, but the AEC management was not reasonable; the management was *good*. They recognized that something new cannot be accomplished without taking risks and we were encouraged to experiment further. The next time we succeeded.

WHAT IS CONTROL?

Control is any process in which a person, group of persons, or organization *intentionally affects* the behavior of another person, group, or organization (Tannenbaum, 1968). As applied to organizations, control must be distinguished from such concepts as influence, authority, and power.

Cartwright (1965) has proposed a useful classification to differentiate these various concepts.

- Influence is considered a basic psychological force which occurs in any interpersonal transaction in which one person acts in some way to change the behavior of another person in some intended fashion. Every influence attempt, however, is not successful. Lack of success does not imply that there is no influence.

- Control involves the distinction between successful attempts at influence and those which are unsuccessful. If one person has control over another in some matter, his influence is sufficiently strong to affect the desired behavior. Lack of control, however, does not imply lack of influence attempts.

- Power is basic to influence and control and is defined as the *capacity* to exercise influence. This means that power is used to refer to some *potential* set of influence transactions.

- Authority is defined as legitimate power, that is, power which accrues to persons by virtue of role or position within the organization.

BASIS OF CONTROL

The ability to exercise influence and, if successful, to control various aspects of organizations stems from various sources of power (French and Raven, 1960):

- *Expert* refers to the individual's ability to affect others intentionally by means of special skill, expertise, and knowledge.

- *Legitimate* refers to the individual's ability to affect others intentionally by means of position in the organization.

- *Coercive* refers to the individual's ability to affect others intentionally by means of the ability to arouse fear.

- *Reward* refers to the individual's ability to affect others intentionally by means of ability to distribute positive benefits.

- *Referrent* refers to the individual's ability to affect others intentionally by means of personal traits and qualities that others consider desirable or admirable.

The manner in which the sources of power and their ultimate effect on control are a function of several factors that characterize health service organizations.

- *Limits of legitimate power:* The nature of decision making among professionals limits the control that managers may exercise on their professional colleagues (Goss, 1961). Regardless of whether managers have professional credentials, they limit their influence to nontechnical aspects of professional work. Here, influence and control focus on allocating and scheduling work rather than on the substantive nature of the task. Health service managers with professional credentials may make suggestions on the substantive nature of the task, but ultimate control resides with the practitioner.

- *Pervasive nature of expert power:* Although there may be limits on legitimate power, expert power is most pervasive and goes beyond the technical nature of the work. Professionals may easily argue that they are unable to function unless provided certain resources and/or structural arrangements. Arguing from a respected area of expertise has a great deal of influence, if not control of decisions beyond those of a technical nature (Freidson, 1970).

- *Limits of professional control:* The ability to influence or control professional practice is limited by its very character. As described by Freidson (1970):

> The system of control was [is] not characteristically either collective or hierarchical in its operation. It was intended to operate like the economist's free market, private individuals being brought into interaction at the points where their individual work interests were involved. This was so in spite of its taking place in a consciously organized group-practice setting. Second, the process worked slowly, for a system of control can work only as rapidly as the information necessary for control can accumulate readily. Finally, the process had a characteristic vulnerability. In the nature of the case, in order to be effective the sanctions used required that all participants be fully responsive to the norms involved. The system was quite helpless in the face of a man who did not depend upon the esteem and trust of his colleagues and who did not respond to the symbolic values of professionalism. Confronted by a man who is not so incompetent or unethical as to be grossly and obviously dismissable and who fails to show any respect for his colleague's opinions, the administration and the colleague group are helpless. He cannot be flattered, shamed, or insulted and so cannot be persuaded to mend his ways or resign: all that can be done is to seal him off and try to minimize whatever damage he is believed to do (pp 152-153).

Moreover, the educational process by which professionals are given the skill for practice contains little opportunity to develop responsiveness to evaluation and direction from others. Training provides an opportunity to develop a personal mastery over basic skills that tends to be self-validating. In a study of professional educational programs involving the postgraduate training of psychiatrists and internists and the graduate training of biochemists, Bucher and Stelling (1977) conclude: "There is nothing in our findings which would support the notion that socialization processes build an effective mechanism for either individual internal control or colleague control among professionals" (pp 281-282).

CONTROL STRATEGIES

The theoretical discussion of control and its various formulations are endless. The real test is whether strategies are available to the health services manager to influence or control the actions of individuals in the organization. Next, we discuss strategies likely to be used by health service managers.

Monetary Rewards

Managers have traditionally placed emphasis on money as a strategy to influence human behavior. Monetary rewards are used to recruit personnel into the organization. Once personnel are recruited into the organization, monetary rewards are used to assure regular attendance. Monetary rewards are also used to influence the performance of individuals, that is, to assure that individuals are functioning up to their capacity vis-à-vis the goals of the organization.

Various types of payment schemes are well developed in industrial organizations and are beginning to be applied to the health services field. These schemes, ranging from base salary or pay to various incentive programs to supplemental pay schedules, are designed to influence individual behavior. The exact formulation of these schemes is limited only by the imagination of the health services manager, and awaits implementation and subsequent evaluation.

In the application of these programs, the health services manager needs to be aware of several issues generic to any payment scheme.

- *The relationship of pay to performance:* The ability to relate pay to performance is a well-accepted principle in the development of salary and incentive schemes. While the relationship is mediated by various factors, such as the attitudes and background of the employee, group norms, size of work group, and so on, the issue is even more complicated when applied to a health service setting.

  Focusing on physician behavior, Williamson (1978a) states that: "Today providers are paid for what they do, not for what they accomplish." To the extent that we accept the idea that improved health status is the end point of health service activities, there is no payment mechanism to ensure the achievement of these activities. Instead, a great deal of activity goes on within the health services field, explaining much of the rising costs and the often questionable benefits with little impact on the overall health status of the community.

- *Equity:* In a rapidly developing field such as health services, it is often necessary to recruit special types of personnel. To accomplish this, organizations often offer higher salaries to attract certain individuals into the organization. For example, a nurse oncologist and an enterstomal therapist are a few of the new subspecialty practitioners that organizations are attempting to attract. To the extent to which they are successful, such recruitment policies create morale problems among personnel in more traditional roles who think they are being treated inequitably—not because they are underpaid relative to the market for their own skills but because they feel they are underpaid relative to the newly hired personnel. Since the individuals are unable to go onto the market and get better-paying positions, their perceived inequity is expressed in terms of complaints and dissatisfaction.

• *Salary secrecy:* A well-accepted policy of many organizations is that the salaries of individuals should be kept a secret. The rationale for this policy is that secrecy increases satisfaction. In other words, if employees know what other employees are receiving, they may be dissatisfied with their own pay.

A number of studies involving industrial organizations tend to challenge this assumption. Analysis reveals that individuals tend to have incorrect information about the pay of other individuals in the organization and that there is a general tendency to overestimate the salaries of other individuals. This perception undermines any attempt to develop a scheme that relates performance with individual rewards. Although these findings need testing in the health services setting, the implication is that a more open salary schedule would facilitate more accurate performance feedback.

Performance Appraisal

A commonly used control technique applied to nonprofessionals as well as to some professional personnel is performance appraisal. This approach involves a systematic description of the relevant strengths and weaknesses of the individual's job (Cascio, 1978). Information gathered through performance appraisal techniques is used (1) to provide information for staff development and training, and (2) to provide the basis for personnel decisions such as promotion, transfers, termination, and salary allocations.

A wide variety of performance measures are available, and their use in health service organizations represents a fairly straightforward adaptation from industrial settings. Two types of measures are most commonly employed: objective and subjective. *Objective measures* tend to focus on individual behavior, including such personnel data as absenteeism, turnover, and tardiness. The measures suffer from several limitations. Perhaps most relevant to health service organizations is the difficulty of obtaining good objective indicators of performance. Even within industrial settings the theoretical and practical limitations often make this an unsuitable approach.

Subjective measures use a variety of rating formats. Figure 9–1 illustrates one form that was used in the evaluation of nursing personnel. Although the approach is widely used, its most serious limitation is the subjective nature of the appraisal process. Even well-intentioned individuals are subject to various biases which undermine the credibility of the entire appraisal process.

In addition, both measures are often used to achieve multiple and frequently conflicting objectives. For example, the same performance appraisal that may be used for motivating employees, improving performance,

Nurse_____ Joan H. Roberts _____   Appraised by_____ E.D. James _____

Section_____ 3A _____   Date_____ June 30, 1976 _____

Instructions: Indicate your appraisal of the actual performance by circling the appropriate letter for each item. ND = Not Descriptive, MD = Minimally Descriptive, SD = Somewhat Descriptive, VD = Very Descriptive, HD = Highly Descriptive.

Technical Knowledge

1. Prepares a complete nursing care plan for each patient.   ND (MD) SD VD HD
2. Keeps up-to-date on latest nursing techniques.   ND MD (SD) VD HD
3. Often provides technical information to colleagues, i.e., other nurses, aides and other health professionals.   ND MD SD (VD) HD

Interpersonal Relations

4. Is well liked by other members of the nursing team.   ND MD SD (VD) HD
5. Respects other people's ability or judgment, i.e. during peer review.   ND MD SD VD (HD)
6. Is readily accepted by co-workers.   ND MD SD VD (HD)

Resistance to Work Pressures

7. Renders high level professional care without continued supervision.   ND MD (SD) VD HD
8. Makes sound decisions under conditions of stress or pressure.   ND MD SD (VD) HD
9. Accepts additional responsibility without becoming annoyed/upset.   ND MD (SD) VD HD

Rules and Policy Adherence

10. Follows unit policy/procedures for nursing interventions.   ND MD SD (VD) HD
11. Knows and strives to meet written standards of care.   ND MD SD VD (HD)
12. Knows and follows the correct format for recording, i.e. POMR.   ND MD SD (VD) HD

Professional Output

13. Keeps patient nursing care plan complete and up-to-date.   ND MD (SD) VD HD
14. Detects/corrects any inadequacies in patient care.   ND MD (SD) VD HD
15. Meets or exceeds written standards of patient care.   ND MD SD (VD) HD

Motivation

16. Does additional reading/study on an unusual patient problem/condition.   ND (MD) SD VD HD
17. Often does that little something extra.   ND MD (SD) VD HD
18. Assumes professional responsibility for every assignment.   ND MD (SD) VD HD

Overall Performance (check one)

☐ Excellent   ☐ Above average   ☑ Typical   ☐ Somewhat below average   ☐ Marginal or poor

Figure 9-1 Staff nurse performance appraisal form.* [J. C. South, "The Performance Profile: A Technique for Using Appraisals Effectively." *Journal of Nursing Administration.* 8(1) (1978), 27-31.]

*The items comprising the form are for illustrative purposes only and are not intended to represent an actual rating scale.

and identifying educational needs, often serves as the basis for managerial decision making, retention, promotion, dismissal, and salary adjustments. The picture is further complicated by the use of performance appraisals to assess the quality of care provided to patients.

A key to successful performance appraisal programs as diagnostic tools, as well as providing the basis for making critical personnel decisions, is the training of supervisory personnel in the use of performance appraisal methods. Where such training has occurred, performance appraisal programs have less inter-rater variation, and information generated by the program tends to be more consistently used in the overall managerial process.

Management by Objectives

A widely used, misused, and often misunderstood control strategy is management by objectives (MBO). The approach was originally developed in the 1950s and was adopted by many industrial organizations as well as various types of health service institutions.

The approach is often considered a management philosophy as well as a specific managerial technique. Closely aligned to performance appraisal, MBO provides a context within which the manager is able to use performance appraisal methodologies.

Management by objectives is an approach whereby an organization establishes goals and programs. To achieve these goals and programs at the highest level, the organization develops a process of establishing subgoals, programs, and activities at various levels within the organization to ensure the accomplishment of the higher-level goals. Through the process, individuals internalize the overall goals and objectives of the organization, thereby assuring compatibility between individual and organizational goals.

The process involves a close working relationship between superiors and subordinates throughout the organization. The interaction focuses on three major sets of activities:

- Determining the goals that the organizational units or individual will achieve within a given time period.
- Planning activities to achieve the objectives.
- Establishing measures by which goals or programs will be assessed and the date by which the activities will be accomplished.

Although the approach has many testimonials and some empirical evaluation studies (e.g., Tosi et al, 1976; Ivancevich, 1974) to document its overall impact, its application to health service organizations must be approached with caution. Given the nature of health service organizations, several difficult problems must be identified. First, the process of implementing an MBO program is estimated to take three to five years. Most health service managers embarking on the implementation of the program have little patience and abandon the effort midway in the implementation process. Part of the reason for abandonment is the fairly short tenure among health service administrative personnel.

A second factor contributing to the problems of implementation is that the process itself is extremely time-consuming. Successful implementation and establishment of objectives, activity plans, and so on, require a great deal of meeting time between superiors and subordinates, who already have extensive demands for actual service delivery activities. Usually, the process of defining goals and action plans is viewed as an appendage to existing work loads as opposed to an integrated part of activities. An exacerbating factor is that many of the objectives and activities associated with health service organizations are difficult to define, thus compounding the problems of establishing goals and specific activities.

A final problem is the inability of the organization to involve the most critical actors (i.e., physicians) in the process of defining objectives and activity plans. There is always the likelihood of a break in the goal-setting chain at some level of the organization. This, coupled with the fairly short time perspective that most employees have within the organization and their concern that this activity takes away time and resources from the major service delivery activities of the organization, limits the use of MBO within many health service activities.

Feedback Strategies

The idea of feedback as an organizational development strategy was discussed in Chapter 6. Feedback is also a strategy capable of enhancing control, particularly among professionals within the organization. As described above, one of the limits of the professional control system is that information about care provided by individual physicians is not readily visible to their colleagues because of the autonomous nature of professional practice. Even among the most conscientious physicians, assumptions develop over time that optimal care is provided when, in fact, there may be a considerable gap between care provided and recommended therapy. Because of the autonomous nature of medical practice, the individuals most capable of exerting influence (i.e., clinical colleagues) are not likely to be aware that influence is required.

The availability of formal feedback processes about patterns of care provides a mechanism whereby other clinicians are systematically made aware of significant deviations in an objective and unbiased manner. This information permits clinicians to exercise influence among themselves and permits individual practitioners to adjust their own behavior accordingly. In a sense the data feedback mechanism provides the profession with an opportunity to control itself. An added advantage of control based on data feedback is that administrators can actively participate and, in fact, facilitate the development of a feedback mechanism. However, only the clinical colleagues themselves exercise control once the information is made available.

Bi-cycle Approach to Quality Assurance

The basic principle of data feedback has been applied to the problems of quality assessment and quality assurance. As seen in Figure 9-2 the development of patient care research is combined with continuing medical education to enhance the overall control affecting quality assurance. The process involves a series of distinct stages beginning with (1) establishing priority areas, (2) developing audit criteria, and (3) measuring actual performance against the established criteria. Based on these comparisons, specific educational programs are designed to correct empirically documented deficiencies. As seen in the figure, the process is a continuous activity providing an opportunity to evaluate educational efforts.

This approach is the assumption underlying most PSRO programs. While the overall effectiveness of PSRO activity remains to be determined (Goran, 1979), several published studies report significant drops in surgical rates for specific procedures as a result of feedback and review (Wennberg et al., 1977; Dyck et al., 1977; Lembcke, 1956). The use of data feedback has also shown significant effects on the use of antibiotics (Brown and Uhl, 1970).

Group Process Strategies

Individuals in most organizations spend a great deal of time in groups, providing an infrastructure through which control is exercised. Within the groups each individual has a substantive contribution to make. It is important to devise a method to channel constructively the individual contributions of each of the members. In health service organizations, participants may have varying degrees of status, with one or two individuals dominating the group. One such approach, channeling individual contributions, is the *nominal group technique.*

The nominal group technique was first developed by Delbecq et al. (1975). The technique involves a structured group meeting in which individuals are given a specific task. This task usually requires a judgmental decision characterized by a lack of agreement or incomplete state of knowledge concerning the nature of the problem or the components to be included in the solution. Participants are asked to respond to this task not by speaking to one another but by writing their ideas on a pad of paper. At the end of five to ten minutes each member of the panel presents his or her ideas in a round-robin process. These ideas are recorded so that they can be seen

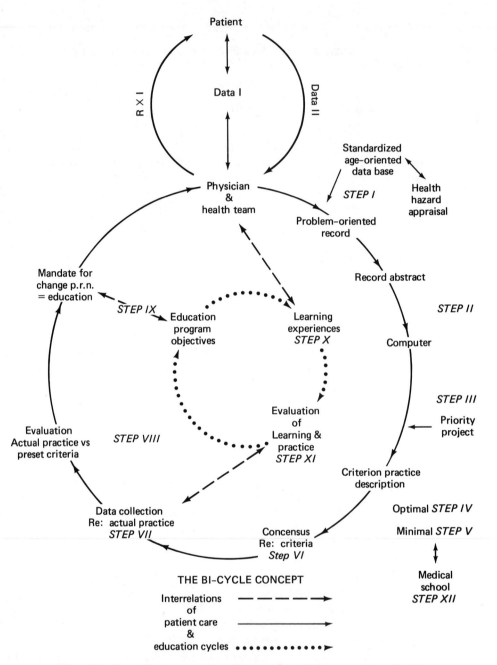

Figure 9-2 The bi-cycle in quality assurance. [C. R. Brown and H. S. M. Uhl, "Mandatory Continuing Education: Sense or Nonsense." *JAMA,* 213 (10) (Sept. 7, 1970), 1660-1668; copyright 1970, American Medical Association.]

by the entire group. However, the ideas are not discussed as they are recorded. Once all the ideas are presented, a discussion follows in which the ideas are clarified and evaluated. Following the discussion, there is a vote on the priority of areas with the group decision derived from the ranking of ideas on the basis of the vote. The process provides a systematic basis whereby all individuals, regardless of their status, are able to present their ideas before the entire group.

An Application to Quality Assurance*

The nominal group approach is used to help establish priority areas where improvements of health or any other target outcomes will most likely be achieved. The approach involves a series of sequential tasks in which individuals are asked to list problem areas characterized as "achievable benefit not achieved" (ABNA). Such problems are listed on a flipchart in a series of rounds until 10 or 11 topics are recorded. Following the listing of these topics, each is discussed by the group to clarify as precisely as possible the problems of patients, providers, and health care changes needed to affect improvement of the target benefit. Based on this discussion the topics are scaled by each of the individuals according to his or her judgment of efficacy, feasibility, and cost effectiveness. The weighting must be estimated in terms of (1) adequacy of evidence that the target benefit is achievable, (2) necessity and practicality of quality assessment to verify current outcome deficiencies, and (3) likelihood that the improvement to be achieved would be worth the time and expense. Finally, the group considers each topic separately, analyzing priority weights in terms of ABNA. Following the discussion, each member records a final scale weight. The individual weights are collated to obtain an arithmetic total weight for each identified problem area. The total for each item represents cost effectiveness of the item for quality assurance activity.

The approach has undergone tests to assess its reliability and validity (Williamson et al., 1978, 1979). Reliability in this context is defined as whether a given group judgment procedure will produce similar results when applied by independent groups within the same institution. Analysis for eight different institutions revealed (1) agreement on topic content, (2) agreement on scaling of similar topics generated by the team independently, and (3) agreement by one team and scaling the topics generated by another team.

Validity focused on the extent to which the approach (1) accurately identifies health deficiencies or strengths, (2) properly identifies correctable causes, (3) develops programs to improve health deficiencies, and (4) could be credited for any improvement that was initiated by the assess-

---

*See Williamson (1978a,b).

ment process. Analysis of data obtained in six medical institutions revealed that predictive validity was achieved for all criteria.

Leadership Style

Leadership is usually defined as the process of influencing the activities of individuals or groups in efforts toward goal achievement in a given situation. Although a great deal of attention has been given to the various facets of leadership in terms of specific behavioral traits such as intelligence, personality, and physical features, the critical question facing most managers is the appropriate way in which these influence attempts should be made and under what conditions they are most appropriate.

A number of approaches have been developed to consider the various types of leadership activities and the conditions under which they are most appropriate. For example, the initial models of leadership focused on two basic activities: task direction and consideration (Bales, 1958). Task direction refers to activities directed at getting the job done: that is, defining responsibilities and relationships, and establishing clear patterns of work. Consideration refers to activities reflecting friendship, mutual trust, and respect. Although the two sets of leadership activities need not be performed by the same individual, both sets of activities are important to the overall effectiveness of the group.

This formulation has led to an extensive research program that has attempted to relate task and consideration activities to various aspects of performance (Stogdill and Coons, 1957) as well as research to identify the conditions under which each type of behavior is more effective. These approaches are presented which provide the basis, or at least the guidelines, upon which to build managerial attempts at leadership.

Contingency Theory

One approach with a great deal of intuitive appeal is to match the type of leadership style with various types of situational variables (Fiedler, 1973). The underlying hypothesis is that the better the fit between the style and the situational factors, the more effective the performance of the groups.

Three situational variables are considered:

- Leader/member relationships (the extent to which the interpersonal relationships are friendly, trusting, etc.).
- Task structure (the extent to which the job to be accomplished is highly structured).
- Position power (the degree to which the leader has control over hiring, firing, discipline, etc.).

Analysis suggests that task-oriented leaders will be most effective under either the most favorable or the least favorable conditions: that is, conditions where leader/member relations are good, the task is structured, and the leader has a strong position of power; or when the member relations are poor, the task is unstructured, and the power position of the leader is weak. As described by Fiedler (1973):

> In very favorable conditions, where the leader has power, informal backing and a well structured task, the group is ready to be directed on how to go about its task. Under very favorable conditions, however, the group will fall apart unless the leader's active intervention and control can keep the members on the job. In moderately favorable conditions . . . a relationship-oriented nondirective, permissive attitude may reduce member anxiety or intragroup conflict and this enables the group to operate more effectively. [p. 165]

This general approach has a great deal of appeal to practicing administrators. First, it raises the possibility of training administrators to diagnose situations and modify their basic leadership styles to meet the situational variables. A second possibility is to manipulate situational variables to enhance the basic style of the administrator or to train the administrator to recognize situations that best fit his or her own leadership style. Table 9-1 outlines the type of situational factors that can be manipulated. Fiedler himself feels that the latter approach is the most feasible, since leadership style is a basic part of personality, not easily susceptible to change.

Although the approach has received a great deal of attention in the research as well as in applied literature, it has been challenged increasingly on a number of empirical methodological and theoretical grounds. The most frequent criticism is that the model fails to explain the process by

TABLE 9-1 *Manipulation of Situational Variables*

Variables Being Manipulated	Task Orientation (Leader Given)	Relationship Orientation (Leader Given)
Leader/member relationship	Members different from self	Members similar to self
Position power	Final authority High title All relevant information Expertise in the area	No final authority No more information than member No unique expertise in the area
Task structure	Time limit Set of methods/guidelines to be followed	No time limit No guidelines

SOURCE: Fiedler (1973).

which leadership style has an effect, given the various situational variables. We now turn our attention to one such approach which has attempted to outline the process whereby leadership style has an impact on individual activities.

Path Goal Model

The path goal model builds upon the general contingency ideas outlined above (i.e., the interrelationship of leadership style and various situational variables). However, the model goes beyond these ideas and attempts to incorporate the individual attitudes and expectations into the overall influence process. Under this model, leadership styles are affected because they enhance the ability of the individual to perform effectively or to facilitate job satisfaction (House, 1971).

The approach outlines four basic kinds of leadership behavior:

- *Directive leadership,* in which the leader lets subordinates know what is expected of them, gives specific guidance as to what should be done and how it should be done, makes his or her part in the group understood, schedules work to be done, maintains definite standards of performance, and asks the group members to follow standard rules and regulations.

- *Supportive leadership* is characterized by a friendly and approachable person who shows concern for status, well being, and needs of subordinates. Here the leader does little things to make work more pleasant, treats members as equals, and is friendly and approachable.

- *Participative leadership* is characterized by a leader who consults with subordinates, solicits their suggestions, and takes these suggestions seriously into consideration before making a decision.

- *Achievement-oriented leaders* set challenging goals, expect subordinates to perform at their highest level, continuously seek improvement in performance, and show a high degree of confidence that subordinates will assume responsibility and put forth efforts in the accomplishment of these goals. This kind of leader constantly emphasizes excellence in performance and simultaneously displays confidence that subordinates will reach high standards of excellence.

The theory also outlines two classes of situational variables. First are personal characteristics of subordinates, with attention given to such characteristics as authoritarianism and ability. A second situational variable consists of environmental pressures and demands with which subordinates must cope to accomplish work goals and to satisfy their needs. Here consideration is given to the basic nature of the task, the formal authority system, and the primary work group within which the individuals function.

The interrelationship of the leadership-style variables and the various situational factors (as they affect individual motivation and satisfaction) are presented in the following hypotheses (House and Mitchell, 1974):

- *Leader directiveness* has a positive correlation with the satisfaction and expectations of subordinates who are engaged in ambiguous tasks, and has a negative correlation with the satisfaction and expectations of subordinates engaged in clear tasks.

- *Supportive leadership* will have its most positive effect on the satisfaction of subordinates who work on stressful, frustrating, or dissatisfying tasks.

- *Achievement-oriented leadership* will cause subordinates to strive for higher standards of performance and to have more confidence in their ability to meet challenging goals. For subordinates performing ambiguous, nonrepetitive tasks, positive relationships can be expected between the amount of the achievement orientation of the leader and the subordinates' expectation that their efforts will result in effective performance.

- When subordinates are highly ego-involved in a decision or task, and the decision or task demands are ambiguous, *participative leadership* will have a positive effect on the satisfaction and motivation of subordinates regardless of the subordinates' predisposition toward self-control, authoritarianism, or a need for dependence. When subordinates are not ego-involved in their task and when task demands are clear, subordinates who are authoritarian and who have high needs for independence and self-control will respond favorably to participative leadership; opposite personality types will respond less favorably. That is, nonauthoritarian personality types working in non-ego-involved situations where the tasks' demands are clear will not benefit from participative leadership style.

In essence, the path goal model proposes that leader behavior is motivated by the extent that it helps subordinates cope with situational uncertainties. Leaders who are able to reduce uncertainty are considered effective because they are able to increase the subordinates' expectation of desirable rewards. The test of these relationships is embryonic, and work to date has failed to account for leadership behavior in settings characterized by collegial rather than superior–subordinate relationships. This is a particularly important limitation for health service managers since many of the issues, such as quality assurance and cost containment, require leadership vis-à-vis health professionals who are characterized by a collegial rather than a subordinate relationship. Yet the ability of managers to have some guidelines as to what leadership style is appropriate to a given situation and to understand why their behavior is effective is an important contribution.

Motivational Strategies

An often-heard criticism of both contingency and the path goal model is that the measures of leadership are too abstract relative to specific managerial activities. Oldham (1976) has attempted to specify the managerial activities on a continuum of individual control over critical organizational resources and policies. Six strategies are identified:

1. *Personally rewarding or punishing:* refers to those interpersonal rewards or punishments directly distributed to subordinates by superiors in response to subordinate behavior. Examples of personal rewards a supervisor might use are a pat on the back or a simple congratulations for a job well done. Examples of punishment may be verbal criticism, a disapproving frown, or possible personal punishment.

2. *Setting goals:* refers to the supervisor actually establishing specific performance objectives, goals, or standards for subordinates to achieve.

3. *Designing feedback systems:* refers to the development of mechanisms whereby previous performance data are provided to individual workers on a regular basis. Since many organizations have systems that convey previous performance data to individual employees, the supervisor may enhance this by discussing and analyzing these data thoroughly with subordinates or getting feedback to subordinates more frequently than is required.

4. *Placing personnel:* refers to the supervisor's assignment or allocation of subordinates to existing jobs or tasks that challenge their operational and/or interpersonal skills.

5. *Designing job systems:* refers to supervisors designing, changing, or developing subordinates' existing jobs so that jobs become more challenging. For example, a supervisor may increase the autonomy of a subordinate beyond that required by the job description, or enhance the individual's overall supervisory responsibilities.

6. *Design reward systems:* refers to supervisor's ability to distribute monetary rewards to subordinates in response to their behavior. For example, material rewards include giving a monetary bonus or an

afternoon off with pay. Materially punishing activity would be suspending an individual for a day without pay.

Although the approach has not been tested in the health service setting, commercial organizations reveal that the more frequently managers use each of these strategies, (1) the more effective his or her rating in motivating subordinates, and (2) the greater the subordinates rated productivity. Obviously, the approach requires testing in the health service situation together with additional research to specify the situational variables that would designate the most appropriate behaviors for a particular situation.

Job Orientation Programs

Health service organizations are characterized by their recruitment and dependency on personnel trained outside their own operations. The individuals arrive in the service organizations with a set of expectations and orientations which may or may not fit the general orientation and objectives of the respective service organization. One approach to ensure the commitment of individuals is to develop job orientation programs to socialize new employees into the operations of the organization. Socialization involves a process in which the individual passes through a number of stages, ultimately resulting in some level of organizational commitment, as reflected by the individual's overall job satisfaction, mutual influence, internal work motivation, and job involvement.

Most job orientation programs are short. The program begins with a one-day orientation by the personnel office to benefits, working conditions, hospital regulations, and the physical plant. Then, depending upon the department, new employees receive on-the-job training from some senior employee or supervisor for various lengths of time. There is usually a probationary period of three months, followed by a formal evaluation which results in either a continuing appointment or termination. During the next few months employees are closely scrutinized by more senior employees. There may or may not be additional in-service training.

A study of the effects of job orientation programs on various types of personnel was performed in a medium-sized community hospital (Feldman, 1976, 1977). Occupational groups included accounting personnel, nurse technicians, engineers, radiological technicians, and registered nurses. Analysis reveals that the various occupational groups experienced significant differences throughout the socialization process. In general, the less professional personnel have the greatest difficulty in the early stages of the socialization process. Professional nurses have the most difficult time in defining suitable roles for themselves within the organization and reaching some agreement with their supervisors with respect to evaluation.

A second finding suggests that the ultimate impact of job orientation programs is not in the direction often expected. Hospital administrative personnel often hope that the job orientation program will increase the motivation of employees and help employees better communicate with their coworkers and supervisors. Although these are desired expectations, data analysis reveals that the orientation program has a greater impact on general satisfaction and mutual influence than on internal work motivation and job involvement. As described by Feldman (1976):

> What socialization programs do affect are the general satisfaction of workers and the feelings of autonomy and personal influence workers have. This is important because general satisfaction consistently relates to decreased turnover and absenteeism and because mutual influence may increase the number and quality of creative suggestions which are made by the workers. Employers need to consider more carefully just what they want to accomplish in the development of individuals and tailor their programs more carefully to those ends. Socialization cannot do everything alone.

Psychological Contracts

An important aspect of a well-designed orientation program is to arrive at a match of expectations between the organization and the employee. This contract is particularly important for professional employees who bring to the organization a set of expectations which may or may not match those of the organization. Table 9-2 is a list of expectations held by the individual and the organization.

Although there is no "cookbook" approach to the development of psychological contracts, several important points should be noted.

- Recruiting efforts provide opportunities for both employer and employee to exchange accurately stated expectations.
- Supervisors responsible for new employees have the necessary skills and knowledge to create sound psychological contracts.
- Opportunities exist throughout the early period of employment to reassess expectations on the part of both employer and employee.

Obviously, the range of expectations on the part of both employer and employee is infinite. Nevertheless, the extent to which it is possible to articulate these expectations has a significant impact on important characteristics of job satisfaction, productivity, and turnover. For example, data suggest that where psychological contracts are made in which there are a significant number of matches and expectations, there is a greater likelihood of job satisfaction, productivity, and reduced turnover than in situations where there are fewer matches or a greater number of mismatches (Kotter, 1973).

TABLE 9-2 *Psychological Contracts: Types of Expectations*

The following thirteen items are examples of areas in which an individual has expectations of receiving and an organization has expectations of giving. That is, for each item in this list, the individual will have an expectation about what the organization will offer him or give him in that area. Likewise, the organization has an expectation about what it will offer or give the individual in that area.

1. A sense of meaning or purpose in the job.
2. Personal development opportunities.
3. The amount of interesting work (stimulates curiosity and induces excitement).
4. The challenge in the work.
5. The power and responsibility in the job.
6. Recognition and approval for good work.
7. The status and prestige in the job.
8. The friendliness of the people, the congeniality of the work group.
9. Salary.
10. The amount of structure in the environment (general practices, discipline, regimentation).
11. The amount of security in the job.
12. Advancement opportunities.
13. The amount and frequency of feedback and evaluation.

The following seventeen items are examples of areas in which an individual has expectations of giving and the organization has expectations of receiving. That is, for each item in this list, the individual will have an expectation about what he is willing or able to give or offer the organization in that area. Likewise, the organization has an expectation about what it will receive from the individual in that area.

1. The ability to perform nonsocial job related tasks requiring some degree of technical knowledge and skill.
2. The ability to learn the various aspects of a position while on the job.
3. The ability to discover new methods of performing tasks; the ability to solve novel problems.
4. The ability to present a point of view effectively and convincingly.
5. The ability to work productively with groups of people.
6. The ability to make well-organized, clear presentations both orally and written.
7. The ability to supervise and direct the work of others.
8. The ability to make responsible decisions well without assistance from others.
9. The ability to plan and organize work efforts for oneself or others.
10. The ability to utilize time and energy for the benefit of the company.
11. The ability to accept company demands which conflict with personal prerogatives.
12. Social relationships with other members of the company off the job.
13. Conforming to the folkways of the organization or work group on the job in areas not directly related to job performance.
14. Further education pursued off-company time.
15. Maintaining a good public image of the company.
16. Taking on company values and goals as one's own.
17. The ability to see what should or must be done, and to initiate appropriate activity.

SOURCE: Kotter (1973). (Copyright 1973 by the Regents of the University of California. Reprinted from *California Management Review*, volume XV, no. 3, p. 93 by permission of the Regents.)

Management by Objectives in a Large Medical Center*

In 1973, St. Vincent's Hospital completed a 20-year transition from a medium-sized community hospital to a large 813-bed medical center. During this time the hospital had always been noted for its excellent organization and its effective management. Although St. Vincent's was a large institution, the pyramid of control was always well defined.

However, the hospital was affected by many internal and external forces. For example, cost-control legislation passed by the state resulted in severe financial cutbacks in all areas. Although the hospital had always operated on a very thin financial basis, financial pressures were increasing at the same time that demands for expansion and modernization were being recognized.

More recently, the hospital has been subject to many changing internal forces, including the loss of the administrator, who had been the chief operating officer in the hospital for many years, and the appointment of a new executive director. There were changes among members of the administrative staff which also resulted in a change in the style of leadership within the hospital.

As a result of the external and internal changes, all elements of the hospital were under pressure to change and adapt. The board of trustees endorsed retaining outside consultants to prepare a long-range plan to replace some obsolete facilities.

To obtain their information, the consultants had to look to the management staff in each department, who were expected to define the long-range goals for their departments. Before long-range goals could be defined, it was recognized that short-range goals must be defined and achieved by the board of trustees and all the staff involved in managing the hospital. To provide a formal and organized system of formulating goals and objectives from the board of trustees down to each individual employee, it was decided to implement a management by objectives program.

At the same time, the hospital was complying with legislation which required that a three-year budget for capital expenditures be prepared rather than a one-year budget. As a total planning program, the three-year budget would provide financial planning, and the management by objectives program for each year would provide organizational and administrative planning with timetables for implementation.

Implementation of the MBO Program

The implementation of the MBO program followed several steps:

Step 1: *Preparation and Education of Hospital Staff for the Program*

The executive director explained the program to the administrative staff, emphasizing that management by objectives is a system of management relating to the planning and the accomplishment of short-term and long-term goals. It ties together financial and non-

---

*Adapted from Sweeney (1977).

financial objectives and it is results-oriented. To be successful, the administrative staff must provide the leadership.

Each member of the administrative staff was to discuss the program with department heads and medical directors for whom they were responsible. A written outline of the entire process was prepared for distribution. A department-head meeting was devoted to an open discussion of the program to assure that everyone understood it.

Step 2: *Formulation of Hospital-Wide Objectives by the Executive Director; Approval by the Board of Trustees*

The executive director requested the administrative staff to submit what they considered the hospital-wide objectives for 1974. They were urged to establish motivational objectives that were realistic, attainable, broad enough to be relevant to the entire hospital, few in number, and consistent with the hospital's philosophy.

Step 3: *Agreement on the Objectives*

A meeting was planned and lengthy dialogue took place between the executive director and the administrative staff to agree on the hospital-wide objectives. The most difficult tasks were setting priorities and limiting the number of goals agreed upon for the year.

When this was completed and the objectives were established, they were submitted to the board of trustees. The board accepted them with minor changes. The goals were then distributed to the department heads and the objectives program was ready to be built.

Next, agreement had to be reached by the division heads and the department heads. They had to discuss what the goals would be, agree on them, and set priorities.

Because of financial cutbacks, the following limitations were attached to all objectives:

1. Capital money is not available.

2. No additional staff can be added.

Step 4: *Putting the Goals Down on Paper*

To facilitate the writing of the goals and to provide some uniformity in their preparation, a form was prepared. The form made it possible for the objectives to be simply stated; the methodology and responsibility noted; the starting and completion quarters recorded; the resources needed or saved; and the hospital-related objective number established. In addition, an implementation schedule was provided which spelled out the timetable for implementation.

Step 5: *The Quarterly Review*

In this process, the department head and the division head meet, discuss, and evaluate how well the program is going. This is done on a quarterly basis after the written progress report is submitted to the division head. The completed form allows the division head to determine whether the goal is behind target, on target, or ahead of target.

A time schedule is prepared so that department heads know when they should submit their progress review schedule.

The division heads as a group meet with the executive director at a formal meeting. A brief narrative report is given by each division head on departmental progress. This is also done on a quarterly basis.

At a department-head meeting, a brief assessment of the progress of the goals is presented.

Operation of the MBO Program

Each member of the administrative staff submitted the hospital-wide objectives for 1974 which they thought should receive priority. Some of the goals submitted were similar, and many of the 28 were related to the achievement of financial stability and communications.

After extensive discussion twelve objectives were agreed upon which were related to fiscal responsibility, patient care, employee attitudes, and community relations (Exhibit A). The objectives were stated clearly and concretely so that all levels of staff could understand them. The number of goals was purposely kept low to assure that they could be achieved within the year. Where possible, objectives were chosen which could be measured and quantified.

EXHIBIT A: HOSPITAL-WIDE OBJECTIVES, 1974

1. Increase hospital revenue.
2. Improve the hospital's cash flow.
3. Establish and implement departmental productivity standards.
4. Implement the J.C.A.H. recommendations.
5. Reduce total utility consumption (electric, steam and telephone).
6. Improve the image of the hospital in relation to the community, patients and visitors. Instill among employees that the hospital is judged by the manner in which they conduct themselves.
7. Improve the personal approach to patients. Reinforce among all employees the concept that patients are to be treated as individuals and that each patient needs personal attention.
8. Develop a more cooperative and professional approach in those employees for whom we are directly responsible.
9. Improve lines of communication with hospital employees on all levels.
10. Develop stronger organizational ties with agencies and community groups who are mutually interested in health affairs.
11. Develop a mechanism for educating the community about their own health and the medical services offered at St. Vincent's.
12. Strengthen among all employees the importance of confidentiality. Discussions regarding patient care and other hospital matters must be conducted discreetly. All medical information must be safeguarded.

After the hospital-wide objectives were approved by the board of trustees, they were distributed to the department heads at their regular meeting. The executive director explained the rationale in the choice of each goal and made the application of each goal as specific as possible. The reaction of the department heads was apprehensive at first but became much more favorable after they saw the objectives and realized that they could both identify with them and participate in their implementation.

The division heads proceeded to meet with their respective department heads to formulate the individual departmental objectives. In some cases this was a process of eliminating objectives which were not feasible because of lack of space. Other goals were not included because they could not be achieved without additional staff. In general, the objectives proposed by department heads were very realistic and capable of achievement without additional staff or capital expense.

The objectives submitted by the departments indicated much thought and planning by the department head with members of the staff. Most department heads worked with their assistants and supervisors in the formulation of the objectives. The division heads agreed with the objectives being proposed by the department heads with very few changes.

After all the objectives were received by the management by objectives coordinator, they were compiled into book form and distributed to each department head. In this volume, 181 objectives were presented, representing 22 departments' plans for the coming year.

Each department head perused the volume. There was considerable discussion among them regarding objectives, particularly if a proposed objective of one department directly affected another department. For example, the director of nursing service had proposed the consolidation of transporter service for all departments and the development of a transporter/messenger service. This proposal would directly affect the Communications Department under which the transporters functioned, as well as Radiology and Rehabilitation, which had their own transporters. This objective immediately initiated dialogue among four department heads who may not have been in close communication before this time. As a first step, it was agreed that a survey be taken of transporter activity to determine whether the function should be located.

Discussion Questions

1. *What were the fundamental problems that the MBO program attempted to solve? Speculate how successful the program was in solving these problems.*

2. *How adequate are the hospital-wide objectives?*

3. *What is the relationship of the objectives defined for specific departments (e.g., nutrition) to the hospital-wide objectives?*

4. *What was the role of the medical staff in the formulation of hospital-wide and departmental objectives? What problems do you anticipate when you attempt to involve physicians in MBO activities?*

CASE 2

Monetary Rewards and Performance Appraisal*

The 1966 Fair Labor Standards Act required hospitals to prepare for large increases in salaries, especially for nonprofessional employees. Bakerville Hospital was no exception. This 300-bed facility, with a long history of meeting the long-term needs of patients in the community, attempted to develop an innovative wage and salary program. The development of the program occurred within the following context.

- The hospital had very few department heads with managerial training or experience.

- The salaries of all employees, including the middle-management staff, was very low and not competitive with industry or other hospitals in the area.

- The wage and salary guidelines used at the hospital were instituted by a few major hospitals of the metropolitan city and promulgated for all the hospitals to adopt.

- The executive director of the Metropolitan City Hospital Council was not receptive to new ideas, especially if they were not accepted by the three hospitals in the area, which had approximately 500 to 900 beds per hospital. Some of the board members of the hospital were also board members of the Metropolitan City Hospital Council and they were advised by the executive director against new approaches to the wage and salary program traditionally implemented in all the area hospitals.

- Some union activity was occurring in hospitals approximately 20 miles from Bakerville Hospital.

- Hospital personnel working in the hospital considered themselves as "one happy family" dedicated to the care of elderly and long-term patients.

- Within the past two years the patient mix changed from long-term care to 80% acute care. Many members of middle management started to work in the hospital before the shift of patient care from long-term to acute care. Their training was not updated to handle the new services needed for acute-care patients or to manage the professional staff along with these services.

- Seniority seemed to be the prevailing criteria for merit increases and promotion to the management staff.

- The MBO program at the hospital stressed evaluation of employees for their development and growth at their jobs or to prepare them in the career mobility program that was being implemented at the hospital.

---

*Adapted from Sister M. Jean Link, FACHA Fellowship Case Reports, 1979.

The following recommendations were presented to the board of trustees through their personnel committee:

1. The hospital should formulate a new wage and salary program with board approval.

2. The hospital should upgrade job qualifications, specifications, and wage ranges of each category of employees to reflect their responsibilities.

3. The hospital should implement a career mobility program which promotes employees from within the hospital only after they receive the proper education, training, and experience needed for the promotion. The hospital would provide assistance through tuition refunds and grants to employees in the program.

4. The administrator will report back to the board within two months with a recommended formal wage and salary program and a listing of pros and cons for the proposed program versus the traditional program now in existence at all the other area hospitals.

A task force of several administrative council members (associate administrator, finance director, personnel director, public relations director, and legal counsel when necessary) was charged with the following tasks:

1. To review all discussion and research data previously obtained by the members.

2. To formulate a wage and salary program with polices and procedures for implementation and present it to the council within one month.

3. To write a plan for communication, education, and training for the implementation of the new program if and when board approval is granted.

Two weeks later, the task force presented its report with recommended plans for the wage and salary program and for implementation of the program. The proposed wage and salary program differed from the existing program in the following ways:

Proposed Program	**Traditional Existing Program**
• Wage increases are given to all employees at the same time annually. Cost-of-living increase given to all employees.	• No cost-of-living increase is given and the wage increase given on the anniversary date of hire is based on merit.
• Wage increases, given in the first quarter, are based on merit and a job market factor.	• A long-form evaluation is used to document employees' performance to determine if they receive a merit wage increase on their anniversary date of hire.
• A short-form evaluation is used for documenting a nonmerit and no increase.	

- Market surveys are conducted and used in determining the various base rates. It is the function of the wage program administrator to review periodically (at least every six months) wages and wage trends in the community, review new positions, etc.

- Annual performance evaluation of each employee is completed on each employee's anniversary date of hire on the long form. The purpose of this evaluation is to note the employee's improvement as a worker.

- An allotment of dollars is budgeted for merit increases and given to each department. This allotment is calculated according to a specific amount per employee. It is left to the discretion of each department head (with certain controls) to reward their top performance employees with the amount determined by the department head for each employee of the department. Not all employees receive a merit increase nor do they receive identical increases.

- Job ranges are updated only when it is apparent through *informal* means that salaries are out of line with the industry in the community. To avert a crisis or to rectify the cause of the crisis, the salary range for a particular job category is changed.

- On each employee's anniversary date, a performance evaluation is done. The purpose of this evaluation is to determine whether or not they receive a merit increase. Almost 90% of all employees receive merit increases, regardless of their actual work performance.

- The same salary increase in dollar amount is given to all employees who have a signed performance evaluation form stating that the department head recommends a merit increase for the employee.

The board of trustees approved the new proposed wage and salary program and the plan for implementation. The communication phase of the plan was immediately put into effect as follows:

1. The major points of the new program, with discussion of problems in the existing wage and salary program, were presented to the executive committee of the medical staff. The medical staff, through their committee structure, was constantly involved in administrative decisions especially on all major issues of the wage and salary program administration.

2. The task force, which dealt with the wage and salary program, conducted educational training and problem-solving sessions for all department heads and all middle-management staff. These sessions were conducted within a two-week period. Each manager received a copy of the approved wage and salary administrative manual with all the policies, procedures, and necessary forms.

3. Department heads (with the director of personnel) held communication sessions for all their employees to communicate the plan, its merits and how it would affect them individually, and to explain when the program would be put into effect. Although some increases would be delayed during the transition period, all the employees were pleased with the prospect of receiving two increases a year.

4. The public relations department published aspects of the program in various written newsletters. A "hot line" was established for questions, answers, and comments on the subject.

The employees' fears, concerns, objections, and questions were heard and responded to by all of the management staff as quickly and effectively as possible.

Current Status of the Program

The implementation of the newly adopted wage and salary program was initiated with all employees receiving a performance evaluation on their anniversary dates, without the evaluation being tied directly to their receiving a merit increase. This evaluation emphasized performance development as a worker. In July of the first year of the program, all employees received an increase based on a factor called a "cost-of-living increase." Any necessary job market increase was given simultaneously with the merit increase to those employees whose merit was documented on the short evaluation form. The amount of money given for merit increases depended on the department head's decision and agreement of the employee as documented on the short evaluation form. In the case of no merit, the employee's status was discussed on an individual basis by the department head with the employee, and a signed agreement or disagreement was submitted to the wage and salary administrator.

Immediately after the increases were given, the following results were evident:

1. The majority of employees and department heads were satisfied that the more productive employees of each department received a larger salary increase than did the less productive employees. All employees received at least some salary increase from the cost-of-living and/or job market factor. Many employees sent letters to the administrator expressing appreciation for their salary increases.

2. The increased cost was budgeted and prepared for by wisely investing the cumulative amount until the money was needed for the increase. The increase in salary cost shown on the financial report given to the Board was more discernible to the board members.

3. The hospital found itself competitive for professional and nonprofessional jobs, especially the nonprofessional jobs within the industrial area.

Several months later, especially around October of the first year, it was realized that two increases per year would be needed instead of the one planned. It was observed in the professional job field that the other hospitals had six months to surpass the wage increases. This problem was recognized by the administrative council, and the wage and salary program administration was modified to give the merit factor and the job market factor increases at the end of the first quarter and to reserve the cost-of-living increase for the last quarter. Since the last-quarter increase was given to all the employees, it allowed the hospital to be competitive, especially within the professional category. The other procedures of the new wage and salary program administration, especially regarding performance evaluation, were not changed with the modification.

The wage and salary program, as modified the first year, has been used by the hospital the past six years or more with only minor revisions of the procedures. And two of the other major hospitals adopted a similar wage and salary program a few years later. Union activities have never been initiated in the hospital, although they have been in some of the other area hospitals.

The overall result was the increased good morale of both nonmanagement and managerial employees. It provided merit dollars to the better employees. In turn, they were motivated to stay and to improve their production because they knew they would be compensated for their efforts. Simultaneously, the program encouraged the less productive employees to leave the hospital. Also, the department heads could concentrate on plans of employee development through the use of the employee's "anniversary date" performance evaluation because it was no longer tied to a merit increase.

Discussion Questions

1. *What problems would you expect in the implementation of the revised wage and salary program?*

2. *Since many of the managers have limited formal management training, design a one-day training program to develop a minimal level of competence in performance appraisal.*

3. *What is the anticipated effect of cost-of-living verus merit increases?*

FURTHER READING

BRAGG, J. E., and I. ANDREWS. "Participative Decision Making: An Experimental Study in a Hospital." *Journal of Applied Behavioral Science* 9(6) (1973):727-733.

PRICE, J. L. and C. W. MUELLER. *Professional Turnover: The Case of Nurses.* Jamaica, N.Y.: Spectrum Publication, Inc., 1981.

RUBIN, I. M., R. E. FRY, and M. S. PLOVNICK. *Managing Human Resources in Health Care Organization: An Applied Approach.* Reston, Va.: Reston, 1978.

SKINNER, K. "Burn-Out: Is Nursing Dangerous to Your Health." *Journal of Nursing Care* 12(12) (Dec. 1979).

VENINGA, R. *Health Administration: Interpersonal Effectiveness.* Englewood Cliffs, N.J.: Prentice-Hall, forthcoming (1981).

WEBBER, J., and M. DULA. "Effective Planning Committee for Hospitals." *Harvard Business Review* (May-June 1974):133-142.

10

Quantitative Control and Measurement

273

The manager's success in an organization is tied closely to the ability to achieve organizational objectives. This involves planning the future direction of the organization (planning and design), and the day-by-day, week-by-week, and month-by-month operations of the organization (decision making and implementation). It also involves controlling and evaluating its activities, that is, assuring that the operations of the organization are conforming to the strategies designed in the planning and operation phases.

The concept of management control was introduced in Chapter 9. It emphasized the manager's responsibilities and abilities to influence and control the behavior of organizational personnel. In this chapter, control will be approached from a more analytical viewpoint, and emphasis will be given to several quantitative methods that aid in managerial control of health services organizations.

CONTROL FRAMEWORK

Control and evaluation include two important dimensions. The manager must be able to *measure the performance* of the organization and to compare this measure to preestablished objectives. The second dimension is to *intercede* in the operation of the organization in order to put it back on course if it is not performing as hoped.

It is useful to view the managerial control function from the perspective presented in Figure 10-1 (Griffith, 1972). The central concept of Figure 10-1 is *feedback,* or the circular nature of the flow of information and activities. First, there is a *process* to be controlled (1). Serving as input into the process are certain *resources* designated to serve this process (2), and certain *operational strategies* that govern the process (3). These three items become the *target* of managerial control activities.

In the first step of feedback, *measurements* (4) are taken from the process which indicate how well the process is performing. These measurements are then *compared* (5) with preestablished *performance standards* or objectives (6). If the measurements are within some specified acceptable limits indicated by the standard or objectives, no intervention is called for, and the control process is (temporarily) satisfied.

If the comparison (5) shows unacceptable deviation from the preestablished standards and objectives, *intervention* (7) is called for. This intervention can be directed to the resources dedicated to the process, the operating strategies designed for the process, the process itself, or some combination of these three.

Consider the following process as an example for the control framework.

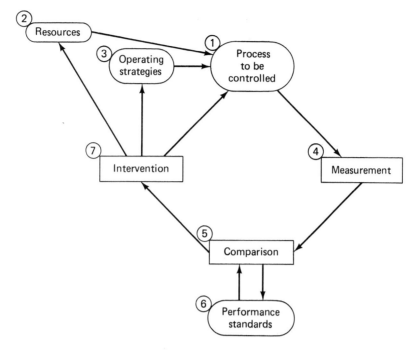

Figure 10-1 The control framework.

The administrator of an outpatient clinic knows that to maintain adequate revenue, the clinic must see a minimum of 350 patients a week. On the other hand, the capacity of the clinic is a maximum of 90 visits a day or 450 visits a week (the clinic is open five days a week). A very simplified control problem is the maintenance of between 350 and 450 clinic visits per week.

The "process" in our example is the admissions process, including the activities that govern the number of patient referrals and walk-ins, and a scheduling function that schedules return visits by patients. The resources involved in this process include such things as the admissions office and its personnel, the existing marketing function, and possibly new marketing programs. The operating strategies include the rules governing when to schedule returning patients, how walk-ins are handled, how many patients each physician is scheduled to see each hour (or day), and so on.

Performance standards or objectives are that there be between 350 and 450 visits per week. This, of course, is highly simplified for our example. Such standards would more likely be specified by type of patient or type of physician seen, or even possibly by the specific physician. It is also likely that the range would be somewhat smaller than between 350 and 450. For purposes of our example, however, these limits suffice.

The measurement function for this process and its performance criteria are straightforward, and could be accomplished by a weekly report prepared late Friday afternoon and/or early Monday morning, showing the number of visits the previous week. A useful report would include the number of visits per week plotted over time since the beginning of the year, such as Figure 10-2.

The comparison function is also quite simple. The task is to establish whether the number of visits last week was between 350 and 450. In a real control problem involving several types of patients and/or physicians, several comparisons would be required, but they would still be easy to perform. A more important consideration for the comparison function is whether an extreme value one week indicates that the process is out of control. For example, if visits remained within limits for the past 16 weeks (ranging between 400 and 425 visits) but last week there were 457 visits, does this require intervention? Probably not. On the other hand, if next week there are 470 visits, the process is more clearly out of control and intervention is more likely required.

Intervention can involve a number of efforts, depending on the situation and on the nature and amount of deviation of the measurement from the standard. In the example, the purpose of intervention is first to determine if the apparent growth trend is a permanent or a temporary phenomenon. If it is temporary, adjustments in scheduling, such as slightly delaying return visits, might cure the problem for the next few weeks.

On the other hand, if long-term growth is anticipated, intervention would call for the planning of expanded service. This could involve either more physicians, longer hours, opening the clinics for a half or full day on

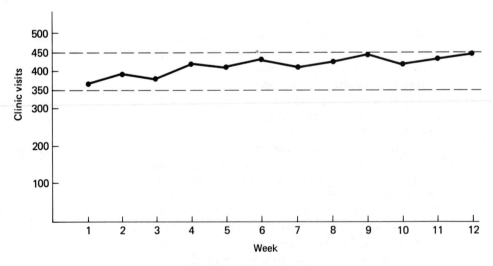

Figure 10-2 Visits per week.

Saturdays, and so on. Other types of intervention may be dictated by the actual situation.

Note an important concept in the feedback process. If the measurement is within the limits of the standard, or the result of the comparison is otherwise determined to indicate that the process is not out of control, the control process (for this aspect at least) stops for the week. This concept allows the "management by exception" principle. This principle argues that if enough control systems are functioning correctly, the manager's time can be focused on just the processes that are out of control or seem to be going out of control. This principle is similar, but not identical, to the principle of management by objectives introduced in Chapter 9.

CONDITIONS FOR SUCCESSFUL CONTROL

For a control system to function successfully, it must be designed in such a way that certain conditions are met (Warner and Holloway, 1978).

Explicit Performance Standards

The performance standards to which the measurement is compared must be explicit enough to make a clear comparison. Usually, this means that the standards must be quantitative, and in the same units of measure as the measurement itself (e.g., number of visits, number of dollars, etc.). For our example, it would be insufficient to specify that visits must be "high enough to attain sufficient revenue." Determining such explicit performance standards can be a major task in itself. In the following section of this chapter, techniques of measurement relevant to such a task are discussed.

Feedback

Feedback is an essential component of a successful control system; without a complete feedback loop the control system cannot function. The feedback must be constant (for our example, *every* week) in order for the control system to monitor continually. Moreover, most problems are not "solved" the first time they are approached, so continual monitoring and intervention in an iterative fashion is usually required. Finally, feedback must be prompt. Late feedback may result in a problem being attacked after it has already cured itself, or worse, it may allow a problem to get so out of control that more drastic means of intervention must be employed. Problems out of control also have a way of causing additional problems. Naturally, the consideration of when feedback is "late" depends on the process being controlled and the speed at which intervention can be successfully employed.

Problem-Solving Capacity

The intervention step assumes that the manager has the knowledge, skill, resources, and authority to intervene. Usually, such intervention requires the types of activities and analyses described in the preceding sections on planning and design and decision making and implementation.

Respect for the System

For a control system to continue to operate successfully, the people involved in each of the functions must believe in its legitimacy. This includes respect for the need to have control systems, belief in the standards of performance, a feeling of responsibility for maintaining control, and a feeling that they do have the ability to intervene when necessary. Essentially, there is the requirement that all people involved—from those in the process to the manager—treat the system as a serious and essential part of the organization.

Forecasting

A less obvious requirement for a control system is that the manager have the ability to forecast when a process is heading for trouble, and once intervention is indicated, what the future holds for the process so that an appropriate strategy can be designed and implemented. An example of predicting when the process might go out of control can be seen in Figure 10-2. From these data, visits per week seem to be exhibiting a steady climb. An observant manager would begin to be concerned about the near future (the first step of forecasting) and attempt to determine the extent of this trend and the reasons for it.

Knowledge of the Environment

The ability to intervene successfully and forecast requires that the manager know the environment of the process under control. In our example, the manager must understand the admissions and scheduling process and know the quality, abilities, and limits of the resources dedicated to the process. Moreover, in order to forecast, the manager must understand the patient referral behavior of physicians, know which communities the clinic patients come from, what unmet needs exist, and where new patients may come from. It would be too late for the manager to try to obtain this knowledge once the process is deemed out of control; this knowledge must be considered a functioning part of the control system.

Backup Support

The last requirement for a successful control system is that there is an organizational structure *behind* the manager which reinforces the manager's authority both to control the process and to step in when circumstances beyond the manager's control cause the process to get out of control. This support structure can be regarded as a "super" control system over the control system itself. That is, the super control system is asked to intervene only when the manager calls for help, or when the whole process (including the manager and the control sytem) appears not to be functioning properly.

Consider what would happen in our example if each of the conditions, one by one, is not met.

MEASUREMENT

Just as forecasting is an essential component of planning and decision making, measurement is an essential component of control and evaluation. It is important for planning and decision making as well, but since it plays such a central role in control and evaluation, a detailed discussion of measurement has been postponed until this point.

In the following discussion, the concept of measurement should not be confused with the function of measurement in the control framework of Figure 10-1. We now consider measurement as an independent concept and as a discipline itself, serving all three functions of management.

There are two general types of measurement: those involving *counting* rules, and those involving *scaling* rules.

Measurements Involving Counting

Counting measurements are usually quite straightforward. In the simplest case, a counting rule requires counting a particular phenomena. For example, measuring the number of clinic visits each week involved a counting rule ("each visit equals one; sum them up"). The number of personnel hours used that week, the number of dollars paid physicians last year, and so on, would also involve a counting rule.

Counting rules become more complicated when it is unreasonable or impossible to count the entire history of an event. In these cases a sample from the past history of the event is used to represent the measure. For example, if a measurement of the average number of visits per day over the last three years is required, to obtain the entire history the number of visits would have to be counted for $3 \times 260 = 780$ days (there are 260 weekdays in a year). Depending on the state of the records from which these data have to be gathered, it may be unreasonable to count all 780 days. A sample of 100 days might be selected as a reasonable and useful representation of the measure. The statistical concepts behind the size of a sample needed and the statistical definition of "reasonable" are beyond the scope of this text. However, the theoretical basis for determining sample size and accuracy of representation has been highly developed and is available to health managers from many sources.

Four steps are involved in constructing a counting measure.

1. Determine exactly which measurement(s) is required (visits per day, visits per week, walk in visits per day, per week, etc.).

2. Determine an unambiguous rule for counting (what constitutes a visit—a patient who sees a nurse but not a physician? or not? etc.)

3. A time (during the year, month) must be determined over which the counting will take place. This usually involves determining a time of "typical" activity, or a combination of "low" and "high" months to reach an average.

4. If less than the full history of data is to be counted, the size of the sample must be determined. This is a highly developed statistical process.

As an exercise, consider which of the measures required in the planning decisions introduced in Chapter 5 require counting rules, and consider how each of these measurements is made. Many of these measurements involve counting things that are not routinely recorded on paper. An example is the counting measure of the amount of time it takes for a physician to see a patient. In this case, a special procedure must be designed to acquire this information. One way is to observe patients with a stopwatch. Clearly, this is a time-consuming and probably disruptive method. A better method might be to use time clocks that print the time a patient arrives for each stage of the process, and the time the patient leaves. A suitable sample of these documents showing all times involved could then be keypunched for a computer to calculate quickly not only examination time, but time for receptionist, wait time, and arrival. A carefully constructed slip or card for each patient to carry through the process would allow most of the measurements to be gathered over one sample period.

Although counting measures appear to be highly accurate, consideration must be made for how well measurements taken in the past (or the present) will represent the phenomenon in the future. If a process is deemed likely to change, it is possible for counting measurements from the past or present to serve as a guide, but the more sophisticated techniques of scaling measurements discussed below should also be considered.

Measurements Involving Scaling

So far we have considered measurements taken on processes that exist in the past and present. Often, measurements are necessary on processes that are proposed or expected and which have no past history. In those cases the measurements must be made by quantifying the subjective opinion of "experts" or the people who are considered the most knowledgeable about the proposed process.

For example, suppose that in planning to expand a clinic, a new service not previously offered is to be included. The planning decision requires that a measure of examination time be determined. If available, it might be possible to use counting procedures at an existing clinic in the community and use these measures for examination time. If this information is not available, or if it is considered unreliable, the opinions of the physicians involved would have to be used.

There is no general method for scaling expert opinion about a future process. The task is to design a method that results in usable quantitative measures. To illustrate a possible method for the example of the examination time for the new service, the following scenario might be one approach.

Looking forward to the desired end result, we might anticipate that what is needed is the proportion of patients that will require 10 to 15 minutes of examination time (assuming that 10 minutes is the minimum), the proportion that will require 15 to 20 minutes, 20 to 25 minutes, and so on, up to the proportion that will require 40 to 45 minutes, assuming 45 minutes to be the maximum. A possible dialogue between the person taking the measure and the physician might be:

Measurer: I've broken down the possible examination times into the following intervals, assuming 10 minutes to be the minimum and 45 minutes to be the maximum:

> 10–15 minutes
> 15–20 minutes
> 20–25 minutes
> 25–30 minutes
> 30–35 minutes
> 35–40 minutes
> 40–45 minutes

First, does this seem to be a reasonable breakdown, and are 10 and 45 minutes appropriate minimums and maximums?

Physician: I guess so—let's try this and see.

Measurer: O.K. Which interval seems the most unlikely?

Physician: Clearly, the 10 to 15 minutes. I'd say only one of a hundred patients would take that short a time. Whereas probably 10% would take 40 to 45 minutes, and, well, I'd say. . . .

Measurer: What is the most likely time?

Physician: I'd say 25 to 35 minutes. Probably 25% of all patients would take that. Probably 20% between 25 and 30 and 25% between 30 and 35.

The results might easily add to over (or under) 100%, such as

10–15 minutes	1%
15–20 minutes	15%
20–25 minutes	20%
25–30 minutes	25%
30–35 minutes	25%
35–40 minutes	15%
40–45 minutes	10%
	111%

This can be adjusted by asking the physician to go back over the numbers to adjust them to add to 100, or by multiplying each number by 100/111, to force it mathematically.

Again, this is only one method of obtaining this type of subjective measurement. An important concept to realize here is the basic difference between this type of measurement and the counting measurement.

A second type of scaling or subjective measurement problem involves measuring not the opinion of what will happen, but measuring a person's preference for what *could* happen. For example, suppose that the manager is trying to determine when to schedule which physicians in the clinic. There are, let us say, five different times the physicians might be scheduled:

Monday/Wednesday	A.M.
Monday/Wednesday	P.M.
Tuesday/Thursday	A.M.
Tuesday/Thursday	P.M.
Friday	All day

In addition, there are three types of physicians:

Ob-gyn
Internists
Surgeons

The task (in our example problem) is to measure each physician's preference for each of the five time slots so that an optimal schedule can be established.

Like the scaling procedure above, there is no one method to make such a measurement. A possible dialogue might be:

Measurer: Can you rank the five time slots according to your preference?

Physician: Sure. I want Monday/Wednesday A.M. most and Friday's the least.

Measurer: How about the other slots?

Physician: Oh, I guess Monday/Wednesday P.M. second, Tuesday/Thursday A.M. third. I really don't want Fridays.

Measurer: Suppose that you had 100 points to distribute among these five alternatives. If you assign all 100 points to Monday/Wednesday A.M. and 0 to the others, it means you want Monday/Wednesday A.M. very much, *but* that you're indifferent between the others as second choice. You get the idea?

Physician: Sure. I'd put 50 on Monday/Wednesday A.M., 0 on Friday. Can I use minus points? No. O.K. 20 each on Monday/Wednesday P.M. and Tuesday/Thursday P.M. and 10 on Tuesday/Thursday A.M. No—40 on Monday/Wednesday A.M., 25 each on. . . .

Averaging this measurement of the preferences of the various types of physicians for the various time slots provides a measurement of the collective preference. This information would, in turn, be useful for determining a schedule suitable to all (or most).

Levels of Measurement

For measurements made by scaling rules, there are four levels of measurement which are increasingly more difficult to quantify but which give increasingly more information.

Nominal Scale. A scale where items are grouped together without regard to one group being relatively higher or lower than another. For example, "measuring" patients by the type of service required—medical, surgical, gynecological, and so on—is a nominal scale, since surgical is not "larger" or "smaller" than medical, only different. Measuring patients by sex—male or female—is another example. Nominal-scale measurements need not (and usually do not) involve the assignment of numbers.

Ordinal Scale. If, in addition to the grouping of items on a nominal scale, a *rank* is given to each group to indicate a relative size, the scale is said to be ordinal. For example, suppose that patients on a nursing unit are measured according to their need for nursing care as either type I (low care), type II (intermediate care), or type III (high care). Type III is "larger" than type II or I, and thus the scale is ordinal. On the other hand, the difference between type III and type II is not necessarily equal to the difference between types II and I. In other words, the "steps" between the types are not necessarily equal. This distinguishes an ordinal scale from an interval scale.

Interval Scale. An interval scale is both nominal and ordinal; plus, the difference between groups (or individuals) is also distinguishable. Dates on a calendar are an example of an interval scale. Day 31 is exactly 6 days from day 37, day 39 is exactly 2 days from 37, and so on. The number assigned to a day allows the difference to be calculated.

Ratio Scale. The most information is contained on a ratio scale, which is an interval scale with a meaningful zero point. This difference is rather subtle and is best presented in examples. If we "measure" patients by their age (in years), we have a ratio scale, since birth (year 0) is a meaningful number for age. We can say that someone who is 60 is twice as old as someone who is 30. This is not true of the measurement of heat with degrees Fahrenheit. That is, we cannot say that it is twice as hot at 70°F as it is at 35°F. This is because zero degrees Fahrenheit does not have any absolute connotation.

In fact, most measurements useful to managers need only be interval in nature, as most decisions involve comparing two or more alternatives, not making absolute judgments. The advantages of interval over ordinal are extremely important for decision making, however, especially when comparing more than two alternatives and/or using several criteria in the comparison.

Reliability and Validity

Two criteria for judging the quality of a rule for a measurement and the measurement itself are reliability and validity. Any unambiguous rule for assigning numbers to a phenomenon constitutes a legitimate measure, so it becomes important to attempt to assess the usefulness of several ways to measure the same attribute of a phenomenon.

Reliability is the extent to which the same number will be assigned to an attribute by different people at different times. The relevant question is: If the same person uses this rule several times, will that person come up with the same number? Or if several people use this rule, will the number they assign be the same? Consider our example of the ordinal scale—the three levels of care for patients—type I, II and III. We would call a rule for assigning patients to one of these three types reliable if we asked several different nurses independently to assign several patients, and they all agreed on the assignments. If there is substantial disagreement, the measurement rule is not reliable.

If unreliable, we might rewrite the instructions (or rules) for assigning patients, or further train the nurses how to make the assignments, and so on. Then a new experiment would be performed to reassess reliability.

A second example is our method (the dialogue) to establish the physician's estimates for the amount of time needed to examine patients in the new service. If the same physician, a week later, assigns essentially the same number to each category, the measure (and the method) is reliable. Or, if several physicians agree independently, the measure can be considered reliable.

There are statistical techniques that are extremely useful for testing the reliability of measures. These are beyond the scope of this text.

Just being able to repeat the assignment of a number to an attribute is not enough to ensure that the measure will be useful to the manager. For a measure to be *valid,* it must indeed measure what it was intended to measure. Usually, counting measures are valid, in that the rules are constructed to count exactly what is to be measured. Visits per week is an example of a measure that would be valid in most cases. However, in our example, what we were really trying to measure was the level of activity on the high side (450) and revenue on the low side (350). It is easy to imagine that simple visits per week is not a valid measure for revenue, as all visits do not generate the same amount of revenue. Thus 350 patients paying $30 a visit do not constitute the same revenue as 350 paying $45, or combinations in between. Using time instead of dollars, the same argument can be made against the validity of visits as a measure of utilization.

In fact, we used visits per week as a *proxy* for revenue, because it is so much easier to measure. If visits per week adequately reflect revenue per week, we can say that it is a valid measure. (This is easy to test. A sample of 20 or 30 weeks where total revenue and visits are compared would indicate if visits adequately reflect revenue.)

Consider a second example. It has been proposed that in order for obstetrical units to be of high quality, over 2000 births a year must be performed in the units. Thus "2000 or more births a year" is a proxy for quality. If you were responsible for establishing if the OB units in your section of the country were of "adequate quality," this would be an extremely useful measure. The alternative would involve assembling a team of experts to visit each facility to establish its quality. This is both expensive and frustrating, especially if there is substantial disagreement among the experts.

The question of validity here is: Does 2000+ births a year represent quality? The validity might be assessed by choosing a small sample of OB units that do between 1000 and 3000 births a year and determining if 2000 is a useful cutoff for quality. Again, statistics would be extremely useful for this type of experiment.

A final example is the validity of asking a physician to estimate the proportion of patients requiring different amounts of time for examination. We could use an existing service in the clinic and measure the actual proportions using a counting scheme. Then we could independently ask a physician in that service to make subjective estimates about this existing service. A comparison of the physician's estimates to the actual would give insight (but of course not conclusive evidence) about the validity of using this, and possibly all, physicians' opinions as a measure for examination time.

In each of the examples above, there exists a *real* measure of which the measure in question was proxy: revenue was real (although harder to get), visits was a proxy; subjective quality was real (but expensive to get), 2000+ births was a proxy. When a real measure exists to which we can compare our proxy measure, we are assessing *predictive validity:* The ability of a measure to reflect the real (known) attribute. Often, there is no real measure with which to compare.

When no real measure exists with which to compare our measure, the validity question becomes one of *content validity*. To what extent does our measure actually measure what we want it to? This is, of course, a very subjective judgment, but an essential one to treat rigorously.

There is no single test for testing content validity, and statistics is not useful. The assessment has to be made along the lines of the user's faith in the people who designed the measure, other peoples' opinion about the measure, and other factors.

THE MANAGER'S ROLE

Control and measurement have been explained with a fair amount of detail in this chapter. Although it is important that managers appreciate some of this detail, it is not the manager's role to be an expert control system designer or an expert measurer. In most cases, people expressly trained in control and measurement will be employed in the design of control systems and in making measurements.

The important responsibilities of the manager concerning control systems are that the manager:

- Make sure that control systems are in place in important areas.
- Make sure that these control systems are designed correctly, so that they control what they are intended to control.
- Motivate the people involved to participate and respect the control system.

- Make sure that the control system gives the manager the right amount of information (not too little and not too much), and that it is timely. The manager's role is not to *run* the control systems but to make sure that they are installed and functioning properly.

CASE

Staffing Pattern in a Primary Care Center

Suppose that you are responsible for designing, implementing, and managing a system for controlling the number of hours of nursing time used in a rural primary care center. The center uses a combination of full-time and part-time nurses, both in the center and through several satellite sites, including nurses that travel to patients' homes.

Required: (a) Discuss briefly the nature of each of the seven *elements* of a control system depicted in Figure 10-1. (b) Discuss briefly what would happen if, *one at a time,* each of the seven *conditions* for successful control were not met.

FURTHER READING

GRIFFITH, J. R. *Quantitative Techniques for Hospital Planning and Control.* Lexington, Mass.: D. C. Heath, 1972.

GRIFFITH, J. R., W. M. HANCOCK, and F. MUNSON. *Cost Control in Hospitals.* Ann Arbor, Mich.: Health Administration Press, 1976.

HARE, V. C. *Systems Analysis: A Diagnostic Approach.* New York: Harcourt Brace & World, 1967.

LOOMBA, N. P. *Management: A Quantitative Approach.* New York: Macmillan, 1978.

MURDICK, R. G., and J. E. ROSS. *Information Systems.* Englewood Cliffs, N.J.: Prentice-Hall, 1975.

SHANNON, R. E. *Systems Simulation.* Englewood Cliffs, N.J.: Prentice-Hall, 1975.

WARNER, D. M., and D. C. HOLLOWAY. *Decision Making and Control for Health Administration.* Ann Arbor, Mich.: Health Administration Press, 1978.

11

Financial Control

┌──────────────────── **OVERVIEW** ────────────────────┐
│   │
│ The financial control of an organization focuses on the protection │
│ of the organization's assets and the reliability of its accounting │
│ records. The objective of this chapter is to provide a framework │
│ for the operation of this control and a discussion of specific strate- │
│ gies appropriate to health service organizations. │
│   │
└──┘

CONTROL FRAMEWORK

Figure 11-1 presents a general model of a basic financial control system. Building on the general control framework described in Chapter 10, Figure 11-1 extends the fundamental perspective for viewing fiscal controls as a *system*.

The model begins with the organization developing plans and procedures. If these plans and procedures are satisfactory, operations may begin. If they are not satisfactory, the plans and/or procedures should be modified. Once operations begin, the control system is concerned with measuring performance or outcomes. If performance is satisfactory and the process is to continue, positive feedback should be forthcoming. If, on the other hand, the measurement of performance or outcomes indicates that performance is not satisfactory, the control system must identify the problems and provide feedback so that plans or procedures can be modified. The feedback in this case is not necessarily *only* negative, since at this stage feedback should have two purposes: (1) to provide sufficient information so that corrective action can be taken, and (2) to provide sufficient motivation so that operations can continue. The sequence of events above continues until it is determined that the process being monitored is complete and feedback is given to those concerned.

As can be seen in this general model (Figure 11-1), planning and operations can be viewed as part of a control system. Planning provides the standards against which the measurement of operations is compared. In this sense, control can be defined as a feedback *system* in which outcomes are measured against standards and adjustments are made as needed.

Control can also be viewed as a *process* by which an organization sets up procedures designed to help it obtain and utilize resources as effectively, efficiently, and economically as possible. In this context, there are two types of financial-related controls: general controls and reporting controls. *Reporting controls* take the form of reports. These include various external reports, known as the *financial statements* of the organization, and internal reports, which focus upon *cost* and/or *variance analysis*. These will be discussed in more detail later in this chapter. *General controls,* on the other hand, focus on laying the groundwork in the organization so that things go as planned

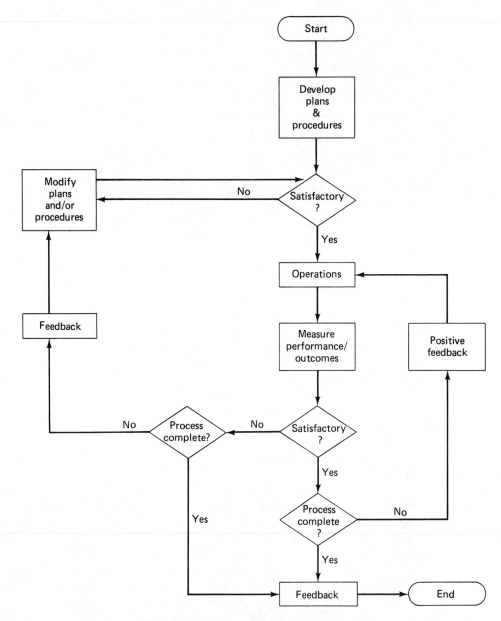

Figure 11-1 Basic service delivery control system.

and records are available to monitor the activities of the organization. Both general controls and reporting controls are shown in part III of Figure 11-2, which presents an overview of the financial management function. The general controls are also listed in Table 11-1.

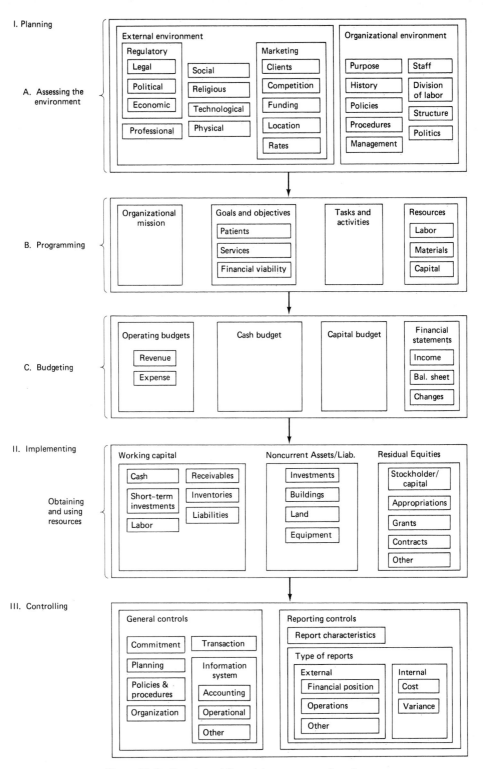

I. Planning

A. Assessing the environment

External environment

Regulatory
- Legal
- Political
- Economic
- Professional

- Social
- Religious
- Technological
- Physical

Marketing
- Clients
- Competition
- Funding
- Location
- Rates

Organizational environment
- Purpose
- History
- Policies
- Procedures
- Management
- Staff
- Division of labor
- Structure
- Politics

B. Programming

- Organizational mission
- Goals and objectives
  - Patients
  - Services
  - Financial viability
- Tasks and activities
- Resources
  - Labor
  - Materials
  - Capital

C. Budgeting

- Operating budgets
  - Revenue
  - Expense
- Cash budget
- Capital budget
- Financial statements
  - Income
  - Bal. sheet
  - Changes

II. Implementing

Obtaining and using resources

- Working capital
  - Cash
  - Short-term investments
  - Labor
  - Receivables
  - Inventories
  - Liabilities
- Noncurrent Assets/Liab.
  - Investments
  - Buildings
  - Land
  - Equipment
- Residual Equities
  - Stockholder/ capital
  - Appropriations
  - Grants
  - Contracts
  - Other

III. Controlling

- General controls
  - Commitment
  - Planning
  - Policies & procedures
  - Organization
  - Transaction
  - Information system
    - Accounting
    - Operational
    - Other
- Reporting controls
  - Report characteristics
  - Type of reports
    - External
      - Financial position
      - Operations
      - Other
    - Internal
      - Cost
      - Variance

Figure 11-2 Overview of financial management functions.

TABLE 11-1 *General Controls*

1. Management commitment and approach
2. Planning controls
3. Policies and procedures
4. Organization controls
a. Structure (responsibility accounting)
b. Personnel control
c. Asset
5. Transaction control
6. Information system controls
a. Accounting system controls
b. Statistical system controls
c. Other

GENERAL CONTROLS

There are six basic types of general controls: management commitment and approach, programming and budgeting, policies and procedures, organization, transactions, and information systems (Table 11-1).

Management Commitment and Approach

Financial management should not be the province of one or two people in an organization. Rather it should pervade the whole organization (Herkimer, 1978). For employees to be committed to controlling costs and protecting the organization's assets, they must perceive that managment has a commitment to those concepts as well. This commitment should be in actions as well as words. That is, management must demonstrate its commitment by facilitating and utilizing the control aspects discussed in this chapter. This may be accomplished by various means, including a suitable organizational structure, adequate information systems, and appropriate guidelines and training. These means will vary considerably by organization, but in each case they are extremely important to the overall success of any control efforts.

With management committed both in word and action to implementing financial management-oriented control, the controls discussed below have a greater chance of being successfully implemented. We now turn to the second general control: planning controls.

Planning Controls

The planning process was discussed in detail in Chapter 4. Two of the major components of planning are programming and budgeting (Vraciu, 1979). These are illustrated in Figure 11-2, part IB and C. To briefly reiterate, the major steps of the programming phase of planning are as follows.

Defining the organizational mission is the first step of *programming*.

After the mission is identified, the next step is to identify the goals and objectives of the organization, including the populations to be served and the services to be offered, and to answer questions related to the financial viability of the organization. Next, tasks and activities should be specified to fulfill the goals and objectives. The final step is to identify the resources needed to complete these tasks and activities. Resources are classified into three major categories: labor, materials, and capital.

Budgeting follows directly from the programming effort. In fact, budgeting is the final step in the planning process and involves identifying the fiscal implications of the programs that are to be undertaken. The result of the budgeting process is the development of an operating budget (including revenue and expense budgets), a cash budget, a capital budget, and *pro forma* financial statements, including the income statement, the balance sheet, and a statement of changes of financial position.

As with overall management, planning controls begin with a commitment by the staff. To get this commitment, it is important for the staff to understand the purpose and the process of programming and budgeting. This is often a major deficiency in building control into the planning process. The lack of understanding of the planning process by the staff may result in a highly ineffective and suboptimally useful set of programming and budgeting activities.

For instance, if budgeting is set forth (as it often is) as a task that must be dispensed with as quickly as possible and which has no future ramifications, it will probably be carried out that way. If, on the other hand, programming and budgeting are set forth as important activities in the course of the organization around which (1) future activities will be based, and (2) around which evaluation will be forthcoming, then these two activities will probably be undertaken in a much more serious vein. However, even with an understanding of the purposes of the programming and budgeting activities, the staff must still have a second type of control available—the resources necessary for the proper commission of their planning activities: time, structure, and information.

Time is often the most difficult resource to supply. Good planning takes time. If the staff is already working near capacity, they may find it difficult to find additional time to devote to the programming and planning process. If such time is not provided for planning, other control efforts may be wasted.

A second control is to provide the *structure* so that planning activities can be carried out appropriately. This involves clearly identifying a responsibility and authority structure for the planning process. The important aspects of this structure have been discussed in other chapters.

A final type of resource control is *information control:* providing the people participating in programming and budgeting with the information needed to carry out their tasks. This begins by providing the *appropriate direction* for the planning and budgeting activities, including a statement of the general objectives of the budgeting process, the policies and procedures of the organization, and the goals and objectives of the organization around which each department is to develop programs and budgets. Similarly, easy-to-follow forms and identification of time lines are also important resources for efficient and effective programming and budgeting.

Other informational controls include providing units in the organization with environmental assessments such as forecasts about the general economy and inflation, as well as more specific forecasts concerning patient demand and staff resources during the coming year. In many large organizations, such information is furnished by a planning department. In other instances, the specific departments are required to develop such information on their own. Considerable time and resources can be saved if such environmental assessments are centralized as the organization grows larger.

Other information that can be provided includes cost and scheduling data. People doing the programming and budgeting should have appropriate information concerning various inputs and outputs, including cost of staff and services.

With the foregoing planning controls in place, an organization should have better control over the efficiency and effectiveness of the planning process, which in turn should help in implementation.

Policies and Procedures

Policies and procedures are essentially the guidelines and rules of the organization. They set forth how decisions or tasks should be approached in various situations. As an organization grows, it is important that all policies and procedures be documented, and periodically updated and revised. All policies and procedures should be clearly written; that is, they should be precise, concise, and written at appropriate levels for those who are going to use them. Policies and procedures that are not intelligible are not likely to be followed.

Even when policies and procedures exist, the staff is not always as familiar with them as it should be. To ensure that policies and procedures are followed, orientation and training sessions should be an integral part of employee development. Furthermore, all policies and procedures should be accessible; employees should know where to go to obtain specific information.

Policies and procedures usually develop over time, incrementally, as situations arise where decisions have to be made. These informal policies and procedures usually become a working part of the organization. Long-time employees feel there is no need, or they do not have the time, to document what they are doing. However, as organizations grow larger, and as employee turnover becomes more of a factor, documentation of policies and procedures becomes necessary to protect the assets and to ensure the efficiency and effectiveness of the organization and the reliability of its accounting records.

In a recent instance, a 700-bed hospital was visited which was noted for its excellence in financial management. The purpose of the meeting was to identify student projects for the coming semester. Much to our surprise, the controller stated that in her tenure she had not had time to commit most policies and procedures to writing. She recognized the importance of this endeavor and was hoping that students would help her in this regard. She said the students would be of great help, as she was the only person in the organization in a position to know all the policies and procedures. Most of the top-level staff were new.

Coincidentally, she was to speak to one of our seminars the following week, but called up the day before and noted that she had twisted her back and would not be in to work for at least 10 days. Athough this caused the hospital problems, imagine the difficulty a hospital would find itself in if its chief financial officer were suddenly to leave permanently and no written policies and procedures existed regarding the financial management of the organization.

Organizational Controls

There are three main types of organizational controls regarding the financial management of the organization: structural controls, personnel controls, and asset and liability controls. Each of these is important for various aspects of sound financial management.

Structural controls refer to the design of the organization to ensure that authority and responsibility are clearly delineated throughout the organization and that staff is allocated for the efficient and effective accomplishment of tasks (Robertson, 1976). The most fundamental element of structural control is to identify responsibility, responsibility centers, and their interrelationship.

As discussed in Chapter 4, responsibility centers are organizational units that are responsible for carrying out specific tasks such as housekeeping, dietary, nursing, sanitary inspections, counseling, and so on. There are four types of responsibility centers in most health care settings. These are outlined in Table 11-2 and are: service centers, cost centers, revenue centers, and investment centers.

Service centers are organizational units that are responsible for providing service. This is the most primitive type of responsibility center, in that there is very little accountability and it involves seeing to it that services are provided at least at minimal quality and volume. Organizations that have only such centers usually do not use the budget as a planning and control mechanism, but as a document to submit to their fiscal authority. Examples of a service center might include counseling teams at mental health centers, in-

TABLE 11-2 *Types and Characteristics of Responsibility Centers*

Type	Responsible for:			
	Quality/ Case Load	Expenditures and/or Costs	Revenues (Profits)	Return on Investment
Service center	X			
Cost center	X	X		
Revenue center (profit)	X	X	X	
Investment center	X	X	X	X

spection teams in health departments, or rehabilitation units in hospitals. Service centers are charged with providing services but do not have a working budget to adhere to and are not monitored for their expenses in any systematic way. They are usually part of an overall organization which is concerned only that it does not exceed its annual budget, but does not closely monitor its departments. As lax as this might sound, numerous service centers exist in health care settings.

Cost centers, on the other hand, are usually responsible both for meeting minimal quality and volume standards and controlling expenditures or costs (Horngren, 1978). In such instances, the persons responsible for a cost center, such as an intensive care or detoxification unit, will know their budget beforehand and are responsible for keeping spending within that budget.

The next type of responsibility is a *revenue center.* Revenue centers are usually responsible not only for meeting minimal quality and volume standards, but are also responsible for controlling their costs and for generating revenues. The difference between revenues and expenses in for-profit organizations is called *profit.* In not-for-profit organizations, it is called "excess of revenues over expenses." Revenue centers provide an important control over both the inflows and the outflows of the organization. They are usually not common in decentralized organizations such as those with geographically distinct clinics.

The final type of responsibility center is an *investment center.* These are fairly rare in the health field, but they may begin to appear in increasing numbers in the for-profit segment of the industry. Investment centers are usually responsible for meeting minimal quality and volume standards, controlling their expenditures and/or costs, generating revenues, and investing their profits wisely to generate a desired return (Horngren, 1978). In investment centers, it is not sufficient for a branch of a for-profit hospital to generate a profit. The head of the branch is also responsible for wisely investing the organization's profits as well.

As can be seen in Table 11-2, each of these four types of responsibility centers provides an increasing degree of financial management control for a health care organization. There are various ways in which responsibility centers can be organized to meet the goals of a health care provider. Four major ways in which this is accomplished are presented in Figure 11-3. On the top tier of this figure, responsibility centers are shown by *functions*. In this example, they are the business function, patient services, consultation, and education. The second tier of Figure 11-3 shows that responsibilities can be set up by *location*. For instance, patient services could be decentralized either within a large centralized medical campus (such as one having different hospitals), or it could be geographically spread out over one or more distinct areas in a *decentralized* organization.

A third way in which responsibility centers can be organized is in regard to *services*. In Figure 11-3, patient services are divided into inpatient, outpatient, and emergency. Although some organizations find it more convenient to include emergency in outpatient or divide emergency among inpatient and outpatient, the organization can be structured whichever way seems to be most suitable. The final way of structuring along the lines of responsibility centers is by *client/patient*. In Figure 11-3, the outpatient service is divided among those focusing on children, families, and adults.

It is not necessary for a provider to organize only along one of these four responsibility center dimensions; rather an organization may use all four of these ways to meet the organization's objectives efficiently and effectively. Responsibility centers should have the authority to accompany their responsibilities; that is, without having the authority to make decisions, a person

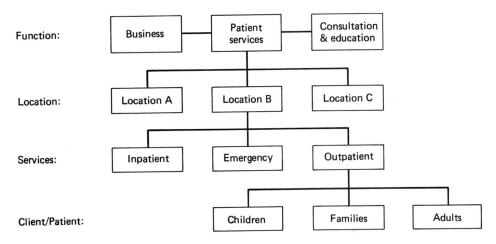

Figure 11-3 Common bases for determining responsibility centers.

should not be responsible for the outcome of any particular activity or process. Similarly, the ultimate authority and responsibility should rest with one person in the responsibility center. To the extent possible, responsibility centers should be small and homogeneous in function. For instance, in a large hospital it would be difficult to have inpatient services as the smallest unit of responsibility. Rather, it might aid control if the inpatient services were broken down into more specific functions such as hematology, neonatology intensive care, and so on. These functions could always be aggregated under a larger responsibility center as needed.

Personnel Control

The second major type of organizational control in the financial management of the organization deals with *personnel*. From the financial management point of view, the major purpose of personnel controls is to hire competent people to carry out various functions which will ensure that the assets of the organization are protected, the goals and objectives of the organization are reached efficiently, effectively, and economically, and the accounting records accurately reflect the transactions of the organization. Given the numerous decisions that employees make regarding these factors, it is extremely important that personnel controls be implemented in an organization. Figure 11-4 presents six of the most important personnel controls.

Personnel controls begin with the *hiring* process. Actually, hiring is the last step of a process that is preceded by a thorough consideration of the duties of the job to be filled and the qualifications the future employee is to have. Writing a meaningful job description is a prerequisite to delineating clearly the duties of the position being filled. There is a great deal of literature available on the hiring process; those interested should pursue selected readings in this regard.

The second personnel control is the *placing* function. This is often a routine activity in organizations that hire a person for a specific position. On the other hand, when there are numerous positions to be filled, and an individual qualified for several of those positions is hired, the organization has the opportunity both to improve itself and to help maximize the goals of the individual. For instance, if an RN is hired and there are several RN positions open throughout the hospital, it is usually advantageous to place the newly hired person in a situation that best fits his or her personality and time requirements. By helping individuals reach their own goals, it is likely that such persons will be more productive and stay longer with the organization. The financial implications of this are discussed below.

The third personnel control is *training*. This is an activity that more and more health care organizations are finding to be an important aspect of personnel. As health providers try to improve their control of costs and the accuracy of their accounting information, both initial training and ongoing

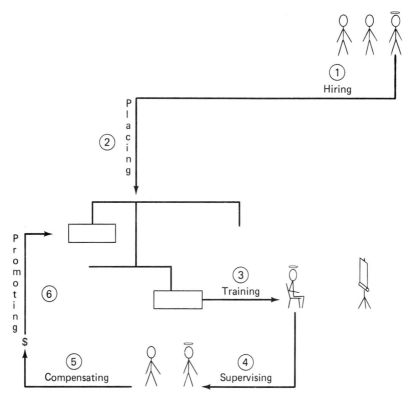

Figure 11-4 Personnel controls.

personnel development become extremely important activities. Such activities may result in more skilled and knowledgeable personnel, as well as increasing the staff's feelings of personal and professional growth and development.

All training does not have to occur within the organization, and many health care organizations are contracting with various training firms or paying their employees to take additional courses in topics of interest. For instance, recent studies have shown that financial management is one of the key areas in which administrators feel they need more background. To this extent, various training entities, including universities, are conducting workshops for health care organizations and for administrators in general. These workshops deal with such diverse topics as basic accounting, budgeting and control, managerial and cost accounting, cost containment, and maximizing reimbursement.

The fourth personnel control is *supervising*. Supervising has long been of interest to management, and voluminous literature on the subject exists. One of the easiest ways to ensure that policies and procedures are being carried out as planned is to supervise properly. Good supervision is greatly facilitated by clear communication and mutual understanding. In Chapters 4, 9, and 10 management by objectives was discussed as an approach that attempts to accomplish this by having the manager and employee sit down and mutually agree upon the goals and objectives and tasks and activities to be accomplished by an employee during the year.

When activities are clearly delineated, the process of supervising becomes much easier. We recently experienced a case where the controller of one hospital was reluctant to monitor personnel in the billing and collections department closely because of the lack of clear job descriptions. He felt uncomfortable monitoring their activities because their duties were not clearly specified. In other words, he was not exactly sure what the employees were supposed to do. Given the large amount of money that was involved in the billing and collections functions, and the possible chances for fraud, this would seem to be a very tenuous position to be in.

The next personnel control is *compensation*. Compensation is one of the most important personnel controls from a financial management point of view. On the one hand, the organization wants to attract and retain good employees and pay them a reasonable salary. On the other hand, it does not want to pay excessive wages and strain the resources of the organization. Compensation is often a point of contention in personnel disputes and one that can often be avoided by good job classification, and by personnel and compensation policies and procedures.

The cost of losing good employees is much higher than it may appear on the surface. Considerable resources have to be devoted to advertising for new positions and conducting hiring, placing, training, and supervising processes. While personnel are spending their time training new employees, they are not delivering services. This can also be very costly. Well-defined personnel compensation policies and procedures can help avoid many problems dealing with turnover.

The sixth area of personnel control is *promoting*. The promotion function is very important both to the individual employee and to the financial management of the provider. On the one hand, it is desirable to give employees an opportunity to move up in the organization. This may provide them with motivation and can save training-related resources. In addition, the organization has administrators who are familiar with the "nuts and bolts" of the organization. On the other hand, it is important to avoid promoting people beyond their level of competence.

From a financial management point of view, the six personnel controls described above are among the most important controls in the organization. Many of the inefficiencies in health care organizations are not due to poor-quality materials, but rather to problems that occur with personnel. To the extent that various units of the organization are understaffed or employees are undertrained, undersupervised, or undercompensated, they do not work as productively. This results in inefficiencies. Because of the labor-intensive nature of many health care providers, these problems cannot be overemphasized. Financial management is greatly concerned with the efficiency and effectiveness of the organization. Time and again when the reason for inefficiencies are discovered, they have to do with disgruntled employees, vacant positions, or high turnover. Poor morale is reflected in poor productivity.

One final point should be mentioned under personnel controls: the concept of segregation of duties. *Segregation of duties* implies that a person should not be placed in a position where they can circumvent good management practices concerning protecting the assets of the organization. This implies separating jobs to build in control. For instance, the following is a list of business activities that normally should be performed by different individuals: those who deliver services should be different from those who collect cash for service delivery; those who collect cash by mail should be different from those who make up/or send patients' bills; those who receive patients' payments by mail should be different from those who deposit cash receipts; and those who record amounts to be paid should be different from those who send cash disbursements.

Similar controls should exist in other functions as well. For instance, in the purchasing area those who identify purchase needs should be different from those who actually do the ordering; those who do the ordering should be different from those who initially receive the goods; and those who initially receive the goods should be different from those who pay for the purchase. An example in the purchasing area is drugs in a hospital. There should be tight control over who identifies the need for additional purchases. The person who identifies the need should not have direct access to ordering the drugs; all ordering should go through the pharmacy. Similarly, a person in the pharmacy should not be able to order unauthorized drugs; all purchase orders should be authorized by the appropriate personnel. To ensure that people do not keep drugs for their own use, the receipt of drugs should be authorized by a person other than those who ordered them. Finally, the drugs should be paid for by someone other than the person who received them, and then only when authorized.

The segregation of duties described above is quite difficult to implement in small organizations, but still extremely important.

Asset control is the final type of organizational control. It is similar to segregation of duties. In asset control, one is trying to restrict access to assets (Stettler, 1977). For instance, only certain people should be able to deposit or withdraw money from bank accounts, requisition drugs, or have access to supplies such as syringes, blood plasma, and drugs. Hospitals often find segregation of assets to be a particular problem due to the nature of providing health care. That is, those providing health care services want access to thermometers, syringes, and drugs when they need them and want such items kept readily available on the floor. On the other hand, these service deliverers are so busy that they often prefer not to sign out for such items when they use them. The hospital should try to take into account the amount of loss and waste that may occur due to such poor practices and attempt to correct these situations within the constraints of providing good-quality medical care and monetary resources.

Transaction Control

Transaction control is the bridge between the general controls just mentioned and the information system control discussed below (see Figure 11-2). Transaction controls are designed to see that all transactions that take place are authorized, carried out as authorized, and recorded appropriately (Stettler, 1977). Essentially, they provide a monitoring of the general controls by ensuring that all things which are recorded on the books have actually taken place: for example, that drugs which have been credited to a patient's account have actually been delivered to the patient. Conversely, transaction control is concerned that all transactions which have occurred are recorded. For instance, if a patient receives medicine, it should be recorded properly on the patient's account. Such records are part of the organization's information system, which is the next topic.

Although the controls listed under segregation of duties, and asset and transaction control, may seem like superfluous red tape, such controls have been developed over time in response to the many problems faced by business regarding inefficiency, negligence, and fraud. The specific controls instituted in any particular organization should be well thought out and implemented with as little disruption to the organization as possible. Many, if not most organizations, would prefer not to have to implement such controls. However, as most organizations grow in size, numerous employees come and go, and the amount of assets purchased increases significantly, it becomes more difficult to rely on personal contact to run and monitor the organization efficiently.

Information System Control

There are two types of information system controls: accounting system controls and statistical system controls. *Accounting system controls* are designed to see that all transactions are recorded properly in the books so that the financial statements that are issued by the organization represent fairly the transactions of the organization (Robertson, 1976).

The first type of accounting control is to record transactions in a set of books. *Books* in this case refers to those books which are common to most businesses for recording their transactions: a journal, a ledger, and subsidiary ledgers (Figure 11-5) (Pyle et al., 1978). The *journal* is often called the book of original entry. It is a chronological list of all transactions that take place in the business. For instance, if John Jones receives a service and pays cash,

GENERAL JOURNAL				P. 1
Date		Account Titles and Explanation	Folio	Increase (+) Decrease (−)
1981 Sept.	1	CASH	110	+50
		PATIENT REVENUES	410	+50
		To record full cash payment for services received 9/1/81 from John Jones		
	2	ACCOUNTS RECEIVABLE	120	+70
		PATIENT REVENUES	410	+70
		To record service delivered to Mary Smith		
	3	CASH	110	+30
		ACCOUNTS RECEIVABLE	120	−30
		To record payment in part from Mary Smith		

GENERAL LEDGER   P. 1

CASH   ACCOUNT 110

Date	Folio	In- crease	De- crease	Bal- ance
1981 Sept.				
1	GJp1	50		50
3	GJp1	30		80

ACCOUNTS RECEIVABLE   ACCOUNT 120

Date	Folio	In- crease	De- crease	Bal- ance
1981 Sept.				
2	GJp1	70		70
3	GJp1		30	40

PATIENT REVENUES   ACCOUNT 410

Date	Folio	De- crease	In- crease	Bal- ance
1981 Sept.				
1	GJp1		50	50
2	GJp1		70	120

Mary Smith   ACCOUNTS RECEIVABLE
                              SUBSIDIARY LEDGER

Date		Folio	Increase	Decrease	Balance
1981 Sept.	2	GLp1	70		70
	3	GLp1		30	40

Figure 11-5 Illustration of major bookkeeping logs.

an entry would be made in the journal which shows that the organization earned $50 and actually received the $50 in cash. The actual entry on the books would increase the cash account by $50 and increase the patient service revenues account by $50. Incidentally, note that in all cases at least two accounts are affected by any transaction. This is standard bookkeeping procedure and serves as a check for errors in recording.

If, on the other hand, John Jones did not pay cash for the service but is to be sent a bill, it would be noted in the books that John Jones owes the organization all $50 of the $50 that was earned. Once John Jones decides to pay his bill, the books would note the amount owed by John Jones decreased by $50, and that $50 in cash was received. With thousands of transactions occurring each day, keeping a chronological list of each and every transaction is extremely important. However, chronological listing has a major disadvantage: since no subtotals are kept, it is difficult to know the results of the transactions at the end of the day. For instance, it would be difficult to know how much was owed the organization without reviewing perhaps thousands of transactions and summarizing them. To overcome this problem, businesses use ledgers.

Ledgers are books that contain specific categories for each of the asset, liability, capital, revenue, and expense accounts of the health care provider. These categories are organized according to a *chart of accounts* that lists each of the asset, liability, capital, revenue, and expense accounts by number. In the example used in Figure 11-6, all assets are numbered 100, liabilities 200, capital accounts 300, revenues 400, and expenses 500. These accounts can be further subdivided. For instance, the asset *cash* could be given the number 110, *accounts receivable* 120, and *marketable securities* 130. Since all liabilities are numbered in the 200s, a chart of accounts might designate *accounts payable* 210, *utilities payable* 220, and *mortgages payable* 230. To standardize and simplify this designation process, hospitals have developed a standardized chart of accounts that all hospitals can use. Similarly, most community health organizations use a standard governmental chart of accounts prescribed by each state.

The final book of relevance here is the *subsidiary ledger*. Subsidiary ledgers are accounts that show the organization to whom it owes money or who owes it money at any particular time. By walking through the transactions on Figure 11-4, the interrelationships between the general journal, the general ledger, and the subsidiary ledger can be seen.

The general journal is nothing more than a book with a series of pages, each one with a title at the top saying "general ledger." The page has a space for the date of each transaction; a middle section entitled "account titles and explanations" in which each transaction is recorded according to the accounts that are affected, and an explanation describing the transaction; a section called "folio," which tells which general ledger account the transaction is also recorded in; and the final columns, which show how much each

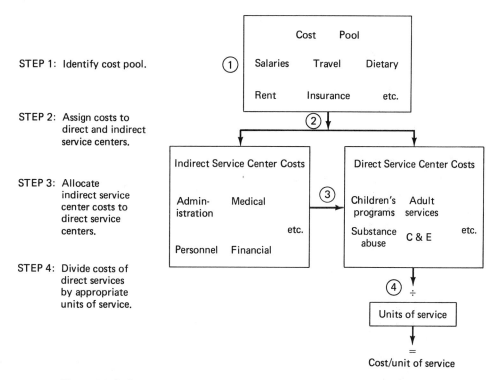

STEP 1: Identify cost pool.

STEP 2: Assign costs to direct and indirect service centers.

STEP 3: Allocate indirect service center costs to direct service centers.

STEP 4: Divide costs of direct services by appropriate units of service.

(1) Cost Pool

Salaries   Travel   Dietary

Rent   Insurance   etc.

(2)

Indirect Service Center Costs

Admin-   Medical
istration

etc.

Personnel   Financial

(3)

Direct Service Center Costs

Children's   Adult
programs   services

Substance   C & E   etc.
abuse

(4) ÷

Units of service

=

Cost/unit of service

Figure 11-6 Steps in determining costs per unit of service in mental health programs.

account is increased or decreased. Debits and credits are used to increase or decrease the amount in any particular account. Since persons often find these terms somewhat confusing, the increases and decreases will be indicated by a + or –, respectively, in the example.

Looking at the first transaction in the general ledger (Figure 11-5), which occurred on September 1, 1981, John Jones received services that cost $50. He paid $50 in cash and the provider earned $50 in revenue. Therefore, cash was increased by $50 and patient revenues were increased by $50. Note that in the folio account, cash has the number 110 by it, and patient revenues has the number 410 by it. Remember, the chart of accounts is organized so that assets are numbered 100 and revenues are designated by the number 400. If you skip down the page to the general ledger, account 110 (cash) has a $50 increase on September 1, 1981. This entry brought the balance in the cash account to $50. In the "folio" section of the cash account, it is noted that this transaction was originally recorded in the general journal, page 1 (GJP1). Similarly for patient revenues, if you skip to account 410 in the general ledger, it can be seen that on September 1, 1981, the patient revenues account increased by $50 and the balance in this revenue account is now $50.

Returning to the general journal, on September 2, 1981, it was recorded that a service was delivered to Mary Smith. As a result of this transaction, the accounts receivable account increased by $70. It was also noted that patient revenues increased by $70. Accounts receivable is an asset and therefore has a 100 number. If you skip down to the general ledger account numbered 120, it is accounts receivable. There it was recorded that accounts receivable increases by $70, giving a balance of $70. However, by only looking at the accounts receivable balance, it is not known who owes the organization $70. Therefore, this transaction was also recorded in a subsidiary ledger to show that it was Mary Smith who owed $70 from the transaction recorded on September 2 in the general ledger page 1. Returning to the second part of the transaction in the general journal of September 2, 1981, besides noting the transaction here, general ledger account number 410, patient revenues was also increased by $70. This brings the balance to $120 in that account. This is because $50 was in the account from money previously earned from delivering service to John Jones. On September 3, 1981, Mary Smith paid $30 of the $70 she owed. Therefore, cash is increased by $30 in the journal, and this is also noted in the general ledger account 110. This transaction brings the balance in the cash amount to $80. Similarly, in the general journal it is shown that Mary Smith owes $30 less by subtracting $30 from accounts receivable. This transaction is also noted in the general ledger, which keeps track of specific accounts. By going to account number 120, accounts receivable, the account is decreased by $30 on September 3, 1981. The balance of money owed is now $40. To show that Mary Smith owes $30 less, the subsidiary ledger account for Mary Smith is decreased by $30. The balance she owes is now $40.

The procedures just described provide the fundamentals for establishing recording controls over transactions. With thousands of patient accounts processed a year, it should be fairly easy to see why many health providers are now automating their accounting systems. It can be expected within the next five to ten years that almost all health care providers will have their accounting records kept by computer. A major advantage of this is that the financial reports which are discussed below can be developed very quickly by using a computer. As well, many of the errors that occur in recording and transcribing numbers can be avoided when computers are used.

One final accounting control that it is important to mention here is a body of rules developed by accountants to assure that all business entities use the same general conventions. These rules are referred to as Generally Accepted Accounting Principles (GAAP). Businesses can turn to the GAAP to find out how to record or summarize transactions where questions exist. A professional body called the Financial Accounting Standards Board (FASB) is in charge of defining GAAP. The FASB is continually expanding and refining GAAP, and issues new opinions throughout the year (Keiso and Weygand, 1977).

It is interesting to note that various industries, such as hospitals and certain governmental entities, are allowed to develop specific accounting conventions when it can be illustrated that there are unusual circumstances regarding the accounting for the industry. A good example is that GAAP suggests that accrual accounting should be used. As we discussed in Chapter 4, accrual accounting states that revenues shall be recognized when earned and expenses recognized when incurred. Many governmental providers, however, are required to record their transactions on a modified accrual basis which is more conservative, and recognizes revenues only when cash is received. The reason they are able to deviate from the GAAP is that government entities have established modified accrual accounting as being more appropriate for their major responsibility, which includes stewardship of assets and budgetary compliance.

We have discussed how the accounting system controls provide standard ways of recording transactions so that financial information can be recorded. Similar input controls have to be developed to describe the services to which financial information is attached. For instance, it is not only important for health care providers to know about the revenues and expenses they generate, but also to know what they have done and who they have served. Therefore, they have to develop a standardized way of recording what they do. This is accomplished through statistical system controls.

Statistical system controls involve the recording of the nonfinancial transactions of an organization. Statistical information usually focuses on patient's characteristics and services delivered to them. Each health care provider must be able to define clearly not only which services it provides, but also how much of each service it provides. The difficulties in doing this are probably best illustrated in the area of psychiatric services.

In psychiatric services it is difficult to differentiate among units of service provided by a psychiatrist, a psychologist, or a social worker, all of whom may have different levels of training. For instance, is a unit of service the same from a physician who is a psychiatrist as it is from a person with a master's degree in clinical social work? Similarly, a definite problem arises as to what service is being delivered. Is it a 15-minute unit, a one-hour unit, or does it have to do with the content of the counseling session? A similar question arises in individual versus group counseling. Is a unit of individual counseling the same as a unit of group counseling? If not, what is the relationship between the two? Such questions are not just pertinent to psychiatric services but are also raised in such areas as vocational rehabilitation, occupational therapy, radiology, and so on.

These and similar questions must be carefully addressed in developing a statistical system. Otherwise, it is very likely that when reports are generated, they will not be as useful as possible. An important information control is a well-designed, user-oriented system. This requires a clear understanding of the organization. The system should be adapted to the organization, as opposed to having the organization adapt to the information system. Such systems should be designed so that they are adaptable to change and can accommodate the interests of various decision makers. The design of such systems should attempt to minimize costs while maximizing utility.

REPORTING CONTROLS

The general controls just discussed are designed to see that the organization has the foundation so that its efforts are carried out as efficiently, effectively, and economically as possible and ensure the accuracy of its accounting records. However, even though these general controls are in place, this is no guarantee that the organization will perform as expected. For people to judge how the organization is performing, reporting controls have been developed. Two major types of reports will be discussed here: external reports and internal reports (Table 11-3). Before getting into the specifics of either of these types of reports, it should be noted that there are certain characteristics of reports themselves which are important: that is, any report should be timely, clear, concise, precise, informative, and pertinent to the decision to be made. Of course, to comply with each of these characteristics costs money and the organization has to carefully weight the costs and benefits of upgrading its information system. For a small organization to put in a large computer-based interactive information system may be foolish. On the other hand, a large health care organization may well be able to function with a manual system if it is well developed. In fact, we know of one case where a large community health organization switched back to a manual system from the computer system it had installed.

External Reports

There are two major reports required of all health care providers: the balance sheet and the income statement (Keiso and Weygandt, 1977). The *balance*

TABLE 11-3 *Reporting Controls*

1. Report characteristics
2. Types of reports
   a. External
      1. Financial position (B/S)
      2. Operation (I/S)
      3. Other
   b. Internal
      1. Cost
      2. Variance
      3. Other

sheet describes the financial position of the health care organization by listing its assets, liabilities, and capital accounts at the end of the financial period (Table 11-4). These numbers come from the accounting books discussed earlier in this chapter. For example, the amount listed for cash, $12,869, is the balance that would be listed in the general ledger account, cash as of December 31, 1981. Similarly, the amount of accounts receivable is the balance that would be listed in accounts receivable, in the general ledger, as of December 31, 1981. The balance sheet gives a snapshot of the financial position of the organization at a point in time.

The *income statement,* on the other hand, describes the results of the operations of the health care provider for the previous year (Table 11-5). Where the balance sheet was a snapshot showing the financial position of the organization at a *point* in time, the income statement shows the results of its operations over a *period* of time. The income statement lists the revenues and expenses of the health care organization.

Just as with the balance sheet, the information on the income statement also comes from general ledger accounts. For instance, the amount in patient revenues would come from the balance of account patient services revenue, as of December 31, 1981.

The information on the income statement and balance sheet is used by creditors and investors to judge how well the health care organization is managed. For example, one may want to look at the current liabilities in

TABLE 11-4 *Statement of Financial Position (Balance Sheet)*

MGP

Pro forma statement of financial position, December 31, 19xx

Assets			
Current			
Cash		$12,869	
Accounts receivable	$40,252		
Less allowance for DA	6,186	34,066	
Merchandise inventory		14,760	
Total current assets			$61,695
Noncurrent			
Fixed assets	23,500		
(Less accumulated depreciation)	6,000		17,500
Total assets			$79,195
Equities			
Accounts payable	1,837		$ 1,837
Fund balance			$ 79,195

TABLE 11-5 *Income Statement*

	MGP		
Pro forma income statement for the quarter ending December 31, 19xx			
Revenues and support			
Staffing grant		$ 37,500	
Patient revenues			
On account	$96,025	116,460	
Cash	20,435		
Total revenues and support			$153,960
Expenses			
Salaries and benefits		$ 61,451	
Cost of goods used		15,020	
Laundry		300	
Maintenance		600	
Doubtful accounts		6,186	
Day care		4,575	
Rent		1,200	
Depreciation		6,000	
Telephone		405	
Travel		520	
Total expenses			$ 96,257
Excess of revenues over expenses			$ 57,703

relation to current assets to find out how likely it is that the organization will be able to pay off its debts that mature in the near future. Similarly, other outside parties may want to look at the relationship between the amount in the capital account and the amount of liabilities to see how *leveraged* the organization is, that is, the extent to which the provider has a high ratio of debts to equity. The higher this ratio, the less outside parties would want to invest any more money.

In addition to these two financial statements, there are various other financial statements that may be required of health care organizations. These include a statement of changes in financial position, a statement of changes in fund balance, and a statement of sources of revenue. Each of these statements reports different information to various users.

Since external reports are required of health care organizations to be used by board members, community creditors, and investors, it is important that they fairly represent the financial position and results of operations of the organization. To verify that this is so, health care organizations are usually required by their funding bodies to be *audited* each year. In fact, the major purpose of an audit is not to detect fraud, as many people errone-ously think, but to verify that the financial statements fairly represent the organization according to GAAP. The auditor is liable for discovering fraud only where it could reasonably be expected to be uncovered in the course of an audit.

There are many types of accountants, including governmental accoun-tants, cost accountants, managerial accountants, and tax accountants. They may or may not be CPAs. The difference between accountants who are certified public accountants and those who are not is that CPAs have been certified by their respective states to have sufficient experience, knowledge, and skill to be called certified public accountants. All states have laws which say that only CPAs may conduct certified audits. This is not to say that non-certified accountants are not experts in their own areas of interests.

Internal Reporting Controls

There are two major types of internal financial reporting controls: those that deal with costs and those that deal with variance analyses. Those that deal with costs usually deal with two aspects of cost: total cost and unit cost. As noted before, the accounting system keeps track of the cost of the delivery of services and the statistical system keeps track of the units of service. This information is put together to determine the cost per unit of a service. For instance, hospitals commonly use the cost per patient day to measure their inpatient costs, whereas they use costs per procedure, such as a shot, x-ray, or laboratory test, to measure their ancillary and outpatient services. As straightforward as this might sound, in the health care profession this is a very difficult task to accomplish. Systems developed to account for these costs are usually done by persons with considerable training in cost account-ing, managerial accounting, or information systems.

Cost determination is important because costs are used in planning, pricing (i.e., services, products, or disciplines), purchasing, controlling, motivating, and reimbursement. The first step in cost determination is to identify the *cost pool* (Figure 11-6). The cost pool contains all costs that are to be included in any total cost or cost per unit calculations. The second step is to identify those costs in the cost pool which can be directly associ-ated with any particular procedure. For instance, we may know which pharmaceutical costs or nursing time were devoted to various inpatient services. To the extent that we can identify labor and materials associated with any particular service, these should be assigned directly to that service.

However, there are numerous material, labor, and overhead costs which are difficult to assign to a particular service. For example, the chief ad-ministrator and administrator's staff, the rent that is paid for all buildings, laundry, and telephone expenses, may be quite difficult to apportion to a particular operation. However, to define the full cost of the service, it is important to distribute these indirect costs among the services that were provided. This process is called *cost allocation* (Berman and Weeks, 1979).

Cost allocation begins by identifying a reasonable basis for allocating indirect costs and then proceeds with the actual allocation of these costs. For example, the total cost of telephones may be distributed to the various departments delivering services in a relation to the relative number of phones a department has. For instance, if a department has one-tenth of the telephones of the organization, it would be allocated one-tenth of the telephone bills. Electrical bills may be distributed by square feet of space attributable to each department, and so on. It should be noted that for determining costs for reimbursement, and for most other purposes, one cannot switch the basis upon which indirect expenses are allocated from year to year.

Once the direct and indirect costs have been attributed to a department or to a service, the only thing that remains is to divide the costs by the units of service to develop a cost per unit of service.

Although all health providers go through these same general steps to determine their costs, there remains a major difficulty in comparing costs among providers. This is because each step has some flexibility as to how it is carried out. It is because of this noncomparability of costs that various states and members of the federal government are attempting to develop uniform accounting and reporting systems. These systems would allow providers in various health care delivery sectors to be compared. There is considerable feeling both for and against uniform accounting and reporting systems. This can be expected to be a major point of dialogue over the next decade. At the present time, hospitals are in the forefront of developing uniform accounting and reporting systems, largely because of initial efforts of third parties to get comparable data for reimbursement purposes.

The final type of internal reporting control is *variance analysis*. Variance analyses look at the variance between actual results and budgeted results to see how close an organization comes to its targets (Table 11-6).

There are several types of variances that can be calculated. Variances can be determined for labor, supplies, and for overhead. The main types have to do with the amount of an item that is used or served, called a *volume* or *efficiency* variance, and the amount paid for an item, called a *rate* or *price* variance. Such information made available on a timely basis can help managers ask questions why variances exist. For instance, when it is found that labor costs are too high, administrators may want to ask questions about the morale or turnover in nursing to see why additional nurses have to be hired in the first place.

It can be seen that the installation of general controls and reporting controls are extremely important for protecting the assets of the organization, ensuring its efficiency and effectiveness, and guaranteeing the accuracy of its financial records. These control procedures should be an integral part of all health care organizations.

TABLE 11-6 *Budget Variances*

MGP				
Budget variances, December 31, 19xx				
Urinalysis	Budgeted	Actual	Difference	
Variable				
Preprinted forms	$ 450	$ 290	$ 160	F
Glassware breakage	300	250	50	F
Supplies	570	400	170	F
Reagents	690	450	240	F
Subtotal	$ 2,010	$ 1,390	$ 620	F
Fixed				
Administration	$ 5,500	$ 5,500	0	—
Maintenance, etc.	7,200	7,200	0	—
Depreciation	3,180	3,180	0	—
Salaries	11,120	10,000	$1,120	F
Subtotal	27,000	25,880	1,120	F
Total	$29,010	$27,270	$1,740	F

F, favorable variance; U, unfavorable variance.

CASE 1

Linen Inventory

Donald Stern was happy with his administrative internship at Good Samaritan Hospital. As part of his rotation, he was assigned to each department for a period of up to two weeks. After his first week in laundry, he and Mr. Thomas White, the new manager of the laundry, had a chance to sit down over coffee and discuss the operations of the laundry. One of Mr. White's major concerns was the total amount of money the hospital had spent for linens over the last three years. Mr. White indicated that according to his records, the hospital should be very well supplied with linens, yet he could not account for all the linen inventory. Mr. Stern indicated that in his previous rotation with the nursing department, he became aware that the nurses kept a considerable amount of linen inventory on the floor. At Stern's suggestion, he and Mr. White went up to the nursing station to look over the situation.

At the first nursing station they visited, they asked the head nurse how much linen was on the floor. She opened up a series of cabinets that were piled high from floor to ceiling with linens. Mr. White then asked the head nurse if there were any other linens on the floor and she directed them to one of the patient rooms. A dresser was opened and was seen to be stocked full of linens.

Wondering how widespread the practice of "stockpiling" linens was in the hospital,

Mr. White and Mr. Stern decided to visit the other nursing stations. Apparently, the word of their visit had traveled quickly throughout the hospital, so that by the time Mr. Stern and Mr. White arrived on each floor, they found nurses moving about the floor quickly with arms full of linens. After discussing the matter with the administrator, Mr. Stern and Mr. White obtained carts and gathered up the excess linen, moving it back to the laundry. Unfortunately, they were so overburdened with excess linen that they had to purchase extra shelving to take care of the overage. In investigating the matter further, they found that although the hospital rule was to have four changes of linens for each bed, there were more than 20 changes of linen per floor. In fact, it was found that there was so much excess linen that some linen that was six years old have never been used.

That evening while walking home, Mr. White passed the home of a surgical resident and noticed a towel with the hospital insignia on it hanging on his clothesline. He asked the resident why he had the towel and the resident replied by noting that "everybody" takes the linens home. Mr. White said, "what do you mean?" The resident responded: "Well, the operating room supervisor lives across the street and look at her clothesline." They went across the street and discovered a clothesline full of hospital linens.

Upon returning to the hospital, the administrator was informed of the matter. Subsequent investigation revealed that a number of nurses were taking linens and selling them in the community and keeping the profits. Other staff were taking linens home for their own use.

Discussion Questions

1. *How does this case illustrate internal control?*

2. *What should have been done to prevent this problem from occurring in the first place?*

3. *What would you do to correct this problem? Why?*

CASE 2

Disappearing Food

As an administrative intern at Good Samaritan Hospital, Herb O'Malley was assigned to each department. This involved not only working in housekeeping, nursing, and the various medical departments, but in the dietary department as well. Although he was very tired from an evening of partying the night before, Mr. O'Malley showed up at 7:00 A.M. in the dietary department to aid Sister Teresa, who had been with the hospital for over 50 years. As he arrived, he saw something he did not expect. There was Sister Teresa handing out packages of food to individuals in a long line of cars. When Herb O'Malley inquired from Sister Teresa what she was doing, she answered "fulfilling the mission of the church." Later that day Mr. O'Malley had a meeting with the Mother Superior of the hospital and discussed with her what had happened that morning. The Mother Superior indicated that it certainly was an unusual circumstance, and that it may very well explain why the hospital had such a high food bill. She suggested that she and Mr. O'Malley visit the kitchen early the next morning.

At 7:00 in the morning, Mother Superior and Mr. O'Malley arrived in the kitchen and witnessed Sister Teresa handing out packages again. They noticed that some of the cars were chauffeur-driven. After the activity ceased, Mother Superior and Mr. O'Malley had a conversation with Sister Teresa. During this discussion, Sister Teresa indicated that, since they belonged to a charitable order, it was the duty of the nuns to see that all the needy received food. Sister Teresa stated that she was helping to fulfill that mission. When asked how often she handed out food, Sister Teresa said "every day." When asked who she gave the food to, she said, "to whoever comes." Apparently, that even included board members of the hospital. In trying to put a halt to the matter, the Mother Superior experienced some difficulty—even considerable animosity from various members of the board.

Discussion Questions

1. *Discuss the general concept of internal control as it relates to organizational dynamics.*

2. *What should have been done to prevent this problem from occurring in the first place?*

3. *What would you have done if you were the Mother Superior? Why?*

FURTHER READING

HERKIMER, A. G., Jr. *Understanding Hospital Financial Management.* Germantown, Md.: Aspen Systems Corp., 1978.

HORNGREN, C. T. *Introduction to Management Accounting,* 4th ed. Englewood Cliffs, N.J.: Prentice-Hall, 1978.

VRACIU, R. A. "Programming, Budgeting and Control in Health Care Organizations: The State of the Art." *Health Services Research* 14(2) (Summer 1979):126–144.

12

Legal Aspects of Control

A lawyer with a long exposure to business as general counsel and later chairman of the Federal Trade Commission wrote this about the challenge of being a chief executive officer:

> In our time businessmen must learn to live with paradox; a complex economy generates demands upon time and energy that often conflict, demands that often seem unanswerable. Not the least of the modern paradoxes is the demand that the senior executive somehow be a generalist in an age of rampant specialization. . . . [A] senior manager . . . must be "THE MAN," capable of exercising competent judgment in situations where a host of special considerations intersect. [Kintner, 1973]

He goes on to discuss the need for a senior executive to know enough law to be aware of its powers and limitations and to know when and how to seek the advice of a specialist in the law.

> No reasonable man can expect the business generalist to develop a close, detailed knowledge of all the disciplines that may impinge upon the area of final corporate decision, but the generalist must be able to recognize the special considerations inherent in a given business operation at an early stage, to know which specialists to call upon, to evaluate properly the recommendations of the specialist, and to formulate plans that give due allowance to all applicable special considerations. . . . Of all the special disciplines affecting business plans, none is more pervasive than the law. . . .

These words are equally applicable to health service administrators. The necessity for broad-based competency is increasingly apparent as health services become more complex and interdependent.

The objective of this chapter is to consider selected aspects of the law and legal process that affect control in health services organizations. Emphasis is given to understanding how the law both constrains and assists managers. Law and legal process are underlying elements and an appreciation of their use and application is necessary for the successful management of health service organizations.

WHY EVERY HEALTH SERVICES ADMINISTRATOR SHOULD KNOW SOMETHING ABOUT LAW: AN ILLUSTRATION

To test the proposition that legal issues are pervasive throughout the organization, consider the experience of Phil Farkas, chief executive officer of Community Hospital, a 250-bed nonprofit general hospital.

Mr. Farkas arrives at his desk at 7:30 on Monday morning to discover that a sheriff is waiting with a subpoena for him to appear at 10:00 the next morning as a witness in a civil trial. The sheriff informs him that the suit involves a counterclaim that a patient has made against a nearby hospital for failure to furnish free care under federal "Hill-Burton" regulations after the hospital had billed the patient for a past-due account. The patient wants Mr. Farkas to testify about the free-care policies in use at Community to compare against the nearby hospital.

Mr. Farkas is interrupted by a phone call from an anonymous caller asking him to come to the employee cafeteria to resolve an argument between a hospital security guard and an unidentified nonemployee who is attempting to hand out union organizing literature. On his way to the cafeteria, Mr. Farkas notices that the corridor in the pediatrics ward is dangerously littered with ladders, toolboxes, and electrical cables belonging to the electrical contractor who is installing new lighting fixtures in the corridor and patients' rooms.

Mr. Farkas's beeper goes off and he picks up a phone to learn that the power is off in the operating room and the emergency generator has not yet started. He recalls that his chief maintenance man has been ill for the past week and, during that week, the emergency generator was scheduled to be tested. He is told that there are two major operations in progress and that the surgeons are using flashlights and manual equipment but that the condition of the two patients is unknown. Before he finishes the conversation, he is told that the generators have been started after a delay of nine minutes.

As he hangs up, an emergency room nurse urgently motions him toward the emergency room and tells him that a semidelerious patient with a bad gunshot wound has been brought in by taxi. He refuses to give permission to treat his open wound or to call the police. While this is happening, a hospital employee from the physical therapy department was sent by Mr. Farkas's secretary to find him but trips over a pile of dirty sheets, suffering an apparent compound fracture of her right arm (she is subsequently unable to return to work in physical therapy because the bones do not heal properly).

Mr. Farkas hurries back to his office to meet the chief of the medical staff, who informs him that the pathologist, on exclusive contract with the hospital, has arrived in the lab in an obviously drunken condition. The chief wants him, as the agent of the board of trustees, to approve the immediate suspension of the pathologist for a 24-hour period. Mr. Farkas replies that he's probably high on drugs as well. A newspaper reporter who had been waiting makes a few notes and slips out the side door. Mr. Farkas works at his desk for a while, signing certificates of completion of training for the hospital's medical technologist program graduates, and reviewing a proposal to extend insurance coverage to volunteers working in the hospital.

He also dictates a letter to the state health planning agency, requesting an appeal of the denied certificate of need application for the wing conversion. The chairman of the hospital board of trustees phones and suggests that the quarterly meeting of the board be again canceled (for the second quarter in a row) because of his business travel schedule; he also suggests that the hospital put campaign literature in the lobby for another board member who is running for city council. As he hangs up the phone, the in-basket on Mr. Farkas's desk spills over and he picks up an item his secretary has marked "Urgent." It is a memo from the director of the dietary department saying that she has filled the vacant supervisor's position with an experienced female from another hospital, but that one of Community Hospital's male cooks, who had wanted the job, has filed an employment discrimination charge with the Equal Employment Opportunity Commission. His secretary has added a note on the memo that the dietary director hired her own cousin.

Mr. Farkas barely makes the 1:00 meeting with the medical records director and one of the new surgery residents who wants to talk about revising the hospital's consent form, an "I consent to anything" type which has not changed in ten years. Mr. Farkas knows that the chief of the medical staff does not want to change it, but that the consent form and protocol was one of the several factors that caused the current one-year JCAH provisional accreditation. The surgery resident mentions during the meeting that there is an 18-year-old football player who was brought in about a week ago with a broken leg and that he has heard that the nurses are complaining about the treatment the boy is receiving from his family doctor. The resident mentions that the nurses suspect that gangrene has already set in. The medical records director said that the football coach had come in this morning and asked for a copy of the boy's medical record, which she gave him.

The phone rings and a distraught mother blurts out that illegal abortions are being performed in Community Hospital, including one on her 15-year-old daughter last week which she just learned about today. She says that she is not going to pay for it and intends to report the incident to the district attorney.

Mr. Farkas's secretary interrupts to inform him that an OSHA inspector is waiting outside to conduct a surprise inspection of all the clinical and dietary areas of the hospital. He wants to see the incident report file and to check the equipment maintenance logs.

Mr. Farkas decides that the day is not going well.

Out of a feeling of desperation he picks up the phone and calls the hospital attorney, who promises to come as quickly as possible. He tells Mr. Farkas to make four columns on a sheet of paper headed, *Event, Legal Issue, Additional Facts Needed,* and *Worst Possible Legal Results* (Table 12-1). He then advises his client to attempt to analyze the legal implications of each of the events of today. Mr. Farkas does so, completing his task just as the attorney knocks on the door. He looks over Mr. Farkas's work and congratulates him on identifying most of the legal issues and some of their implications, commenting that he must have had a course in health law during his formal education in becoming a hospital director. Mr. Farkas smiles and replies that it was Benjamin Disraeli who said: "The more extensive a man's knowledge of what has been done, the greater will be his power of knowing what to do." Nevertheless, the attorney points out some of the missing pieces in the analysis and rejoins with Alexander Pope's words: "A little learning is a dangerous thing." At that the two settle down to a serious attorney–client discussion of the problems and how to begin to deal with them. Table 12-2 lists the suggested steps the hospital attorney advises in approaching each of the problems.

An exaggerated story? Perhaps, but all those events could happen over a period of time in the operation of a typical health services facility. How these problems are handled by the administrator is critical to the effectiveness of

TABLE 12-1 *Community Hospital Case*

Event	Legal Issues	Additional Facts Needed	Worst Possible Legal Results
Subpoena	Obey or not?	Acceptable excuses	Contempt of court
Free-care policies	In compliance with federal regulations?	Current requirements of regulations	Exposure to possible administrative action by federal agency
Union literature	Can distribution of campaign literature be prohibited?	Hospital policies about solicitation	Unfair labor practice charge
Dangerous corridor	Who would be liable?	Contract with electrician	Hospital liable for any injuries
Emergency generator	Negligence?	Extent of patients' injuries	Major lawsuit for deaths or brain damage
Gunshot wound	Treat without authorization? Report wound to police?	Determination of patient's competence; statutory requirements for reporting violent wounds	Lawsuit by patient; statutory penalties; bad publicity
Employee accident	Does workers' compensation apply?	Coverage of workers' compensation statute and hospital insurance policies	Statutory liability in excess of insurance coverage
Drunk pathologist	Authority to suspend summarily?	Confirmation of incapacity to perform; provisions of medical staff bylaws	Liability for wrongful suspension; reinstatement
Appeal of certificate of need	Appeal justified?	Criteria and procedures for appeal	Denial sustained
Board meeting cancellation	Violation of corporate bylaws, state laws, or fiduciary responsibilities	Provisions of bylaws; state's nonprofit corporation statutes	Class action lawsuit by patients or creditors for negligent management
Campaign literature in lobby	Violation of hospital's solicitation policy? Validity of policy?	Provisions of policy; state or city political campaign regulations	Prescribed penalties; invalidation or non-enforceability
Hiring relative for dietary position	Discriminatory employee relations practice?	EEO regulations; requirements of job and qualifications of applicants	EEO complaint investigation; required replacement
News reporter	Defamation?	News story printed? Confirmation of pathologist's condition	Liability for libel or slander
Certificates for medical technologists	Valid certification?	Verification of each graduate's successful completion	Invalid credentials; accreditation questions

320

TABLE 12-1 *Community Hospital Case (cont.)*

Event	Legal Issues	Additional Facts Needed	Worst Possible Legal Results
Insurance for volunteers	Jeopardize status of volunteers?	Other benefits provided to volunteer; type of insurance (liability, health, workers' compensation)	Volunteers be deemed employees and subjected to tax liability
Consent form	Legal sufficiency of consent form?	Hospital protocol for informing patients and inserting in record; state statute; state case law	Unauthorized treatment charges; liability for damages
JCAH accreditation	Legal effect of JCAH accreditation?	Other reasons for provisional accreditation; JCAH criteria for consent	Loss of accreditation; loss of reimbursement
Gangrene in patient	Negligence by doctor? nurse? Corporate negligence?	Referral/consultation policies of hospital	Negligence charges; liability for damages
Copy of medical records to coach	Breach of confidentiality?	Patient's authorization?	Invasion of privacy charges; liability for damages
Abortion	Is abortion on 15-yr. permissible?	Mental competency of patient; state law	No payment; criminal charges
OSHA inspection	Can inspection visit be refused?	Inspector's credentials; OSHA regulations	Search warrant presented

managerial control. The administrator must therefore know something about law.

FAMILIARITY WITH THE LAW

A basic understanding of law by managers requires familiarity with the different types of laws: constitutions, statutes, judicial opinions, and administrative regulations.

Constitutions

Constitutions are documents that set out the organization and powers of the government and the fundamental rights and relationships between governments and the citizenry. The validity of all legislation and regulations is measured against either federal or state constitutional standards, or both,

TABLE 12-2 *Community Hospital Case*

Event	Lawyer's Advice
Subpoena	Notify court immediately of intention to comply; present excuse of lack of fair notice for failure to appear when scheduled.
Free-care policies	Make current hospital practices conform to current federal regulations; seek federal agency advice.
Union literature	Review hospital solicitation policies to ensure that permissible and impermissible purposes are stated clearly, fairly, and consistently; union literature can be banned only if most other solicitation is also banned.
Dangerous corridor	Require independent contractors to minimize risks of accidents and to carry adequate liability insurance coverage.
Emergency generator failure	Conduct an investigation of the cause of the emergency generator failure and take steps to prevent recurrence; offer monetary settlement for any injuries only after consulting insurance carrier.
Gunshot wound	Treat wound only if physicians determine that it is an emergency case and patient incapacitated; describe circumstances in the medical record. Report to police if statute requires it.
Employee accident	Provide medical care for employee; review insurance policies for adequate coverage under statutes.
Drunk pathologist	Revise medical staff bylaws to ensure that authorization for summary suspension includes "drunk on duty" as specific grounds.
Appeal of certificate of need	Review letter requesting appeal for compliance with state requirements.
Board meeting cancellation	Suggest rescheduling prior to end of quarter.
Campaign literature in lobby	Comply with hospital's current policy; suggest review in light of relevant laws and regulations.
Hiring relative for dietary position	Document the hiring procedures followed and the new employee's qualifications.
News reporter	Phone reporter to discuss story prior to publication.
Certificates for medical technologists	Sign them, but if suspicious, consult program director.
Insurance for volunteers	Buy liability insurance for acts of volunteers.
Consent form	Rewrite consent forms and develop new protocol in conjunction with medical staff.
JCAH accreditation	Suggest consultation on deficiencies relating to legal concerns.
Gangrene in patient	File incident report and notify insurance company.
Copy of medical records to coach	Request coach to return records.
Abortion	Explain state law to administrator.
OSHA Inspection	Allow the inspection, accompanied by hospital employee.

322

depending on the issue. For example, workers in state hospitals or county health departments may challenge the application of federal wage and hour requirements on the basis that the U.S. Constitution protects state and local governments from undue intrusion by Congress. In fact, in a 1976 case, *National League of Cities* v. *Usery,* 426 U.S. 833, the U.S. Supreme Court ruled that the federal Wage and Hour Act was inapplicable to state and local government employees because federal–state relations were guided by the Ninth and Tenth Amendments to the Constitution, preserving some degree of state sovereignty over matters "essential to its separate and independent existence."

Statutes

Federal statutes on health are based on the power of Congress to spend tax money for the general welfare and to regulate any activities that affect interstate commerce. An example of funding legislation is the Medicare and Medicaid program. The extensive restrictions on controlled substances (narcotics and dangerous drugs) are an example of the interstate commerce regulation. On the other hand, state governments have the authority and responsibility to promote and preserve the public health, safety, and welfare. Therefore, state legislation on health is extensive in the areas of environmental health, public health, mental health, and the licensing of health facilities and occupations.

Judicial Opinions

Judicial opinions are rulings by federal and state courts which both decide the issue being litigated between the two or more parties in the lawsuit and set a "precedent" or a guide for predicting the outcomes of future similar lawsuits. In the health arena, lawsuits run the gamut from torts and contracts to antitrust and mental commitment (see Table 12-3 for definitions). The amount of litigation affecting health services administration has increased dramatically over the last fifteen years, primarily in the area of medical malpractice, employer–employee relations, and entitlement to health program benefits. The courts have developed "case law" precedent in a number of important areas, such as abortion rights, blood transfusions liability, and "free-care" benefits for the poor. Sometimes litigation narrows or broadens existing legislation; other times it substitutes for the absence of legislation or regulations; still more often it engenders amendments to legislation or even the passage of new laws.

Regulations

Regulations have the same force and effect as laws and can be enforced by an agency through judicial as well as administrative avenues. Health regula-

TABLE 12-3 *Legal Causes of Action*

Battery: Any unlawful beating, wrongful physical violence or constraint, or even a nonviolent touching of another human being without consent or authorization. Performing medical procedures on a patient without his or her consent is a form of battery. Battery is both a criminal and a civil offense.

Breach of contract: The failure, without legal excuse, to perform a contract. A contract is a promissory agreement between two or more persons that creates, modifies, or destroys a legal relationship; or, more simply, an agreement, upon sufficient consideration, to do or not to do a particular thing.

Conversion: Any unauthorized act that deprives an owner of his or her property permanently or for an indefinite time.

Embezzlement: The fraudulent appropriation to one's own use or benefit of property or money entrusted to one by another.

Extortion: Obtaining money or property by means of fear, threat, or coercion.

Fraud: A generic term that embraces all the multifarious means that can be devised by human ingenuity and resorted to by one individual to gain an advantage over another by false suggestions or by suppression of the truth.

Invasion of privacy: An encroachment on the right of privacy or the right to be "left alone" to live in seclusion without being subjected to unwarranted or undesired intrusion. Commonly arises when a patient's medical records are revealed to unauthorized persons.

Libel: Any falsehood that is written or printed and published and that injures the character of another by bringing him or her into ridicule, disgrace, or contempt.

Malpractice: The form of negligence that occurs when a professional, in treating or caring for a patient or client, does not conduct himself or herself with due care or reasonable skill. Sometimes means professional misconduct, generally.

Negligence: The failure to do something that a reasonable person guided by the considerations that ordinarily regulate the conduct of human affairs would do, or doing something that a prudent and reasonable person would not do. Negligence is not a fixed standard but must be determined in each case by reference to the situation and knowledge of the parties and the attendant circumstances.

Nuisance: A legal wrong that arises from the unreasonable, unwarranted, or unlawful use by a person of his or her own property or from his or her own improper or unlawful personal conduct, which causes an obstruction of the rights of another person or of the public or which produces a material annoyance, inconvenience, discomfort, or harm to others.

Slander: Any falsehood that is spoken and calculated to injure the reputation of another.

Tort: A legal wrong committed upon the person or property of another for which the law gives a civil remedy, usually money damages for the resulting injury. Common torts are negligence, assault, battery, false imprisonment, libel, slander, and invasion of privacy.

tions at the federal level are directed at a multitude of objectives but basically are designed to carry out congressional intent as expressed in legislation. Examples of federal regulations affecting health facilities and programs include a wide diversity of topics: Medicare and Medicaid, health planning, human experimentation, occupational health and safety, employment discrimination, food and drugs, medical devices, air and water pollution, radioactive wastes, controlled substances, peer review, collective bargaining, and health education. At the state level, regulations implementing state legislation also cover a broad range, from facility licensure to preschool immunization.

FINDING THE LAW

It is also useful to know something about the form of legal material.

Constitutions are found in the same sets or volumes where statutes are collected.

Statutes are codified, arranged according to subject matter, in sets of volumes or codes that are periodically updated to reflect recent changes. Statutes are also available in a form indexed in the chronological order of their enactment.

Judicial opinions or rulings ("case law") are much harder to locate, but are published in a variety of sets, called "reporters," arranged by state, region, or jurisdiction of the court, and are in chronological order. Since one is generally concerned with the subject matter of an opinion, there are techniques for locating cases utilizing various published indices and the case summaries and headnotes that are found preceding most judicial rulings. This is a relatively difficult area to attempt and exceedingly difficult to master.

Regulations are also published according to subject matter and in chronological order of their enactment. At the federal level they are relatively easy to find; some state governments are inefficient in making regulations available in a timely fashion and, sometimes, making them available to the public at all.

Upon first glance at legal material, it must appear that the legal profession is extraordinarily preoccupied with references and cross-references, to the point where legal literature is particularly cumbersome to read. Actually, the vast amount of material encompassed by years of lawmaking necessitates this phenomenon. A basic introduction to legal references and citations is most useful for health services administrators in both understanding and locating the law.

INTERPRETING LEGAL CITATIONS

Although statutes can be referred to, and therefore located, by their title (e.g., the Administrative Procedures Act or the Social Security Act), they are most often cited by the section and volume of their code. In the case of the Administrative Procedures Act, that would be properly cited as 5 U.S.C. 1000, meaning volume 5 of the *United States Code* at section 1000. For state statutes, the citation is basically the same, although state statutory citations often refer to a section or chapter or title within the state code (e.g., N.Y. Gen. Bus. Law 352, meaning New York General Business Law, section 352). Statutes can also be cited by reference to the number and year of their enactment (e.g., the National Health Planning and Resource Development Act of 1974 is officially P.L. 93-641, the 641st public law passed by the

93rd Congress). Each statute is later placed in the code, where it is indexed by subject matter and more easily found. The section reference in the *U.S. Code* for P.L. 93–641 is 42 U.S.C. 1543–1568.

Regulations are cited in a similar fashion. All federal regulations are published in the *Federal Register,* a weekly publication of federal government notices and regulations, but codified in the *Code of Federal Regulations* by their volume and section number (e.g., 42 C.F.R. 22542).

Judicial opinions or rulings are more uniform in their citations. They will almost always be cited by their page and volume number in the applicable reporter service. For example, 182 U.S. 427 (1901) is a United States Supreme Court case decided in 1901 that appears on page 427 of volume 182 of the *United States Reports.* As another example, 459 F.2d 6 (1st Cir. 1972) is a 1972 case, decided in the U.S. First Circuit Court of Appeals, that can be found on page 6 of volume 459 of the *Federal Reports,* second series.

About the only real difficulty with case citations is understanding the rather complicated system of abbreviations that has developed over the years. One also has to be aware of the fact that most judicial opinions are published in more than one reporter and each case has several citations.

Anyone can find the law from a citation, provided that the citation has been transcribed exactly. It is helpful to know, however, that most public law libraries have reference librarians to assist in the interpretation of citations—a service used quite frequently by lawyers as well as the public.

Why should a health services administrator know about these legal materials? Familiarity with legal citations and references is necessary for the modern manager to keep up with legal and regulatory developments in the correspondence and literature that cross his or her desk. It is essential in discussing problems with attorneys and understanding their advice. As illustrated in the Community Hospital story, some of daily administrative happenings in a health organization may lead to a lawsuit against you or others in the institution, or against the institution itself.

What happens in a lawsuit? For a health services administrator to be prepared to play the proper role in the litigation that may arise, he or she must know something about legal process.

ADMINISTRATOR'S GUIDE TO THE LEGAL PROCESS

The term *litigation* refers to a lawsuit. A lawsuit generally begins by the complaining party (the plaintiff) filing a document, generally called a *complaint.* In the complaint, the *plaintiff* asks for certain relief from the party against whom the plaintiff is complaining. For example, a patient who is unhappy with the treatment received in a hospital and the "excessive bill" may consult an attorney for advice about filing a lawsuit. If the attorney is satisfied that there are reasonable grounds for doing so, he or she will prepare the complaint, listing the allegations against the defendant physicians, hospital, and hospital employees and describing the injuries and damages caused by them. The complaint will state the relief sought by the patient in the form of an amount of money calculated to compensate for the extra medical expenses borne by the patient, other financial losses (such as loss of earning power, in the case of a resultant disability), and "pain and suffering" (a subjective determination of the patient's personal damages).

The party complained against is generally called the *defendant*, although he or she may also be known as the respondent.

Each state has rules governing the *jurisdiction* of the state and local system. These must be carefully observed to avoid summary dismissal of a suit. For example, there may be three different levels of trial courts (such as a magistrate, a district court, and a superior court), each of which accepts different type of suits. Also, each type of action may force other considerations, such as a different statute of limitations which limits the time period during which a lawsuit may be filed.

Under certain circumstances a plaintiff may be eligible to file in either a state court or a federal court. Although there may be procedural advantages in filing in federal court, the right to do so is limited. The plaintiff could file in federal court if interpretation of a federal statute is involved or if there is diversity of citizenship (i.e., the parties are from different states) and the amount in controversy is $10,000 or more.

The complaint is filed together with a *summons,* and a U.S. marshal (in federal courts) or the sheriff (in state courts) serves the summons and a copy of the complaint on all named defendants. Service of the summons on the defendant gives the court jurisdiction over the defendant. The summons advises the defendant that a lawsuit is pending and further advises the defendant what he or she must do and within what time limits.

If the defendant is served with a summons and does nothing, the court, having obtained jurisdiction over the defendant by service of the summons, may enter *judgments* on a default basis against the defendant based upon the uncontested testimony of the plaintiff. An administrator who ignores a summons and allows a default judgment against his or her institution or agency may have difficulty defending this negligence to his or her superiors.

The defendant will normally retain an attorney and file an "appearance," which is a document that prevents a default judgment from being filed. The defendant will then file a response to the various allegations in the complaint. This response is generally called an *answer.* The answer will either admit or deny each of the allegations in the complaint. At the same time, the defendant may also choose to file a cause of action or *cross-complaint* against the plaintiff. In this case the defendant may also be designated as "counter-plaintiff" and the initial plaintiff may now be also designated as "counter-defendant."

In the example, the hospital may choose to deny that the patient was given improper treatment and also countersue for the unpaid hospital bill.

If the defendant raises new affirmative matters not referred to in the plaintiff's complaint, the plaintiff will generally file a *reply*. When all allegations of various pleadings have been responded to and the case is ready to move forward, the parties are said to be "at issue."

At that point, *discovery* procedures are used by both sides to obtain information, including depositions and interrogatories to question witnesses in advance of the trial.

A *deposition* is a proceeding whereby a party to the lawsuit (plaintiff or defendant) or other witness is compelled to give testimony, under oath, normally in an attorney's office based upon oral questioning. *Interrogatories* refer to questions in writing which must be answered by the other party in writing.

In the example, the plaintiff may seek to depose the physicians, the hospital administrator, the medical records director, and selected nurses to obtain valuable information that will affect how the case will proceed.

Very often the defendant's first court filing, or pleading, will not be an answer but will be some form of *motion*, such as a motion to dismiss the complaint. Such a motion, in effect, says that even if it is accepted that what the plaintiff says is true, the plaintiff does not state a cause of action for which the court can grant relief. Other motions include a challenge to the court's jurisdiction, a request for change of venue (place of trial), and so on. Motions must be responded to and the court may request briefs from both sides before ruling on the motion.

In the example, the hospital may file a motion to dismiss, since merely being "unhappy with the treatment" is not a "cause of action," or legitimate basis for a lawsuit. If the motions are denied, the trial proceeds.

Parties to litigation may be seeking either money *damages* or something other than money. That something other is in the nature of "equitable relief." Thus a party may be asking the court to declare a statute unconstitutional or to enter an injunction to prevent enforcement of the statute.

Once the trial judge makes a decision, either party may, as a matter of right, *appeal* to the appellate court. The appellate court does not re-try the case. It receives excerpts of testimony and legal arguments of counsel in the form of appellate briefs. The rulings of the appellate court are written in a form that serves as precedent, so that both an explanation of the reasons and a specific holding are provided.

In the example, if the judge dismissed the patient's suit as not constituting a cause of action, the plaintiff would appeal the decision to the appellate court, which would review the decisions of other courts on similar issues and would refer to any applicable statutes. The court would then decide to uphold the judge's dismissal or reverse the decision and remand the case for further proceedings. The case would go back to the judge and the trial would continue, unless the parties decided to *settle* the case.

This is a very general description of the usual process of litigation. The process can be time-consuming, and there are often numerous and lengthy depositions and literally volumes of documentary proof and information. A great deal of litigation and numerous appeals stem from alleged errors made by the parties or the judges in the process itself, rather than disagreements about the substance of the questions or issues involved in the litigation.

A health services administrator may find himself or herself intimately involved in every aspect of litigation. Knowing the sequence of the process stages enables a competent administrator to be more effective in working with the attorney for the institution or agency.

In addition, administrators are increasingly being called as witnesses in litigation. They will be more effective and professional if they know both the purposes of the litigation and the various steps involved.

THE HEALTH SERVICES ADMINISTRATOR AS AN EXPERT WITNESS IN LITIGATION

As a professional person, a health services administrator may from time to time be called upon to testify in court as to standards of quality of administration, in either his own or some other institution, agency, or other organization.

The expertise of a health services administrator as a witness in a trial or hearing will largely depend upon his or her education, experience, and recognition by colleagues in the field of health services administration. For example, he or she may be called upon to bear witness to the extent of the legal duty that is owed by a hospital, health department, or planning agency and its administrator and agents to the patient, to the employees, to the community, to the news media, to the visitors, and to people with whom the organization does business. In such a case the administrator will usually be asked to testify about the soundness of certain organizational procedures.

In this situation, the administrator is attesting to the degree of control and lack of control in the organization. In a sense it is a test of accountability, just as demanding as an audit or a report to a governing body. The testimony of a health services administrator may have a profound influence on litigation involving his own or another institution or agency.

Darling v. Charleston Community Memorial Hospital: An Illustration

One situation where the testimony of an expert hospital administrator had some influence on the outcome of the litigation was the celebrated case of *Darling* v. *Charleston*

Community Memorial Hospital, 211 N.E. 2nd 253 (1965), which made new law concerning hospital responsibility for the acts of physicians practicing on its premises. The case involved the loss of a lower leg by amputation about 6 inches below the knee, following the development of gangrene resulting from application of a constricting plaster cast and the cutting of the patient's leg in removing the cast. The plaintiff, Dorance Darling, a 17-year-old high school student, claimed that the Charleston Hospital personnel assisted in performing these acts which caused injury to him, that the hospital permitted an unqualified doctor to perform these acts, and that the hospital's nursing staff and administrator failed to take steps to procure competent assistance when trouble was apparent.

In attempting to defend itself, the hospital asked another hospital's administrator to testify at the trial as to what generally accepted practices were routinely followed at similar hospitals. This information would be useful to the jury, hopefully, in deciding that the Charleston Hospital did not fall below the recognized standard of care legally required in such cases. Thus a qualified hospital administrator, Anthony J. Perry, M.S.H.A., F.A.C.H.A., administrator of the Decatur and Macon Hospital in Decatur, Illinois, about 50 miles away from Charleston, was called as an expert witness by the defending hospital. The witness, during direct examination by Mr. Horsly, the hospital's attorney, gave his approval to Charleston Hospital's facilities and procedures.

The witness was then *cross-examined* by Mr. Appleman, the attorney for the plaintiff, Dorance Darling.

Q. Mr. Perry, you stated you took courses at a number of institutions to qualify you to serve as hospital administrator. Is that right?

A. No, this is not correct. I was qualified by virtue of my attendance at Northwestern University.

Q. What textbooks did you study at Northwestern in that field?

A. All of the textbooks described by the university that were necessary for an Associate Master's Degree of Hospital Administration.

Q. What where they?

A. There was Dr. MacEachern's book [*Ed. note:* Malcolm T. MacEachern, M.D., *Hospital Organization and Management,* 3rd ed., Physicians Record Co., 1956]. He was considered to be one of the outstanding authorities in this field; and I studied under him.

Q. Did you consider him as one of the leading authorities in the country in the field of hospital administration?

A. Yes.

Q. Do you have the current edition of that work in your library, Mr. Perry?

A. Yes.

Q. And do you use it in the performance of the duties of hospital administration which you perform?

A. When we feel we must refer to a text.

Q. In other words, you do regard this as an authoritative work forming a part of your background of knowledge in this field?

A. It is one of the recognized texts in the field.

Q. Recognized by you, as well as by others, sir?

A. I would say that, yes.

[Portion of the proceedings omitted.]

Q. Now, was there a Code of Ethics adopted jointly by the American Hospital Association and the American College of Hospital Administrators to direct the conduct of the hospital administration?

A. I am not familiar with what you are referring to, sir.

Q. Well, if you will look in the book right there in front of you on page 1055, I think you will find it. Do you find it there?

A. "Hospital Code of Ethics." Yes.

Q. Were you not given a copy of that to be framed and placed on your wall when you became a Fellow of the American College?

A. Yes.

Q. So you have seen it before today?

A. Yes, I did not know what you were referring to.

Q. If I may borrow that [book] just a moment. With reference to Paragraph 3, does it not state as follows? You may read it with me if you like. "The medical staff should be properly organized. Only qualified doctors of medicine, legally licensed to practice in the state, or surgeons, should be admitted to membership." Then, skipping to Paragraph 4, does it not state as follows: "It is the responsibility of the medical staff and of the governing board of the hospital to safeguard the interest of the public so that no member of the medical staff or other practitioner shall be permitted to undertake any procedure for which he is not fully competent. Reluctance

to interfere, pecuniary gain, must never be permitted to jeopardize the welfare of the patient or reputation of the hospital. For the protection of the patient in all serious or doubtful cases, there should be adequate consultation." Do I read it correctly, sir?

A. Yes.

Q. And, again, going on with this Code of Ethics, does it not provide in Paragraph 12, as follows: "It is the responsibility of all who have anything whatsoever to do with the care of the patient to make every effort to insure that all patients receive the best possible care with minimum delay, with the utmost of skill and efficiency, and with the greatest personal consideration and tenderness." You recall that, do you not?

A. That is correct.

Q. And, in Paragraph 21, in speaking of the administrator, does it not say this: "The relationship of the administrator to the medical staff should be one of sympathetic understanding and helpful cooperation. The administrator should endeavor to have medical problems adjusted by the medical staff or its committees as necessity demands. However, the administrator, as a representative of the Board of Trustees, must act with decision and with firmness consistent with the welfare of the patients and the continued good reputation of the hospital." Does it not so state?

A. Yes.

Q. You subscribe to those views, do you not?

A. As far as administration practices are concerned.

Q. That is what all these paragraphs are talking about.

A. Administration practices, yes; but not medical.

Q. Do you think that I am not referring to medical care, sir, of patients?

A. No. I am qualified to make a statement of the administrator's responsibility.

Q. Are you seeking to divorce your responsibility as a hospital administrator from the medical care of the patient?

A. No, I am not. However, neither the hospital nor the administrator is licensed to practice medicine.

Q. Do you feel that you don't have a duty to the patient because of the low quality of medical care given to the patients within the hospital?

[Defense attorney objected and the plaintiff's attorney withdrew the question.]

[Portion of the proceedings omitted.]

Q. However, you, as hospital administrator with some years of experience, would have some knowledge of what goes on in a hospital, would you not, sir?

A. Administratively, yes.

Q. And, as such an administrator, you rather keep a watchful eye out for problem cases?

A. Not problem medical cases.

Q. Let me give you a hypothetical question, now, Mr. Perry. Assume that an 18-year-old boy sustained a broken tibia fibula in the right leg, which fractures are closed but comminuted; that the wound is extensively trauma-tized, with soft tissue swelling having commenced; that such patient is brought to the hospital emergency room, at which time the only member of the medical staff on emergency duty is a general practitioner who graduated from medical school in 1927; that such person is not the family physician; that no adult member of the boy's family is present. Now, Mr. Perry, would you permit that general practitioner to perform a closed reduction of those fractures and apply a plaster cast without notifying the parents of the boy?

A. Yes, if he was a legal member of the medical staff and his name had been placed on the list of approved physicians to be called in the case of an emergency, and he was aware of the fact that consent had not been obtained.

Q. Assume, further, Mr. Perry, that this general practitioner does not shave or sterilize the patient's leg; and that within three hours of the injury he applied an unpadded plaster cast directly to the broken leg; that within two hours of the application of the cast, the toes are swollen; that within seven hours of the cast application the toes are very edematous; that the toes continue very swollen and within less than 24 hours of the cast application there are blisters on the feet; that within 36 hours of the cast application the foot is very edmatous and dark. Now, Mr. Perry, would you by this time ask the head of the medical-surgical staff to look in?

A. I would not necessarily do it. These are observations that would be made and referred to the attending physician and it is his responsibility to seek consultation if he feels it is necessary.

Q. And you, Mr. Perry, as hospital administrator—

A. I am not qualified as a physician and I would not be qualified to evaluate the management of that case.

Q. Let's continue, Mr. Perry. Let's assume that, all during this period of time, there have been persistent complaints of pain by the injured boy, for which he has been given Demerol, Carbitol, and other pain medications; that such complaints of pain continue until, on the fourth day of his admission, he receives eleven separate administrations of pain medicines; that, on the second day of his admission, the toes are swollen, tight, discolored, and insensitive to touch and the patient cannot move them; that 46 hours after application of the cast the nurses report that the foot is cold to the touch and slightly cyanotic. Now, Mr. Perry, would you ask the head of the medical-surgical department to look in?

A. No, I would not if the attending physician had been seeing the patient regularly and the nursing personnel had been carrying out his orders and I had no evidence or history to indicate that the physician was incompetent and should be referred to medical supervision.

Q. All right. Let's go on, Mr. Perry. Now, assume, further, that the patient continues to have pain in the injured limb although receiving pain medications; that the toes remain swollen, cold, and dark; that 24 hours after such cold condition is reported, the cast is split vertically on both sides of the leg and the patient cut in two places with a Stryker saw; that the following morning the nurses report bright blood on the cast and the pillows, and blisters on the leg which had been in the cast; that just after midnight further bleeding is reported; that there is a pussy discharge or drainage from blisters on the leg into the sides and bottom of the cast; that the patient is reported as crying with pain; that a foul stench is detected in the area of the leg that of rotting flesh. Now, Mr. Perry, would you ask the head of the medical department or surgical department or a qualified staff orthopedist to look in on the case?

A. I would say probably not, because I am not qualified to evaluate the importance of those symptoms.

Q. So, if we understand it, sir, even if this patient should die in the hospital, you would not ask a doctor, other than the attending physician, to look in on the case?

A. At some stage of the game there is a medical staff regulation.

Q. Just answer, sir, as to what you would do. Would you or would you not have another doctor look in on the case?

A. I would say no, unless it was recommended to me.

Q. That's all.

[The expert witness was then questioned on *redirect examination* by Mr. Horsly, the attorney for the defending hospital.]

Q. Now Mr. Perry, you may state whether complaints of pain are or are not commonplace by patient in hospitals.

A. Yes, they are commonplace.

Q. You may state, please, whether, when complaints of pain are made, you ask a doctor other than the treating physician to look in.

A. No, we generally do not.

Q. You may state whether odors, some of them objectionable, in hospital rooms are commonplace in a hospital.

A. Very definitely.

Q. And state, please, whether the presence of foul odors in a room would or would not move you to ask a doctor to look in or take over.

A. Definitely not.

Q. You may state, please, whether blood on a cast or on a pillow may or may not be a common thing in hospital experience or medical treatment.

A. It is common experience.

Q. You may state, please, whether the fact that there is blood on a pillow or on a cast, or otherwise, would or would not move you to tell another doctor to go in and take over or look over the situation.

A. I would not if the attending physician was seeing the patient regularly.

Q. And now I ask you to assume, Mr. Perry, that the attending physician does see the patient regularly, at least twice or three times or more each day during hospitalization, and that the attending physician is a staff member; that he has been from the beginning; that he has been licensed to practice in Illinois for thirty-four years—or for thirty-two years at the time of this occurrence. In what, if any, way would those things affect your decision about what you as hospital administrator, would do.

A. I would construe this to mean that if he has been a successful and capable practitioner this many years, I would assume he was competent and capable of managing his own case, unless he is violating some rule of the hospital.

Q. And, in the hypothetical question asked by plaintiff's attorney, you may state, please, whether you could not see any violation of any rules of the hypothetical hospital.

A. I do not see any violation of the rules.

Q. Mr. Perry, Mr. Appleman [attorney for plaintiff] read you several things from Dr. MacEachern, particularly including the duty of the board to eliminate unethical, unqualified, and unworthy physicians. What is meant by those terms?

[Portion of the proceedings omitted.]

A. My interpretation would be that he would not be qualified to practice medicine in the eyes of the law and that he was unsafe in his practice.

[After an exchange of conversation about the accreditation requirements for hospitals, the expert witness was questioned again on re-cross examination by Mr. Appleman (attorney for plaintiff).]

Q. Mr. Perry, just to be sure we understand you, your position, all of us—the court, jury, and I—

A. Yes, sir.

Q. It is your feeling that, if a man is licensed by the State of Illinois to practice medicine, it is not your province, as hospital administrator, to interfere with what he does? Is that right?

A. No, this is not right. If he is licensed to practice by the State of Illinois and his credentials have been properly reviewed by the committee of the medical staff and they have recommended to the board of directors that he is competent to practice medicine—

[Portion of the proceedings omitted.]

Q. Let me get it very specific. If a man is on the staff of this hypothetical hospital and he is a general practitioner and he undertakes to do open-heart surgery, would you, as hospital administrator, stop him?

A. Generally the—

Q. Just "yes" or "no." Would you or would you not?

[Objection by defense counsel.]

Judge: He may answer "yes" or "no," if he can; and if he can't, he may say so.

Q. You can answer that.

A. I cannot answer "yes" or "no."

[Portion of the proceedings omitted.]

Q. Mr. Perry, just in case we might have misunderstood you. Do we understand from you that it is commonplace in hospitals, where broken legs are placed in casts, to have blood on the cast, blood on the pillow, a foul odor in the room, the foot to be dark, toes to be tight and insensitive to touch, and continuing complaints of pain? Is that commonplace in your opinion?

A. I would not say commonplace. However, I am not qualified to judge the course of events.

Q. That wouldn't scare you?

[Defense objection to the word "scare" sustained by the judge.]

Q. Would those conditions, occurring together, induce you to ask for a consultation?

A. Not necessarily. It may induce me to check to see whether the physician is seeing the patient regularly and is aware of this condition.

Q. And if you found out from your examination that the doctor was seeing the patient regularly and the condition kept getting worse, wouldn't you, as hospital administrator, begin to wonder what kind of doctor—

[Defense objection to the word "wonder" sustained by the judge.]

Q. Would you do anything about it?

A. I said what I would do about it. I would check.

Q. Just check with the doctor and that's all?

A. I would check with my personnel, the nursing personnel, to see if the physician was seeing the patient regularly as required by the medical staff and the hospital.

Q. But, if he was seeing the patient regularly and the complaints kept getting worse, you as hospital administrator would do nothing about it?

A. If I was convinced that the attending physician was a qualified man who had been practicing successfully in the community for a number of years, I would probably not do anything about it.

Q. Assume that the odors kept getting worse, the complaints of pain kept getting worse; you would not go beyond talking to that man, the attending physician?

A. Probably not.

Q. Do you still have this Code of Ethics hanging on your wall?

[The judge sustained the objection of defense counsel to this question.]

Q. You feel you are bound by that, don't you, sir?

[The judge ordered witness to answer the question over the objection of defense counsel.]

A. They are a guide.

Mr. Appleman: That's all.

Lessons from the Darling Case

This skillful series of questions to the administrator by both the plaintiff's attorney and the defense attorney demonstrates the interaction between the actual hospital practices followed by administrators and the ultimate legal requirement of adhering to an *acceptable minimum standard* of care and practice. The law generally recognizes as acceptable legal standards those statements of ethical and desirable practice put forth by persons and organizations representing the profession, in this case the hospital administrator. The plaintiff's attorney in the Darling trial was trying to show the applicable standards by quoting from textbooks, codes of ethics, licensing laws, and other printed material. The hospital administrator serving as a witness, assisted by the defense attorney, was trying to show that in actual practice the standards should not be applied too strictly.

The outcome in the Darling case was dramatic. The court decided that the administrator and nursing staff of Charleston Hospital had fallen below acceptable legal and professional standards in failing to provide minimum hospital services and care for the patient and in not taking steps to initiate a consultation or to review the negligent physician. The physician in this case had already admitted negligence and had settled with the plaintiff out of court for his part of the responsibility.

The new law created by this case has sometimes been described as "corporate liability," meaning that an institution can be held *independently liable* for its own negligence in not providing a system of safe practices suggested by the textbook teachings and "customs of the industry." Thus, if specific administrative processes and policies are described in texts and teachings or are used in customary practices, an administrator who ignores them can cause his or her institution or agency to be found liable for those same errors. Although not all states follow the Darling rule, the trend is clearly in that direction. Suffice to observe, then, that administrators must know the generally recognized good administrative practices and follow them.

Whether the administrator is merely an expert witness whose role is to describe those practices, as Mr. Perry attempted to do, or the defendant whose practices are being questioned, the Darling case is clearly instructive. Litigation is a part of the environment in which health services management functions and students of management can gain valuable insights by examining cases like *Darling.*

RISK MANAGEMENT

One of the lessons from the increase in medical malpractice cases during the past several years has been a new attention to loss prevention and risk management in health institutions and agencies. Although there is a distinction between the two concepts, both are important in addressing malpractice issues. *Loss control* is essentially the cost-efficient settlement of a claim once made and *risk management* refers to the minimization of the chance of claims being made at all. Loss control has become a major program of some insurance companies through the development of claims investigation procedures which emphasize prompt gathering of essential information about a claim or potential claim so that favorable disposition can be made when possible. It includes requiring organizations to operate an internal reporting system and responding to such reports with appropriate legal, engineering, statistical, and managerial expertise. The decision to settle a claim or to defend it in court can best be made when the insurer has a complete and contemporary record of the accident that led to the assertion of a claim by a patient of the insured institution or agency. This record is made for every accident, error, or unusual incident that could lead to legal liability. The record is usually called an "incident report."

Incident Reports

The principal purposes and functions of a prompt reporting system for all accidents and incidents are as follows:

1. To provide a permanent record of the incident.
2. To assist in refreshing the memory of the parties involved.
3. To alert the risk manager of a possible claim situation for subsequent investigation.
4. To allow for a timely investigation.
5. To provide a statistical base for incident patterns from which preventive recommendations can be made.

All unusual incidents qualify, including situations where a slightly unfavorable result follows the performance of a standard procedure. No segment of the hospital's staff is excluded from this responsibility. Insurers attempt to make it the duty of everyone to participate conscientiously in the prompt reporting of acts or omissions and general complaints. The theory is that anything that could result in serious patient dissatisfaction might precipitate formal legal action against the hospital, physicians, and staff.

Risk Management Protocol

A typical hospital risk management protocol might require these steps following the recognition of an accident:

1. The person witnessing, or involved with, the incident promptly describes it on an incident report form, notifies the physician, and secures a medical report from the physician.

2. The physician responsible for the patient provides appropriate care for the patient and then makes a diligent preliminary investigation and completes the medical report portion of the form or dictates an oral report.

3. The incident report that has been forwarded to the risk manager is then reviewed for:

   a. Cause
   b. Severity
   c. Present condition of the injured party.
   d. Pertinent x-ray findings, if applicable; and so on.

4. Should additional medical information be required, the responsible physician will be notified by the risk manager.

5. The risk manager then creates a file on the incident which includes the following:

   a. File creation sheet
   b. Copy of patient's medical record
   c. Reserve computation worksheet
   d. Claims committee review form

6. Based upon this information, the risk manager or the claims committee will immediately evaluate the need for further investigation, patient/relative contact, possible settlement, or other disposition effort, and notify the insurance carrier.

7. The incident will then be incorporated in the monthly summary for the purpose of developing monthly and year-to-date statistical trends.

8. The risk manager will appropriately communicate to the administrators any pertinent information that could dictate corrective measures.

9. The report and all attendant investigative material is maintained in a pending file for periodic review until the matter is considered re-

solved. This file is kept in the risk manager's office as part of the confidential records of the hospital's attorney.

Confidentiality of Reports

One of the important legal issues not resolved across the country is the degree of confidentiality of incident reports. Since it may be the first written statement for a potentially litigable event, the question of whether a plaintiff's lawyer has a right to obtain a copy is very important. Despite the apparently common practice of overlooking this source of useful information, some lawyers have sought copies, been refused by hospital administration, and brought suit to compel release.

Generally, any document relevant to a lawsuit can be sought by either party unless the document is privileged. The most common privileges are communications between physicians and patients and between attorneys and clients. The latter privilege includes the concept that a lawyer's "work product" in connection with preparation of a lawsuit is confidential and not discoverable. The question in regard to incident reports is obvious: was the report prepared for the purpose of assisting the hospital's attorney in defending against a lawsuit?

The few courts that have considered the question have arrived at different conclusions. One state supreme court in 1978 found that the incident report was not privileged and was therefore discoverable because it had not been prepared by the hospital attorney and was used primarily by hospital administration. In another state the incident report was held to be privileged since it was prepared for the insurer to be used by the insurer's attorney. Still another state court found privilege on the ground that the reports were prepared by the hospital at the direction of the insurer and the hospital did not retain a copy.

The cases on this issue seem to be decided on the individual facts and the state's privilege statutes.

Willis argues that public policy should favor maintaining the confidentiality of incident reports. He asserts:

> With increasing medical and hospital litigation and rising medical care costs, courts may well view with tolerance the argument that the interest of the public is served by allowing hospital administrators and medical staffs to analyze and review the quality of the health care provided by their institutions without fear of having their internal administrative reports used against them in court. [Willis, 1979]

This argument is buttressed by the recent adoption in most states of statutes that provide confidentiality of the records of peer review committees.

Some hospitals have already taken the practical step of having incident reports prepared at the request of the hospital attorney, given only limited circulation, and stored in a file marked "confidential." This special handling of the reports promotes a management-wide trust that they will be used in the legal defense of the hospital rather than offensively by a patient's attorney.

Quality Control

Quality control has achieved new priority since 1975 as one response to the malpractice problem. Commercial insurers have at long last taken an interest in it by giving increased attention to incident reports, sending engineer and nurse teams to insured hospitals to advise on risk management, and providing more useful literature on claims experience. Perhaps the publicity given to malpractice has challenged the managerial instincts of hospital administrators, producing a more receptive market for risk management programs.

A system developed in California focuses on 18 events which usually indicate that there has been a serious threat to patient safety. For example, if a patient has an operation repeated, his or her record is automatically scrutinized. Effective risk management programs use incident reports as a management tool to monitor problem areas. Other related programs include quality control, personnel indoctrination, safety and hazard checks, human engineering (e.g., providing appropriate hygienic clothing), and management information systems.

It may also be that the creation of doctor- and hospital-owned insurance companies has made an impact on risk management and quality control. Nationwide, 1022 hospitals now belong to one of the 40 mostly offshore insurance companies set up since 1975, and about 1500 other hospitals insure themselves. Self-insurance has naturally promoted loss awareness.

Quality control through risk management has now become the responsibility of administrators in every type of health organization. Moreover, this phenomenon reinforces the necessity for mastery of effective control techniques and strategies at all organizational levels.

CONTRACT LAW IN HEALTH SERVICES

Central to any relationship between an institution or person rendering a service and a person receiving it is a binding tie, known in the law as a contract. The contract may be either explicit or implicit, and it can exist even when the parties do not realize the full legal import of their relationship. It commonly exists between persons doing business together: employer and employee, landlord and tenant, hospital and doctor, health agency and patient, and doctor and patient. Every health organization is a party to numerous contracts, most of which affect the exercise of control by managers.

There is a common notion that contracts are legal documents, necessarily written down on paper, and containing the signatures of the persons involved and of duly present witnesses, together with whereases, herewiths, some heretofores, and a proviso or two. Additionally, it is assumed that there is an exchange of money and a handshake. This type of neat protocol is not generally the rule, however useful it may be in dramatizing a contractual transaction.

Many of a health organization's contracts are ordinary business contracts, often contained only in memoranda or telephone messages relating to supplies and services or controlling its fiscal affairs. Some are less obvious and not even found in written form. For example, the relationship between provider of health services and a patient is in fact a contractual one, although none of the formalities just described may have occurred. A close look at the patient-provider relationship reveals some insight on contract law.

Initial Agreement

A contract is an agreement between parties to do or refrain from doing a certain act. A person who decides that he needs medical attention brings himself to a health institution or medical person and presents his symptoms. If the patient is not rejected, the practitioner takes some action, either providing assurance or prescribing treatment, or both. The person, now a patient, accepts the practitioner's decision and responds to his or her actions. The symptoms and causes are dealt with and the patient is satisfied. A bill for services is sent and the patient pays it. The practitioner is now satisfied. The contract is completed. But what are the problems for a health service administrator? Most contractual controversies center around misunderstandings and unfulfilled expectations.

Defining Expectations

Before any contractual relationship is established, it becomes critical to delineate the terms. Nothing causes more contractual confusion than mistaken expectations by either or both parties. There must be a "meeting of the minds" as to exactly what the contract is about in order for it to be valid. This is true for business contracts and also for patient care relationships. Although most health institutions and agencies do not think in terms of a contractual undertaking with their patients, the proposed terms of a contract are contained in the explanations of the need for tests, the nature of the diagnosis, the therapeutic options, the prognosis, and the estimated cost. By allowing the patient to raise questions and express concerns, the provider can bring about the needed "meeting of the minds." Open communication in the provider–patient initial encounter facilitates a clearer contractual relationship, just as it does in arms length business negotiations.

Unfortunately, many valid and enforceable contracts result in dissatisfied parties. Although there may have been an overall understanding, some of the details of the agreement or process of giving care may not have been fully articulated. These provide the subjects for business contract arbitration and litigation as well as, perhaps, the cause of patient noncooperation during diagnosis, poor response during treatment, bad manners during a dispute, and allegation of breach of contract, which may take the form of a malpractice suit.

In summary, business contracts form the basis for much of the daily grist in the administrative mill and an experienced health services administrator will have garnered a considerable quantity of contract law through on-the-job training. For example, administrators quickly learn the five generally accepted requirements of a valid contract: offer and acceptance, competent parties, valid legal purpose, evidence of "consideration" or something of value being exchanged, and acceptable legal form for the agreement. It is, however, beyond the scope of this chapter to present a short course on contract law, while still respecting its importance for exercising managerial control in most health care settings.

THE CONCEPT OF INFORMED CONSENT

Even apart from contract law, the law provides a prophylactic against unfulfilled expectations and unhappy sequelae in health services transactions. It is sometimes called "informed consent" but is better described as valid patient authorization for care. When the matter of lack of consent is introduced in a lawsuit against a provider, it is legally characterized as an element of tort liability rather than as a breach of contract. But the two are clearly related in origin, both being based on patient dissatisfaction. In fact, the legal principle here is that a patient has the right to say what may or may not be done to his body. If another person proceeds to touch a person without his consent, he has committed battery. In the health care setting this touching generally takes the form of the invasion of a scalpel, a medication, a hand, or some other instrument into or onto a patient's body without his having expected it. Thus when a patient is told either nothing or too little about what treatment he will be receiving, he or she may later make an allegation of technical battery. This is possible even if there was not resultant pain or harm to the patient. An essential element of a successful tort claim, however, is the demonstration of some damage. In a suit for a technical battery without more than inconvenience or surprise as the damage claim, the probability of an ultimate victory by the patient is slim, although technically a court could give a nominal monetary judgment based on "principle."

On the other hand, it is serious business when a mistake is made on a patient who has not understood or truly agreed to the procedure performed by a practitioner. Even if the mistake was a medical accident not attributable to the negligence of the practitioner or institution, and therefore not grounds for a malpractice suit, the patient can still bring a successful tort suit and claim all the damages directly resulting from unauthorized treatment. When a patient couples allegations of unauthorized treatment together with negligent care resulting in considerable immediate and long-term damage, the defendant provider is clearly in an uncomfortable position.

A number of questions are presented by the doctrine of informed consent: Who can authorize treatment? What is the legal age for consent? What does the doctrine say about patients who are unconscious, delirious, confused, or incompetent? Must the authorization be in writing? If so, what should the document say? Should there be witnesses to the signing? Are there certain treatments that need the concurrence of the patient's spouse or a consulting physician? How much should be told the patient about the alternative modes of treatment that are medically feasible? Who chooses the mode—the physician, because of his or her superior knowledge of the situation, or the patient, because he or she ultimately has the responsibility for his or her own body? How about the risk—should the patient be told about a 50% risk? A 1% risk? "Negligible risk"? What if the patient refuses to listen to the explanation and simply gives the provider carte blanche? What is the role of the administrator in all of this?

Much to the consternation of physicians and administrators, the answer to questions about informed consent cannot be set out in a simple, precise, and universal fashion. Only the general principles can be stated and reference made to relevant cases in which the principles have been applied. The next step, applying the principles effectively in the doctor–patient relationship, is a mutual responsibility of the doctor and patient, but the doctor must take the lead on many occasions and the administrator should facilitate the process.

Rules of Informed Consent

An administrator with responsibility for any patient services should know these rules of law relating to informed consent.

1. Every person has the right to do with his or her body what he or she chooses; otherwise, the constitutional right of privacy is violated.

2. A person must authorize, or consent to, the touching of his or her

body by another person; otherwise, this touching may in law be assault and battery.

3. A person may manifest consent by words, action, or operation of law in emergencies and other special situations.

4. Consent does not have to be in writing, but a consent or authorization document is worthwhile preservable evidence.

5. Other records of expressed consent may include a notation in the medical record, a recorded telephone call, and a note written by the provider at the time of the event, in addition to the memory of the provider or the remembered observation of a witness.

6. Implied consent may be given nonverbally by a patient in any number of ways: appearance at the clinic or office seeking treatment of an obvious medical condition, cooperation during the administration of tests and treatment, failure to object when a course of action is undertaken, or passivity in a situation in which consent could readily be refused.

7. Authorization for treatment is provided by operation of law in several instances:

   a. In a medical emergency, when there is insufficient time to obtain the consent of the patient in order to save his life or treat a serious condition.

   b. When the patient is unconscious or otherwise unable to consent for himself (because of confusion, mental or physical incompetency or incapacity, legal incompetency by being under 18 years of age, or inability to speak the language), and there is no spouse or next of kin reasonably available to consent on his or her behalf, and his condition would deteriorate substantially lacking immediate attention.

   c. Upon issue of a court order regarding a patient whose case has been filed with the court on the basis of parental neglect, parental religious objection, or parental absence.

   d. In compliance with specific statutory duties, such as examination for venereal disease, tuberculosis, or other communicable disease, examination of prisoners or mental patients, and immunization of children. (However, a parent or guardian can still object vigorously even to such mandatory treatment and may challenge the mandatory treatment or immunization statutes on constitutional grounds.)

8. To give informed consent, the patient must be apprised of his or her medical condition, the reasonably available alternative modes of treating that condition, the expected risks associated with the treat-

ment procedure (both general and those specific to that patient), the prognosis of the condition, any special or unusual factors to be involved (the use of experimental drugs or techniques, the conducting of teaching or research, the use of cameras, etc.), and the name of the person in charge of the treatment.

9. Implicit in an acceptable informed consent procedure is the opportunity for the patient to ask questions and to receive honest answers in understandable language.

This, then, is the protocol the law provides for accurately defining in advance the contractual expectations of both the patient and the practitioner. Adherence to the law of informed consent has more rewards than mere avoidance of a lawsuit. It may be useful in enhancing mutual respect between doctor and patient, or institution and patient.

CONFIDENTIALITY OF INFORMATION

One of the health services administrator's traditional dilemmas is how to handle information discovered in the process of diagnosing and treating a patient. The problem arises with medical information that would be useful or interesting from the standpoint of a present or potential employer, a health or life insurance company, banks, lending institutions, or the news media. The problem presents itself sometimes more dramatically with information not directly related to medical treatment but of special interest to a spouse, a law enforcement agency, or, again, the news media. For example, if the mayor and his girlfriend are slightly injured in an auto accident, whom should the treating physician inform? The rules of law are relatively clear, but the application is becoming increasingly difficult.

Basically, the law reinforces the tenet of the Hippocratic Oath to "keep silent thereon, counting such things to be professional secrets," and the AMA's Principles of Ethics:

> A physician may not reveal the confidences entrusted to him in the course of medical attendance, or the deficiencies he may observe in the character of patients, unless he is required to do so by law or unless it becomes necessary in order to protect the welfare of the individual or the community.

Litigation

All but 12 states recognize a "testimonial privilege" in the rules of evidence in court-related proceedings. This means that a physician must not disclose information he has learned in the course of treating a patient, unless the patient permits it. It is a rule established for the protection of the patient, not the physician or institution, so that the patient may feel free to be open and frank about his condition or history. There are numerous exceptions to the rule, such as the following:

1. Communications made to a doctor when no doctor–patient relationship exists.

2. Communications made to a doctor that are not for the purpose of diagnosis and treatment or are not necessary to the purposes of diagnosis and treatment (e.g., who inflicted the gunshot wound and why).

3. Actions involving commitment proceedings, issues as to wills, and actions on insurance policies.

4. Actions in which the patient brings his or her physical or mental condition into question (e.g., a personal injury suit for damages, an insanity defense, and a malpractice action against a doctor or hospital).

5. Reports required by state statutes (e.g., gunshot wounds, acute poisoning, child abuse, motor vehicle accidents, and, in some states, venereal disease).

6. Information given to the doctor in the presence of another not related professionally to the doctor or known by the patient (e.g., another patient).

Other Situations

This testimonial privilege is a statutory rule varying slightly from state to state but always applying only to the giving of testimony in a court action. What about the numerous other situations? There is no comprehensive federal or state statute outlining a patient's right to confidentiality and privacy, but court decisions and commentators provide guidance. A provider who reveals information that a patient does not wish to have disclosed may be subject to a civil action for damages based on one of four grounds:

1. Breach of a common law duty not to reveal confidences obtained through the doctor–patient relationship unless prompted by some supervening societal interest.

2. Invasion of a patient's constitutional right to privacy by unauthorized disclosure of initmate details of the patient's health.

3. Breach of an implied contractual obligation to keep a confidence.

4. Disclosure of false and defaming information, which constitutes libel (if written) or slander (if oral), by the provider, even if the inaccuracy is disclosed in good faith.

The difficulties in implementing these rules have been accentuated by the computerization of medical records. Nevertheless, they apply and must be respected. The role of the administrator is to establish a system in the institution or agency that will enable both outside practitioners and inside employees to follow these rules of confidentiality.

In a larger sense, the role of the administrator is to be sufficiently knowledgeable about the law of contracts and torts (as well as tax, antitrust and other special areas) and to be adequately familiar with judicial procedures and legal practices in order to carry out the level of leadership and accountability appropriate in the health organization.

EXERCISE

Testing Your Legal Knowledge

The following statements illustrate many of the points involved in any application of legal principles to problems of managerial control. Some are true and accurate statements; some are false or inaccurate. Read each statement twice and try to assess whether it is true or false. For each of the false statements, think about what change in the statement would convert it to true.

This exercise is intended to emphasize how acquired legal knowledge, together with common sense, can be applied to familiar managerial issues. It also demonstrates how mistaken impressions of legal principles can cause confusion for a manager and why counsel should be sought in complex situations such as occurred on Monday for Mr. Farkas. On any possibly important legal matter, large or small, legal counsel should be sought whenever any manager is in doubt about the appropriate response or decision.

T F 1. Hospital administrators exercise the delegated powers of the governing body of the hospital.

T F 2. In many states nursing home administrators must be licensed.

T F 3. Failure of a board to remove an incompetent administrator is a breach of the duty of due care.

T F 4. Hospital records are generally not excluded by the hearsay rule if they are prepared in a customary manner.

T F 5. Administrators will be personally liable on contracts they make on behalf of the hospital even when acting within their authority to contract.

T F 6. The duty to select members of the medical staff is legally vested in the governing board.

T F 7. Nurses who are hospital employees are not personally liable for negligent acts in the course of their duties.

T F 8. A clearly visible "slippery when wet" sign will insulate a clinic from paying claims for visitor falls on wet floors.

T F 9. A hospital must have the latest models of diagnostic equipment to avoid liability when a patient is injured by the equipment.

T F 10. The ACHA Code of Ethics has been used by courts as an indication of the standards required of an administrator.

T F 11. The medical staff has the ultimate legal responsibility for the quality of the hospital and for providing patient care.

T F 12. Hospital emergency rooms can turn away patients who are uncooperative.

T F 13. Shared service organizations will be ruled tax exempt by the IRS only if they do not compete with local commercial services.

T F 14. A public health officer may exercise either express or implied authority.

T F 15. The Darling case requires governing boards to establish mechanisms for medical staff review and consultation to avoid harm to the patient.

T F 16. Courts will generally decline to intervene in medical staff appointment matters in private hospitals.

T F 17. The most important single source of law applicable to institutional governing boards is the state incorporation statutes.

T F 18. The law of agency provides that agents will not be personally liable on contractual obligations created within the scope of their authority.

T F 19. Failure of an administrator to obtain a permit from the health department for operation of the cafeteria could result in a criminal fine against the administrator.

T F 20. Nonprofit hospitals cannot conduct profitable activities.

T F 21. Public health department records are exempt from subpoena.

T F 22. An assistant administrator of a state mental health hospital who discloses a patients' records to a news reporter may be liable to the patient and the patient's physician.

T F 23. Most community hospital governing boards are self-perpetuating community representatives.

T F 24. The net proceeds of a nonprofit institution cannot be shared by any individuals even upon corporate dissolution.

T F 25. A release form must be signed before a patient can be safely permitted to leave the hospital against medical advice.

T F 26. Unions are not permitted in nonprofit nursing homes.

T F 27. The authority of federal hospitals stems from acts of Congress and the regulations of federal agencies.

T F 28. The maker of the medical record physically owns it but the patient has a property right to know the information contained in it.

T   F   29. NLRB rulings have narrowed its exclusion of jurisdiction regarding governmental hospitals.

T   F   30. Title VII of the Civil Rights Act requires free care for all indigent patients.

T   F   31. Informed consent can be proved by entries in the medical record.

T   F   32. Medical examiners and coroners cannot order autopsies over the objections of surviving close relatives.

T   F   33. An intoxicated employee would nonetheless be eligible for workers' compensation for injuries "arising out of an accident in the course of employment."

T   F   34. Blood drawn by a physician at the request of the police but without patient consent has been held by the U.S. Supreme Court to offend the "sense of justice."

T   F   35. Hospital trustees may be held personally liable for failing to require adequate fire insurance.

T   F   36. The courts have held that the Fourteenth Amendment prohibits appointments to the staff of a public hospital based on a racially discriminatory policy.

T   F   37. A nonprofit hospital cannot waive or discount charges for patients.

T   F   38. Workers' compensation laws permit injured workers to choose whether to sue the employer for negligence or to file a claim for damages under the laws' special provisions.

T   F   39. Malpractice is a form of negligence.

T   F   40. Assault and battery is a basis in a suit for lack of consent to an immunization.

Answers:					
(1–5)	T	T	T	T	F
(6–10)	T	F	T	F	T
(11–15)	F	F	F	T	T
(16–20)	T	T	T	T	F
(21–25)	F	T	T	T	F
(26–30)	F	T	T	T	F
(31–35)	T	F	F	F	T
(36–40)	T	F	F	T	T

FURTHER READING

AMERICAN HOSPITAL ASSOCIATION. *Federal Regulation: Hospital Attorney's Desk Reference.* Chicago: American Hospital Association, 1980.

ANNAS, G. J. *The Rights of Hospital Patients, The Basic ACLU Guide to a Hospital Patient's Rights.* New York: Avon, 1975.

CORLEY, R. N, R. L Black, and O. L Reed. *The Legal Environment of Business,* 5th ed. New York: McGraw-Hill, 1981.

GRAD, F. P. *Public Health Law Manual.* Washington, D.C.: American Public Health Association, 1973.

HAYT, HAYT, and GROESCHEL. *Law of Hospital, Physician, and Patient,* 4th ed. Berwyn, Ill.: Physicians Record Co., 1972.

POZGAR, N. *Legal Aspects of Health Care Administration.* Germantown, Md.: Aspen Systems Corp., 1979.

SOUTHWICK, A. *Law of Hospital and Health Care Administration.* Ann Arbor, Mich.: Health Administration Press, 1978.

WARREN, D. G. *Problems in Hospital Law,* 3rd ed. Germantown, Md.: Aspen Systems Corp., 1978.

WARREN, D. G. *A Legal Guide for Rural Health Programs.* Cambridge, Mass.: Ballinger, 1979.

WING, K. R. *The Law and the Public's Health.* St. Louis, Mo.: C. V. Mosby, 1976.

THE ENVIRONMENT

I once asked a worker at a crematorium who had a curiously contented look on his face, what he found so satisfying about his work. He replied that what fascinated him was the way in which so much went in and so little came out. [Cochrane, 1972, p. 12]

The visual demonstration of the gap between input and output is increasingly apparent in the field of health services. Increased resources are being allocated with only a modest change in mortality and morbidity indicators. The objective of this section is to describe the basic components of the health system which are involved in the transformation of resources into health service activities and the future changes likely to affect service delivery. Chapter 13 describes the major components of the health system, characteristics of the population it is attempting to serve, and the larger social-political-economic-legal environment in which it functions.

Chapter 14 discusses the future of health services. Future trends and issues are presented as they confront the health system, the health service organization, and the health service manager.

13

The Health Services System

┌─────────────────── **OVERVIEW** ───────────────────┐

The management of health service organizations does not occur
in isolation, but in a complex arena composed of different types
of organizations involving thousands of individual actors. In addition, the arena interfaces with a larger socioeconomic, political,
and legal environment which affects the behavior of both individuals and organizations. The objective of this chapter is to describe
the basic components of the health system and explain their relationship to the larger society.

└───┘

WHAT IS THE HEALTH SYSTEM?

At first glance, the health system does not look like a system at all, but rather
a bewildering array of organizations and people going off in separate directions. In fact, the provision of health services is often termed a "nonsystem."

On closer inspection, however, this array of organizations and professionals takes on a pattern of interrelationships that do operate in a predictable
and systematic fashion. Although its efficiency and overall effectiveness is
often questioned, the pattern provides a mechanism for handling recurrent
problems that disrupt basic social functions. Children need to be born; scarce
goods and services need to be allocated; authority and power need to be
regulated; appropriate social conduct needs to be rewarded and deviant behavior needs control and punishment. Without the orderly performance of
these tasks, society as we know it would be inconceivable. Illness at its
simplest level interrupts the individual's ability to perform social roles and
interferes with the life of society. The health services system is a social in-
vention in which people arrange themselves in some orderly fashion to control and regulate the hostile world of disease, disability, and premature death
(Darsky and Metzner, n.d.).

In the United States, the development and maintenance of the health
system has taken on gigantic proportions. As seen in Figure 13-1, the approximately $244.6 billion allocated to health service activities in 1980
represents 9.5% of the gross national product (GNP). Perhaps as important
as the 1980 total is the general trend. In 1965, health expenditures totaled
$43.0 billion, representing 6.2% of the GNP. It is projected that in 1990
health expenditures will increase to $757.9 billion and represent 11.5% of
the GNP.

How are these expenditures allocated among the various health service
activities? Figure 13-2 indicates that the greatest expenditures are for hospital care, followed by physician services. Trends are equally important in this
area. For the past 50 years the proportion of expenditures for hospital care
has increased and it is expected that this increase will continue into the

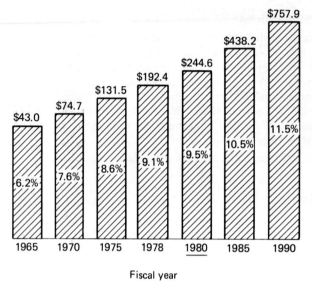

Figure 13-1 National health expenditures and percent of gross national product, selected fiscal years 1965-1990 (in billions of dollars). [R. M. Gibson, "National Health Expenditures." *Health Care Financing Review*, 1(1) (Summer 1979), 1-36. M. Freedland et al., "Projections of National Health Expenditures, 1980, 1985, and 1990." *Health Care Financing Review* (Winter 1980), 1-27.]

1980s. Similarly, the proportion of expenditures for nursing home care has been increasing and this trend is also expected to continue into the 1980s. The proportion of expenditures for drugs, physician services, dental and other professional services and other health services has shown a steady decline since 1929, and this decline is expected to continue. The largest decline is in the proportion of health expenditures allocated to other health services.

POPULATION

What are the major diseases and illnesses affecting the population? Figure 13-3 suggests that the types of problems have changed dramatically over the past 50 years. There has been a steady decline in tuberculosis, influenza, and pneumonia as the major causes of death and a steady increase in cardio-vascular disease and cancer as the primary causes of mortality.

The rates for these diseases vary by age as well as by ethnic background. Figure 13-4 provides a guide to some of the major causes of mortality for various age groups. With the exception of the 65 and older group, whites have a significantly lower mortality rate for all major causes of death.

Significant differences are also reported in the patterns of diseases that are important causes of mortality for the various age groups. Accidents represent the major problem for the age groups of 1-14 years and 15-24 years. For the age groups 25-64 and 65 years and over, heart disease, cancer, and stroke represent the major causes of death.

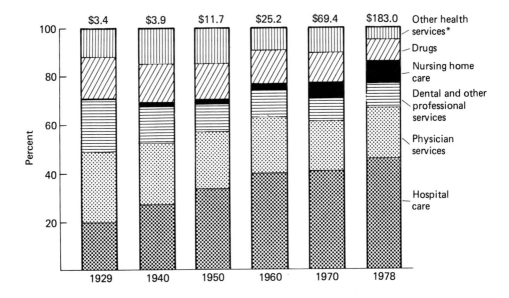

*Other health services includes: public program expenditures for health services not classified as to type of service covered; industrial inplant services; school health services; and medical activities in federal units other than hospitals.

Note: Numbers above bars are total expenditures for health services and supplies.

Data obtained from Robert M. Gibson, "National Health Expenditures, 1978," *Health Care Financing Review*, 1 (1), (Summer 1979), Table 3, 23-24.

Figure 13-2 Percent distribution of national health expenditures by type of expenditure, selected fiscal years, 1929-1978 (in billions of dollars). [Source: A. Donabedian et al., *Medical Care Chart Book,* 7th ed. (Ann Arbor, Mich.: Health Administration Press, 1980)].

COMPONENTS OF THE HEALTH SYSTEM

- How has our society chosen to deal with the problems of illness and disease?
- What are the components of the system, and what are their relationships?

A clue to understanding the components of the system and their interrelationships was outlined initially in Chapter 2. In that chapter we identified the basic components of any social system: production, maintenance,

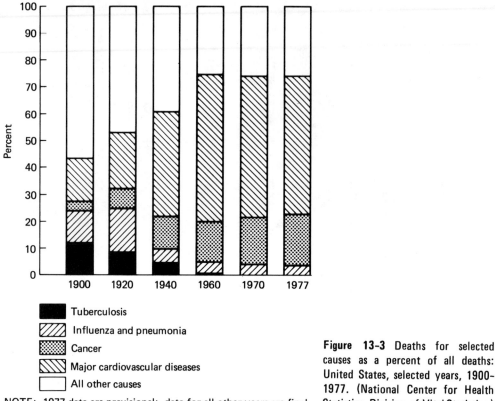

Tuberculosis

Influenza and pneumonia

Cancer

Major cardiovascular diseases

All other causes

Figure 13-3 Deaths for selected causes as a percent of all deaths: United States, selected years, 1900–1977. (National Center for Health Statistics, Division of Vital Statistics.)

NOTE: 1977 data are provisional: data for all other years are final.

adaptive, and management (Katz and Kahn, 1978). These components provide a scheme to classify the many organizations and activities in the health system:

- *Production:* organizations and activities concerned with the provision of services.
- *Maintenance:* organizations and activities concerned with training and rewarding people for their roles in the larger health system.
- *Adaptive:* organizations and activities concerned with monitoring change in the larger social system (e.g., disease patterns and expectations) and translating this information to the operation of the existing health service system.
- *Management:* organizations and activities concerned with coordinating, controlling, and directing organizations and activities associated with the other components.

Figure 13-5 presents the four components and their interrelationships as a framework for considering the many activities and organizations involved in the provision of health services. Classification of particular health service activities and organizations is based on their major contribution to the overall health system. Many organizations make contributions in more than one component. However, our task is to judge their primary contribution to the larger system.

Production Subsystem

The organization and professionals primarily concerned with the direct provision of health services are part of the production subsystem. Four major sets of activities can be identified: public health, hospitals, major professional providers (physicians, dentists, chiropractors, optometrists, and podiatrists in various practice arrangements), and self help/care groups. Below is a brief discussion of the function, structure, and financing of each activity.

Public Health

The primary objective of public health is to ensure the health of the public. As defined by the Milbank Memorial Fund Commission on Higher Education for Public Health [Sheps, 1976], it is

> the effort organized by society to protect, promote and restore the people's health. The programs, services and institutions involved emphasize the prevention of disease and health needs of the population as a whole. Public health activities change with changing technology and social values, but the goals remain the same: to reduce the amount of disease, premature death, and disease-produced discomfort and disability.

Although the best method of achieving this objective is currently under discussion, the historical focus of public health has been (1) the control of infectious agents, (2) emphasis on preventive services, and (3) the community as the primary focus of activity. Despite public health's glorious history, changes in the health care problems of the population and in the composition of the population traditionally served by public health departments have raised serious questions about future functions of public health. Some of the options are presented below.

Comprehensive Services. The American Public Health Association (APHA) has suggested that health departments should offer the following types of services contingent on the needs and demands of local communities:

1. Community health services, including communicable and chronic disease control, family health, dental health, substance abuse, accident prevention, and nutrition.

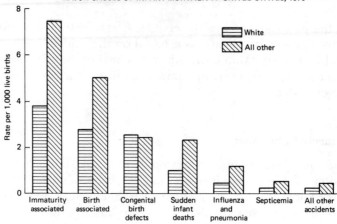

MAJOR CAUSES OF INFANT MORTALITY: UNITED STATES, 1976

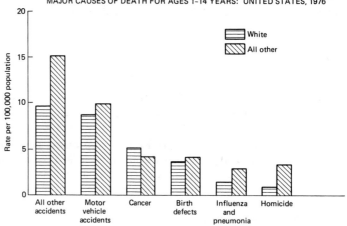

MAJOR CAUSES OF DEATH FOR AGES 1-14 YEARS: UNITED STATES, 1976

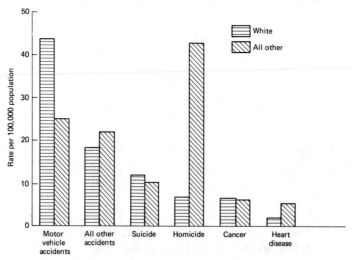

MAJOR CAUSES OF DEATH FOR AGES 15-24 YEARS: UNITED STATES, 1976

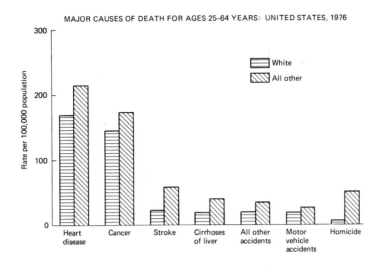

MAJOR CAUSES OF DEATH FOR AGES 25-64 YEARS: UNITED STATES, 1976

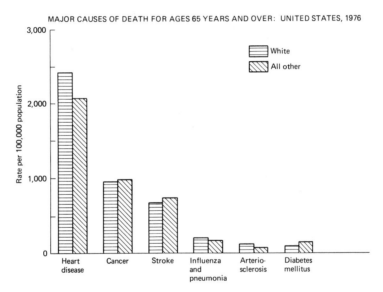

MAJOR CAUSES OF DEATH FOR AGES 65 YEARS AND OVER: UNITED STATES, 1976

Figure 13-4 (on facing page and above) Major causes of death, by age group. (Based on data from the National Center for Health Statistics, Division of Vital Statistics.)

2. Environmental health services, including food protection, liquid waste and water pollution control, swimming pool and water supply sanitation, occupational health and safety, radiation and vector control, housing conservation and rehabilitation, and related services.

3. Mental health services, such as prevention, consultation, diagnosis, and treatment via outpatient, emergency, and short-term hospitalization.

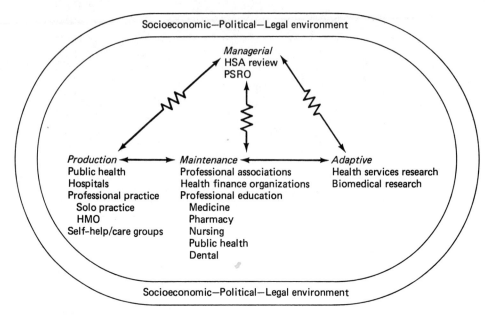

Figure 13-5 Major components of the health system.

4. Personal health services in cases where an individual cannot assume personal responsibility or where specific types of care are otherwise unavailable.

More recently, concern has been expressed about the constituencies traditionally served by public health departments. Data suggest that populations requiring services provided by public health agencies have markedly decreased with expansion of public and private health insurance (Gibson, 1979). Also, individuals receive public services for shorter periods of time and are less committed to the maintenance of public institutions (Aaran, 1978). These factors have eroded the traditional rationale and constituency for public health services.

If public health is to endure, it must expand its function and its constituency (Blandon, 1982). First, public health should extend its responsibilities to include citizens who suffer from "medicalized" social problems (problems reflecting the responses to stress of contemporary life, which affect *all* segments of our society). These problems include overuse of alcohol, substance abuse, violence, child abuse, rape, and marital and sexual problems. A second group, which is more consistent with the traditional focus of public health, should serve those segments of the population which are not served by private arrangement due to areas of geography, language, culture, or poverty.

Preventive Services. A more restrictive but aggressive position was presented by Milton Terris (1976), who suggested that a new emphasis is needed on the prevention of noninfectious diseases. In identifying the 10 leading causes of death, it is apparent that a significant decline in mortality is possible only through primary prevention, a role unique to public health departments. This activity would require health department involvement in (1) control of the environment through both regulation and financial measures, (2) screening for the detection and correction of impairments, and (3) health education focusing upon behavior change.

Management Services. A third possibility is for public health to discard the provision of personal health services because of opposition by organized medicine, unenthusiastic support by government, and indifferent use of service by recipients (Bellin, 1977). Under this scheme, the primary role of public health is to control the quality of health services provided in the community by promulgating, monitoring, and enforcing standards of health care. In addition, public health would be responsible for communicable disease contact, follow-up and statistics, and environmental health concerns such as occupational health and safety. All activities involved with the direct provision of personal health services would be transferred to private agencies.

An even more limited role is suggested by Milton Roemer (1975). Under this definition all programmatic responsibilities would be transferred to agencies other than the public health department. All personal health services would be handled by health maintenance organizations and environmental programs would be reallocated to regional environmental quality control boards. Local health departments would plan, control, consult, and evaluate services provided by other agencies in the community.

Structure and Financing. Public health activities involve both state and local government agencies. At the state level, public health activities take a number of organizational forms, ranging from separate departments reporting directly to the governor to subunits of larger departments.

Local public health agencies have an equally complex variety of forms and have been defined in the following way (ASTAHO, 1979):

> An official (governmental) public health agency which is in whole or in part responsible to a sub-state governmental entity or entities. The latter may be a city, county, city/county, federation of counties, rural township, or any other type of substate governmental entity. In addition, a local health department must meet these criteria: (a) it has a staff of one or more full-time professional public health employees (e.g., public health nurse, sanitarian; (b) it delivers public health services; (c) it serves a definable geographic area; and (d) it has identifiable expenditures and/or budget in the political subdivision(s) which it serves.

The relationships of local health departments to the state agencies vary among the 50 states. Three types of organizational arrangements have been identified (Miller, 1977):

- Centralized organization in which the state health agency operates local health departments directly under the state's authority.

- A decentralized organization in which local governments operate health departments while the state health agencies provide technical assistance and consultation.

- A shared governmental control arrangement in which local governments operate departments which may also be subject to some authority of the state health agency.

Both state and local health departments are funded primarily from tax revenues and the major expenditures are allocated to providing personal health services. Figure 13-6 presents the sources and the expenditures of funds for programs of state health agencies. Seventy-two percent of all expenditures is allocated to the provision of personal health services. Fifty-five percent of all funds for state activities is generated by state tax revenues, 10 percent by fees and reimbursements, and 35 percent by federally funded categorical programs.

Figure 13-7 illustrates the expenditures and sources of funds for public health programs of local health agencies. The greatest proportion of expenditures is again allocated for personal health services; state funds are the primary source for program activities.

Hospitals

The recognized center of the health system is the hospital. It is a repository of sophisticated medical technology and provides the basic facilities of practicing physicians. Historically, the organization has been viewed as the "physician's workshop," and although this primary focus remains in many institutions throughout the country, many hospitals are designing programs and special arrangements to provide a comprehensive array of services with an explicit recognition of the health needs of the community.

Figure 13-8 presents the distribution of short-term general and other special beds by type of ownership over the past 40 years. There have been significant increases in both the number of beds and the number of hospitals. Moreover, the figure reflects a series of changes in the type of ownership of hospitals. Perhaps the most significant change is the early decrease in the proportion of for-profit hospitals and beds and the more recent stabilization of that trend.

An equally important area of concern is the distribution of beds by geographic area. As one can see in Figure 13-9, there are significant differ-

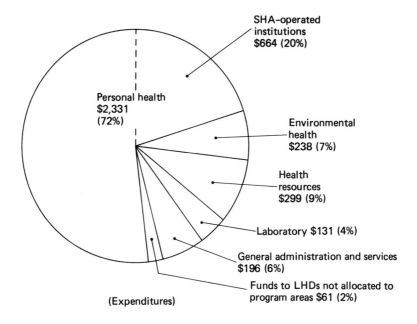

SHA-operated
institutions
$664 (20%)

Personal health
$2,331
(72%)

Environmental
health
$238 (7%)

Health
resources
$299 (9%)

Laboratory $131 (4%)

General administration and services
$196 (6%)

Funds to LHDs not allocated to
program areas $61 (2%)

(Expenditures)

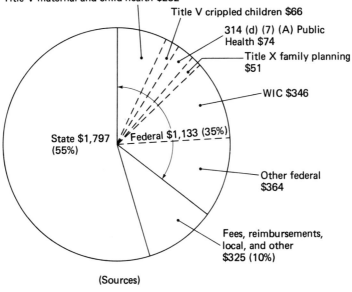

Title V maternal and child health $232

Title V crippled children $66

314 (d) (7) (A) Public
Health $74

Title X family planning
$51

WIC $346

State $1,797
(55%)

Federal $1,133 (35%)

Other federal
$364

Fees, reimbursements,
local, and other
$325 (10%)

(Sources)

Total: $3,256 million
for 57 SHAs

Figure 13-6 Expenditures and sources of funds for public health programs of
state health agencies, fiscal year 1978 (in millions of dollars). (Association of
State and Territorial Health Officials, *Comprehensive NPHPRS Report: Services,
Expenditures, and Programs of State and Territorial Health Agencies, Fiscal Year
1977:* ASATHO, 1979.)

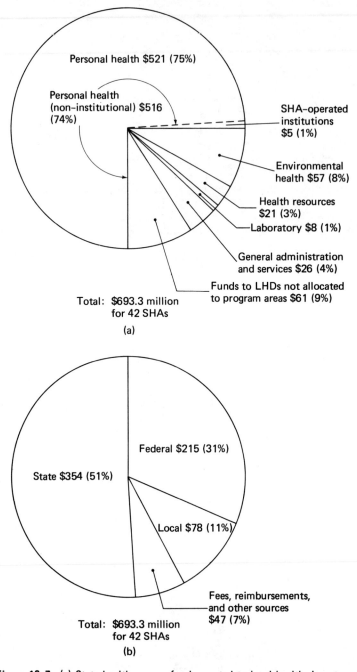

Figure 13-7 (a) State health agency funds granted to local health departments, by program area, fiscal year 1978 (in millions of dollars). (b) State health agency funds granted to local health departments, by sources of funds, fiscal year 1978. (Association of State and Territorial Health Officials, (*Comprehensive NPHPRS Report: Services, Expenditures, and Programs of State and Territorial Health Agencies, Fiscal Year 1977:* ASTHO, 1979.)

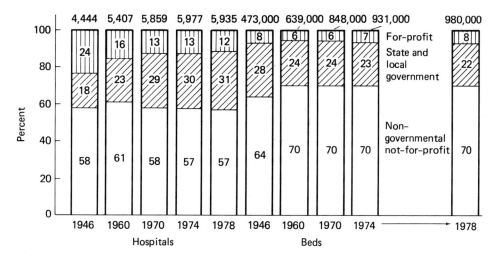

Data obtained from American Hospital Association, "The Nation's Hospitals: A Statistical Profile," *Hospital Statistics,* 1975, 1979 ed., Chicago.

Figure 13-8 Percent distribution of short-term general and other special hospitals* and of hospital beds, by type of ownership (United States, selected years, 1946-1978). [Source: A. Donabedian et al., *Medical Care Chart Book,* 7th ed. (Ann Arbor, Mich.: Health Administration Press, 1980)].

ences among the various regions of the country. The West North Central states have the greatest beds per population ratio and the Pacific and Mountain states have the least. Also, there has been a decrease in the bed–population ratio for all areas of the country between 1973 and 1978.

Multi-Hospital Systems. A significant development in the organization of hospitals is a growing trend toward shared services and other multi-hospital arrangements. Multi-hospital arrangements have taken a number of corporate forms (DeVries, 1978):

- *Formal affiliation:* close association under formal agreement commonly conducting joint education programs (e.g., medical school affiliation with community hospital for residence programs).

- *Shared or corporate services:* formal or informal arrangement to share one or more administrative or clinical services which can be provided by a hospital or group of hospitals or through a separate taxable or tax-exempt organization (e.g., shared service organization providing purchasing services).

- *Consortium for planning or education:* voluntary alliance of institutions, usually in the same geographic area, for a specific purpose (most often planning or education).

---

*Registered by the American Hospital Association. Federal hospitals excluded.

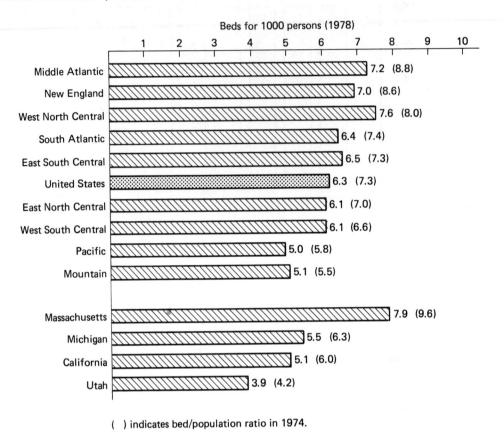

Beds for 1000 persons (1978)

( ) indicates bed/population ratio in 1974.

Figure 13-9 Hospital bed population ratio, by geographic area and selected states (1973-1978). (U.S. Bureau of the Census, *Statistical Abstract of the United States,* 1929 edition. American Hospital Association, *Hospital Statistics,* 1979 edition, Chicago.)

- *Contract management:* total responsibility for management of a health facility contracted to a separate entity for a specific period of time.
- *Lease of a condominium:* for transfer of property under a contract for a special rental fee for a specific period of ownership of shared and unique space in a single facility.
- *Corporate ownership separate management:* assets are owned by a single organization but management responsibilities are delegated by the owner.
- *Integrated ownership in management:* assets are owned and controlled (managed) by a single entity.

The true extent of the movement is not known. However, available data suggest that significant numbers of hospitals are participating in multiple arrangements in various ways. For example, in 1978 the American Hospital Association reported that 84.4% of all hospitals were sharing at least one service. At a more formal level of cooperation in which incorporated systems exist, it is estimated that there are more than 370 hospital systems representing one in every four short-term community hospitals and one in every three beds in the country (Brown et al., 1980; Brown, 1980).

Financing Hospital Services. The primary source of hospital funds is through third-party payment. In 1978 it is estimated that approximately 90% of the population had some form of hospital insurance. This insurance covers approximately 86% of all services provided by hospitals (Health Insurance Institute, 1980).

Practitioners*

The third element of the production subsystem is independent practitioners—that is, physicians, dentists, chiropractors, optometrists, and podiatrists. The primary function of this element is to provide professionally competent and ethically obligated service on an individual basis.

The largest number of independent practitioners is physicians (377,468), followed by dentists (117,890), optometrists (21,798), chiropractors (18,164), and podiatrists (7121). As seen in Figure 13-10, the number of independent practitioners has changed over time. The number of physicians has recorded a sizable increase, whereas only a slight increase is reported for dentists. There has been a slight increase in the number of optometrists, but the number of chiropractors and podiatrists has declined over the past 20 years.

The primary mode for providing professional services is through private practice. Approximately 60% of all active physicians are in office practice, 20% in house-staff capacity, and 12% are full-time hospital based. Of those physicians practicing outside the hospital, 95% are in private practice, with the balance in some form of organized care (e.g., prepaid group practice and neighborhood health centers) (AMA, 1979).

Figure 13-11 represents the number of medical groups and the number and percent of physicians in group practice for the past three decades. As

---

*Other types of health care providers are often termed allied health and include dependent practitioners and supporting staff. Dependent practitioners are allowed by law to provide a limited range of services under the supervision of appropriate independent practitioners. Dependent practitioners include nurses, psychologists, social workers, pharmacists, physician assistants, dental hygienists, and therapists (e.g., speech, physical, and occupational) although some of these practitioners are also permitted to perform a range of independent functions. Supporting staff provide a range of services under the supervision of an independent or dependent practitioner and include clerical, maintenance, housekeeping, and food processing personnel, nurse aides, dental assistants, and technicians (Hanft, 1977).

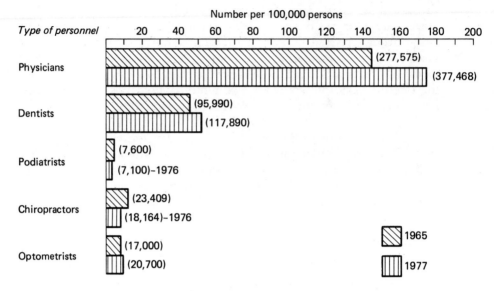

Figure 13-10 Numbers and number per 100,000 persons of independent practitioners in the United States, 1965 and 1977. [Health Insurance Institution, *Source Book of Health Insurance 1978-79,* p. 79. U.S. National Center for Health Statistics, *Health Resources Statistics, 1976-1977.* Public Health Service Pub. No. 79-1509, Table 154 (and *Health Resources Statistics, 1965*). American Medical Association, Center for Health Services Research and Development, *Profile of Medical Practice, 1978,* pp. 145, 147. Department of Health, Education, and Welfare, *Supply of Optometrists in the U.S. Health Manpower References,* October 1978, Pub. No. (HRA) 79-8, p. 1. U.S. Bureau of Census. *Statistical Abstracts of the U.S.,* 1979, pp. 10-11.

one can see, the number of physicians in group practice represents a relatively small percent of the total number of active physicians. However, the figure demonstrates a steady growth of the number of groups as well as the proportion of physicians in some form of group practice.

Health Maintenance Organizations. One form of group practice that has been expanding since 1973 is health maintenance organizations. These organizations are formally organized systems of health care delivery that combine the delivery and financing function and provide comprehensive services to an enrolled membership for a fixed prepaid fee. HMOs have taken a number of forms (Zelten, 1979).

- *Model I:* HMO owns or controls its hospital facilities, and the physicians who render services to the HMO members are salaried employees of the HMO.

- *Model II:* HMO owns or controls its hospital facilities, but physicians

Year	Number of groups	Number	Percent of all active physicians (Federal and non–Federal)
1946	368	3,084	2.6
1959	1,546	13,009	5.2
1965	4,289	28,381	10.2
1969	6,162	38,834	12.8
1975	8,483	66,842	16.3

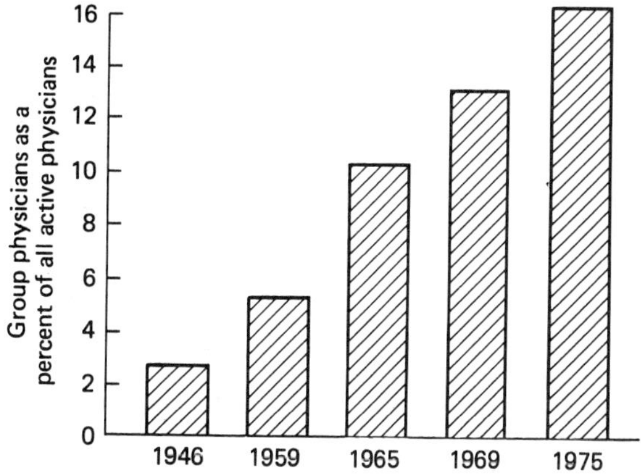

Figure 13-11 Number of medical groups, and number and percent of physicians in group practice, by years (United States, selected years, 1946–1975). (American Medical Association, Center for Health Services Research and Development, *Profile of Medical Practice, 1975-76.*)

Note: As defined by the AMA Council on Medical Service, group medical practice is the application of medical service by three or more physicians formally organized to provide medical care, consultation, diagnosis and/or treatment, through the joint use of equipment and personnel, and with income from medical practice distributed in accordance with methods previously determined by members of the group.

are not employees of the HMO. Physicians are a separate legal entity (a group practice) which contracts exclusively with the HMO to provide medical services.

- *Model III:* HMO contracts with hospitals for inpatient services. Physicians are salaried employees of the HMO.

- *Model IV:* HMO contracts with both hospitals and physicians. The physicians are members of the group practice and are reimbursed on a per capita basis.

- *Model V:* HMO contracts with both hospitals and physicians. The physicians are members of a group practice and are reimbursed by fee-for-service.

- *Model VI:* HMO contracts with both hospitals and physicians. Physicians are members of separate and already existing fee-for-service multi-specialty groups. Hospital contracts are arranged with those hospitals regularly used by existing medical groups.

- *Model VII:* HMO contracts with both hospitals and physicians. The physicians are engaged in solo practice and single-specialty group practice.
- *Model VIII:* The HMO contracts with hospitals and individual physicians. The physician's contract is negotiated through a separate physician association called the Individual Practice Association (IPA).

Financing Professional Care. Professional care is financed through a complex arrangement of third-party as well as private expenditures. The percentage of people covered through third party insurance and the percentage of expenditures covered varies for different types of provider services. For example, in 1976, 70% of the population had private insurance to cover physician, office, and home visits compared to only 22% of the population having private health insurance for dental care. Whereas the percent of population covered has substantially increased over time, the proportion of expenditures covered by third-party payors is significantly less and has remained relatively stable over time. For example, in 1976 only 46% of consumer expenditures for physician services was met by private insurance, an increase of 2% over 1970.

Allied Health Personnel. The allied health occupations are an extremely heterogeneous group of personnel and their exact numbers depend upon the definition of allied health. Excluding nurses and nurse auxiliaries, allied health personnel comprise over 1.8 million health workers, about 36% of the entire health services work force of 5.1 million (NCOAHE, 1980).

Figure 13–12 lists selected dependent and supporting-type allied health personnel. Nurses represent the largest category (1,018,000) and together with medical and psychiatric social workers, they report a substantial increase in the number of personnel since the 1960s. All forms of personnel report an increase except for pharmacists and midwives.

Self-Help Groups*

A growing set of activities affecting the provision of health services is self-help organizations. These organizations take a variety of forms and may

---

*It is important to differentiate between self-help and self-care. Self-help connotes a group activity. It involves concerted effort by some organizations of people to participate together toward the solution of some mutual problem. Self-care, on the other hand, emphasizes the individual's own ability to function effectively on behalf of his or her own health promotion and prevention and disease detection and treatment (Kronenfeld, 1980).

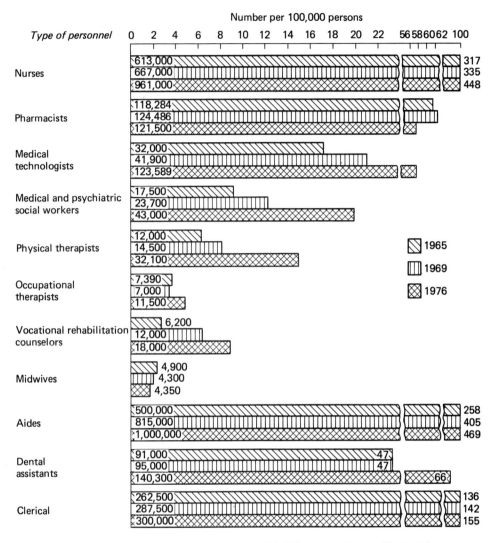

Figure 13-12 Numbers and numbers per 100,000 persons for specified health personnel (United States, 1965, 1969, 1976). (U.S. National Center for Health Statistics, *Health Resource Statistics, 1976-1977,* Public Health Service Pub. No. 79-1509. Health Insurance Institute, *Source Book of Health Insurance,* 1978-79.)

be defined as:

> A voluntary small group effort for mutual aid and the accomplishment of a special purpose. Self-help groups are usually formed by peers who have come together for mutual assistance in satisfying a common need, overcoming a

> handicap or life destructing problem and bringing about desired social and/or
> personal change. The initiators and members of such groups perceive that
> their needs are not or cannot be met by or through existing social institutions.
> Self-help groups emphasize face-to-face social interactions and the assumption
> of personal responsibility by members. They often provide material assistance
> as well as emotional support: they are frequently "cause" oriented and
> promulgate an ideology or set of values through which members may obtain
> and enhance sense of personal identity. [Katz and Bender, 1976]

These groups provide direct services to patients (and relatives) in the
form of education, coping skills, peer encouragement, and other supporting
activities which help the individual deal with some medical problem. Examples of self-help groups include such organizations as Emphysema Anonymous, Mended Hearts (open-heart surgery), Stroke Club, International
Association of Laryngectomies, Reach to Recoveries (mastectomy), and
United Ostomy Club.

Reliable information on the number of groups or chapters in any particular year is difficult to obtain. One survey (Tracy and Gussow, 1976),
however, describing their growth patterns since 1940 reports that these
organizations had an average rate of growth of about 3% over the three
decades (1942–1972). These data represent minimal patterns since new
groups are constantly forming.

The primary function of the self-help groups is to provide mutual aid and
assistance to members in dealing with adaptive problems resulting from disability due to illness, disease, or other health-related disorders. The disease is
usually a chronic one. Although the emergence of self-help groups is a testimonial to the failure of medicine in providing certain types of services to
patients, available information on the operation of these groups does not
reveal individual criticism of the quality of technical medical care received.
The primary focus is one of coping with problems of outlook and functioning with family, friends, and employers. It is in the latter area that institutional medical care facilities and providers have been least responsive.

The operating structure of these self-help groups is usually loosely organized and informal, with small or nonexistent operating budgets. Although
little information is available on the operations, the data suggest that the
groups are characterized by a great deal of variability and diversity in approach. Moreover, the membership cuts across various demographic social
strata of the community (Levy, 1976).

Another form of self-help group is the voluntary health association. This
form of self-help group is more foundation-oriented and is defined as an
organization that is administered by an autonomous board which holds
meetings, collects funds for its support primarily through private sources,
and expends money, whether with or without paid workers, in conducting
a program directed primarily to furthering the public health by providing

public health services or health education or by advancing research or legislation related to health or by a combination of these activities.

Voluntary health agencies may be classified as one of four basic types:

- Agencies concerned with specific diseases: for example, National Cancer Society, National Tuberculosis and Respiratory Diseases, the National Foundation (Polio and Birth Defects), American Diabetic Association, National Cystic Fibrosis Research Association, and the National Multiple Sclerosis Society.

- Agencies concerned with certain organs/structure of body: for example, National Society to Prevent Blindness, American Society for Hard of Hearing, National Society for Crippled Children, and American Heart Association.

- Agencies concerned with health/welfare special groups and society: for example, National Association for Retarded Citizens, and National Easter Seal Society for Crippled Children and Adults.

- Agencies concerned with particular phases of health/welfare: for example, Planned Parenthood Federation of America and the National Hospice Association.

These organizations are funded primarily by citizens' contributions and donations. A 1977 survey by the American Association of Fund Raising Council (1975) reports that more than $½ billion was contributed to 23 national health agencies in 1976. This represented an overall increase of nearly 8.7% from the previous year.

Maintenance Subsystem

The primary objective of this subsystem is to ensure stability and predictability in the provision of health services. Several organizational activities can be identified as fulfilling this objective: professional associations, professional schools, and financing mechanisms (e.g., Blue Cross/Blue Shield and other commercial insurance).

Professional Associations

Service delivery organizations and individual health care providers have associations to protect their interests. An association—whether composed of health manpower (physicians/AMA, administrators/ACHA and AGMA, dentists/ADA, nurses/ANA, allied health/ASAHP), or institutions (hospitals/AHA, group health organizations/GHAA, medical schools/AAMC, Blue Cross/Blue Shield Insurance/BCA)—is an organization of health providers who band together to perform functions which they cannot perform as individual units. Although associations perform many functions, perhaps the most immediate is to make as much money as possible for the individual providers of institutions they represent. This is accomplished through various types of legislative activities designed to increase revenues by enhancing the market power of members of the association.

One study (Feldstein, 1977) has attempted to document the role of various types of health provider associations and their demand for health legislation favoring policies that (1) increase the demand for services of health professionals and organizations to be reimbursed for the services as a price-discriminating monopolization (i.e., providers are able to charge different purchasers different prices for their services based on each purchaser's willingness and ability to pay); (2) lower the price of comparable provider inputs; and (3) increase the price of substitutes for their services and restrict additions to the supply of health professions and organizations represented by the professional association.

The structures of professional associations differ. They may be closely controlled from a central office or they may allow considerable autonomy to local branches of the association. The model most frequently emulated is the American Medical Association. The AMA is composed of local county medical societies which elect representatives to a state body. The state medical association house of delegates, in turn, elects representatives to the National House of Delegates. The major power is vested in the board of trustees elected by the National House of Delegates, since the delegates themselves meet only for a few days twice a year. The board of trustees functions in an autonomous fashion and the relationship between the trustees and the AMA members is similar to that which exists between boards of directors and stockholders of corporations. The trustees are supplemented by an extensive staff that is able to exert a great deal of influence on social legislation affecting all phases and aspects of professional activity.

Professional Schools

The provision of health services requires a predictable flow of independent practitioners as well as dependent practitioners and supporting staff. Below is a brief discussion of selected professional schools.

Medical Schools.* In the fall of 1979 there were 124 schools conducting accredited or provisionally accredited programs to award the M.D. degree in the United States and two schools conducting an accredited or provisionally accredited program for the first two years of the M.D. degree. In addition,

---

*Material based on Ruhe (1980).

plans were continuing for the development of the medical school at two other universities.

Existing schools employed 46,598 full-time faculty in 1979 and enrolled 62,754 medical students. These figures reflected a continual increase in both the number of full-time faculty as well as the number of medical students since 1971 while maintaining an approximate medical student full-time faculty ratio of approximately 1.3. In addition to providing instruction to medical students, the medical schools are responsible for the instruction of a variety of other students. For example, medical school faculties were responsible for providing instruction to 12,597 dental students, 8645 pharmacy students, 20,891 nursing students, 1810 physician assistants, as well as graduate and postgraduate students and allied health personnel.

Applications to medical schools have been generally increasing since 1957. In 1978-1979, the total number of applications was 36,636. This represents a 14% decrease from the peak year of 1974-1975, in which there were 42,624 applicants. In 1978-1979, 2.2% of the total number of applications were accepted. Considering the geographic as well as sociodemographic characteristics of applicants, analysis reveals that 78% of those accepted were residents of the state in which the school was located. Further analysis reveals that the number of women entering medical school increased slightly while the number of women applicants decreased. In 1978-1979, 26% of the total applicants were women, with approximately 25% admitted to the entering class. This is twice the percentage recorded in 1971-1972.

The proportion of minority enrollment remains relatively constant. For example, in 1978-1979 blacks represented 5.8% of the first-year enrollment as well as 5.8% of the total enrollment. Twenty-eight percent of this enrollment is accounted for by three schools: Howard, Meharry, and Morehouse, which admit black students predominantly.

The financing of medical schools has shown a dramatic shift over the past 10 years. In 1967-1968, $2 of every $5 of medical school revenues supported the general operations of the institution. By 1977-1978, these activities required almost $3 of every $5 in revenues. The shift is further demonstrated by the fact that federal dollars for the support of specific programs, such as research, targeted teaching, and training, accounted for more than one-half of the medical school revenue 10 years ago and now provide only 30%. Federal research funds are now less than one-fifth of the total revenue, compared with one-third in 1967-1968.

The long-term changes in financial support can best be characterized by the increased relative proportion of the total funds derived from medical school health and community service activities (i.e., income provided through medical services plans and clinics in hospitals and by the increased support provided by state and local governments). This shift in funding will have a significant impact on future revenues as well as on the role of the medical school in community services activities.

Public Health Schools.* Most public health personnel are trained in one of 21 schools of public health, with a combined enrollment of approximately 6800 students and a total faculty in excess of 1750. The schools provide instruction in 10 specialty areas, including biostatistics, epidemiology, health and hospital services management, environmental health, nutrition, biomedical laboratory sciences, maternal and child health, population studies, health education, and occupational health.

Students in public health have a significant amount of previous work experience before beginning their professional training. It is estimated that more than 25% of the students have more than 3½ years of actual work experience in the public health setting. Moreover, one out of every three students enrolled already has a prior master's degree and one in 10 students has an M.D. or D.D.S.

Applications to schools of public health have had a continual rise since the 1960s. However, there has been a moderate decline in the ratio of admissions to applications. Analysis of sociodemographic characteristics of students reveals that there is an equal number of male and female students, with more than 77% of the students enrolled being white, 7% black, 7% Asian (Hawaiian background), and 6% Hispanic.

Public health schools have had a long history of federal funding for both teaching and research programs. However, since 1975, there has been some major reallocation of federal funding, requiring increased support from institutional sources. For example, the financing of schools of public health has shown a major shift since 1974. A review of the percentage of federal-versus non-federal-funded expenditures reveals that in 1974, 55% of all expenditures were federally funded, whereas in 1977 this amount had been reduced to approximately 50%. Although this represents a fairly significant decrease, the proportion of decrease is not equally distributed by type of school. This proportion of federal funding remained relatively constant (48%) for state schools of public health, whereas private schools of public health recorded a decrease from 63.2% of expenditures federally funded in 1974 to 53.4% expenditures federally funded in 1977 (U.S. DHEW, 1980a).

Although schools of public health constitute an important educational and training mechanism for public health personnel, there are several other sources for such training. These include training programs in health administration and health planning, public or community health education, environmental health and nutrition, as well as programs in health statistics and epidemiology. These training programs are conducted by a range of institutions, including schools of medicine, dentistry, business and public administration, allied health, sciences, engineering, education, and home economics.

---

*Material based on U.S. DHEW 1980a,b.

Nursing Schools.* In 1978 there were 1374 basic nursing programs and 1329 practical or vocational nursing programs in the United States. The basic nursing programs are composed of three types: associate degree, diploma, and baccalaureate. The associate degree programs are usually conducted in junior or community colleges and require a two-year program of study. The diploma programs are conducted by community hospitals. The programs usually require 24 to 36 months to complete training. The baccalaureate degrees are located in universities or colleges and require four years of academic training.

The practical/vocational nursing programs are usually offered by vocational schools in public educational systems or by hospitals or junior community colleges. The program requires one year of training and emphasizes clinical practice.

Unlike medical schools, which have been increasing, the number of nursing and practical nursing programs has remained relatively stable over the past few years. It is expected that the number of total programs will decline during the next several years.

Nursing programs enrolled 91,393 students and the practical/vocational programs enrolled 36,957 students in 1978. These numbers represent a significant decline in admissions since 1974, in which 95,389 students were admitted to RN programs and 40,098 were admitted into practical nursing programs.

The number of applicants also declined in both RN and practical nurse programs. In 1978 there were 231,423 applications for RN programs, compared with 274,785 applications in 1977. Similarly, 75,095 applications were received for practical nurse training in 1978 compared to 99,755 in 1977.

The proportion of minority enrollment has remained stable since 1975. In 1978, for example, 6.3% of the class admitted into RN programs and 4.5% admitted into practical nurse programs were male, in contrast to 6.9% males admitted into RN programs and 5.9% into practical nurse programs in 1975. Similarly, in 1978, 7.2% of the class admitted to RN programs and 11.1% admitted to practical nurse programs were black, in contrast to 7.7% and 12.5% in 1975.

Allied Health Schools. Allied health personnel are trained in a variety of postsecondary educational programs. In 1976 it was estimated that there were 14,000 formal postsecondary programs preparing allied health personnel (NCOAHE, 1980). It is estimated that 52 to 54% of allied health programs are housed in collegiate settings, 33 to 35% in hospitals, 10 to 12% in post-

---

*Material based on National League for Nursing (1978), and Vaughn and Johnson (1979).

secondary noncollegiate institutions (e.g., public vocational technical institutes, private career schools) and 1% in the armed forces.

A 1975-1976 American Society of Allied Health Professions survey revealed 280,531 students enrolled in collegiate allied health programs. The mean number of students per program was about 50, but half the programs had 20 or fewer students. Women predominated among students, with the highest proportion of women enrolled in medical records, rehabilitation (occupational), dental services, dietetic and nutritional services, nursing related services, and veterinary services. Women were in the minority in allied health activities associated with biomedical engineering, environmental services, emergency services, vision care, and physician assistant programs.

One out of every 10 students enrolled in basic occupational programs was black, but there was wide variation in curriculum areas. Black students composed only 8% of the enrollment in basic occupational allied health programs in four-year colleges and universities, compared to 12% in two-year college programs. Thus they tend to be underrepresented in allied professions requiring more training and overrepresented for those occupations requiring less training.

Financing Organizations

The provision of health services requires a predictable flow of funds from the consumer to the providers of care. Our society has created several complex organizational mechanisms to assure the predictable transfer of these monies: government, private insurance companies, and nonprofit insurance companies.

Government. The single largest governmental-based financing mechanism is provided by Medicare and Medicaid, primarily viewed as cost-based reimbursement programs. These programs, known as Title XVIII and Title XIX, respectively, were initiated as part of the 1965 Social Security Act.*

Medicare provides a range of benefits for persons 65 and older who are already covered by Social Security. The program is uniform throughout the United States and is divided into two major components. Part A is financed

---

*Numerous other federal financing programs for health care also exist for designated purposes or groups, such as pregnant women and disabled adults. Not to be overlooked is the Internal Revenue Code, which in effect partially subsidizes personal medical expenses. In addition to simply providing reimbursement-type financing mechanisms, the federal government has developed funding and specific service activities for selected population groups. These include the Veterans Administration (veterans), the Department of Defense (military), Public Health Service (merchant marine, federal employees), and Indian Health Services (native Americans). States also have funding and service activities of various types, such as rural health programs.

Funds are also available for medical expenses and income loss resulting from occupationally related diseases and injury. These are provided by state government through workers' compensation programs, which vary by state.

by payroll taxes collected under Social Security and provides coverage for care rendered in hospitals, extended care facilities, and patient homes. Part B is a voluntary supplemental program which pays certain costs of physician and other medical expenses and is operated by general tax revenues and private contributions.

Neither Part A nor Part B provides fully comprehensive coverage. Both have a series of deductions and coinsurance features as well as specific limits on the amount of coverage provided.

Medicaid is a joint federal–state program guaranteeing medical services to welfare recipients. Federal funds from general tax revenues are allocated to states on a cost-sharing basis according to the state's per capita income. The program provides full payment for services given to the aged poor, the blind, the disabled, families with dependent children, and for early and periodic detection treatment of diseases for persons under 21. The program focuses on six types of services: (1) inpatient and outpatient hospital care, (2) other laboratory and x-ray services, (3) physician services, (4) skilled nursing care, (5) home health agencies, and (6) family planning services. Other types of services, such as prescription drugs, dental services, and eyeglasses, are allowable options that may be provided at the state's discretion.

Private Carriers.* A second financing arrangement assuring the predictability of funds within the health system is made up of private carriers, non-profit and profit. Blue Cross/Blue Shield represents a nonprofit component characterized by the various state-based Blue Cross/Blue Shield Plans. Blue Cross is responsible for reimbursing the costs of hospital services; Blue Shield is responsible for reimbursing the costs of physician-type services. The various state plans are loosely coordinated through a national association—The Blue Cross/Blue Shield Association.

The reimbursement of the cost of hospital and physician services by Blue Cross/Blue Shield traditionally consists of two major characteristics: payment of service benefits to hospitals rather than cash benefits to the individual insured, and community rating. Community rating provides benefits to all members of the community at the same rate rather than at a higher rate for high-risk groups.

A more recent function assumed by the Blue Cross/Blue Shield providers is to act as financial intermediaries between federal and state government in Medicaid/Medicare programs. Under Medicare, for example, Blue Cross/Blue Shield as an intermediary (1) determine how much the provider is to be paid, (2) make the payment, (3) audit the provider, and (4) assist in the development and maintenance of utilization review systems.

---

*In addition to providing a financial mechanism, a number of private insurance programs are combined with service delivery activities to form health maintenance organizations—see pages 370-371 for a description.

Commercial insurance companies (e.g., Metropolitan, Prudential, and Aetna) provide health insurance coverage together with other types of insurance coverage, such as life, accident, and automobile. The companies provide a wide range of coverage. In addition, various plans can be purchased to cover major medical expenses and catastrophic illnesses. Insurance premiums under the commercial insurance plans are specifically tailored to the risk associated with various age groups within the population. Another distinguishing feature is that payment is to the insured individual in a flat sum of money per day of hospitalization or per visit to the physician, as opposed to direct reimbursement to the provider, as in Blue Cross/Blue Shield.

Adaptive Subsystem

The primary objective of this subsystem is to monitor changes in the larger environment and suggest modifications in basic technology, functions, and structure of the health services system. Through these changes, the system will be better able to survive and function in a changing environment. Health services and biomedical research are basic activities within the subsystem.

Health Services Research

Health services research is the systematic study of health service delivery programs and structure. The objective of this study is to affect actual delivery of health services. Health services research may be divided into several components or functions: (1) collection and diffusion of information and statistics, (2) development and evaluation of new health services systems and processes, (3) research and training, and (4) policy analysis (U.S. DHEW, 1972). These functions represent major problem areas in which the basic disciplines of epidemiology, economics, sociology, and the management sciences are applied in an effort to resolve important health services delivery issues. The work itself is conducted by a number of public and private research organizations.

The National Center for Health Services Research and Development. The mission of the National Center is to undertake and support research, demonstration, and evaluation of problems in the organization and delivery and financing of health services; to serve as a focal point for the coordination of health services research within the public health service; and to disseminate the findings of health service research to policy and decision makers in the public and private sectors (USDHEW, 1978(b)). Priority areas include the following types of services:

- *Health care costs and cost containment:* analysis of the factors underlying the increase in health care costs and the structural reforms and incentives which might modify these costs.

- *Health insurance:* analysis of the sociodemographic, economic, and administrative implications of various health insurance initiatives.

- *Planning and regulation:* development of techniques to make cost-effective investment and production decisions in the health sector and and the analysis of market- and regulation-based strategies for shaping such decisions.

- *Technology and computer science applications:* analysis of technology-based approaches to modify the organization and delivery of health care services, with particular emphasis on the uses of computer science and medical information systems.

- *Health manpower:* analysis of the economic and behavioral aspects of health manpower education requirements, distribution, utilization, and development.

Research in these as well as other issues are conducted through the intra-mural program of the National Center and through research conducted in various universities and private research organizations throughout the country. Although these organizations may differ in terms of focus and structure, they all share the characteristic of attempting to apply the basic disciplines of the social and behavioral sciences to important health service delivery questions.

The National Center for Health Care Technology. * The mission of the center is to undertake and support a variety of programmatic activities directed at improving the understanding and consequences associated with the development and application of technology in health care. Technology is broadly defined to include "any discrete and identifiable regimen or modality used to diagnose and treat illness, prevent disease, maintain patient well-being or facilitate the provision of health care services." Two areas of activity are given emphasis (NCHCT, 1980):

1. Development and testing of methodologies for assessing the safety, efficacy, and effectiveness of particular health care technology and their social, economic, and ethical impact.

2. Focus assessment or analysis of particular aspects of a health care technology (e.g., its effectiveness or social, economic, or ethical implications).

---

*Beginning in the 1982 fiscal year, functions of the National Center for Health Care Technology are to be incorporated into the National Center for Health Services Research and Development.

The National Center for Health Statistics.* The mission of the National Center is to develop and maintain data systems capable of providing reliable, general-purpose, national, descriptive health statistics on a continuing basis and to disseminate these statistics to provide a factual basis for planning national programs designed to advance the health and well-being of the American people.

Data collection systems include:

- *Vital registration system:* collects and publishes data on births and deaths in the United States.

- *Vital statistics follow-back survey:* periodic data collection based on samples of births and deaths occurring during a calendar year. Provides a national estimate of births and deaths by characteristics not available from the vital registration system.

- *Health interview survey:* continuing nationwide sample of households, providing data on the incidence of illness and accidental injuries, prevalence of disease and impairment, the extent of disability, utilization of health care services, and hospital utilization.

- *Health and nutrition survey:* collects data that can be obtained only by direct physical examinations, clinical and laboratory tests, and related measurement procedures. Two kinds of data are collected: (a) prevalence data for specific diseases or conditions of ill health, and (b) normative health-related measurement data, which show distributions of the total population with respect to particular parameters such as blood pressure, visual acuity, or serum cholesterol levels.

- *Master facility inventory:* provides a comprehensive file of inpatient health facilities in the United States. These facilities include hospitals, nursing and related care facilities, and other custodial or remedial care facilities. Information is collected about the ownership, major type of services offered, number of beds, admissions, inpatient days of care, discharges, patient census, revenues, expenses, assets, and staffing.

- *Health manpower inventory:* baseline statistics about health manpower in the United States. Data derived from professional associations as well as state licensing agencies include basic information on the numbers, characteristics, and distribution of various health occupational groups.

- *Hospital discharge survey:* continuing nationwide sample survey of short-stay hospitals in the United States. The survey provides information on the characteristics of patients, the lengths of stay, diagnosis

---

*Based on personal communication with M. G. Kovar, National Center for Health Statistics, n.d.

and surgical operations, and the patterns of use of care in hospitals of different size and ownership in various sections of the country.

- *National nursing home survey:* a biannual series of nationwide sample surveys of nursing homes and their in-staff residence.
- *National ambulatory care survey:* a continuing nationwide probability sample of ambulatory medical encounters. The survey covers physician-patient encounters in physician offices. Information is gathered about the types of patients seen in terms of their sociodemographic and medical care characteristics as well as the disposition of the visits.

Biomedical Research

Biomedical research is the development of new technology to deal with the health problems of our society. This represents a broad spectrum of activities and includes:

1. *Basic research:* activity and pursuit of new fundamental knowledge in the biological sciences and related fields with a high level of uncertainty.

2. *Applied research and development:* activity drawing upon basic information to create solutions to problems in prevention, treatment, or cure of disease.

3. *Clinical investigation:* studies of human beings to increase knowledge in such areas as etiology, pathophysiology, and epidemiology of disease.

4. *Clinical trials:* research activities to test and evaluate prophylactic, diagnostic, and therapeutic agents in human beings under varying degrees of control in a more defined population.

5. *Demonstration programs:* activities to show the efficiency of verified clinical techniques or procedures in a practical clinical setting in a specific region population group, etc.

6. *Control programs:* activities to prevent or control disease that span major categories of effort from prevention to demonstration of improved treatment.

7. *Education programs:* activities to disseminate and communicate to the health professions and the public new and existing information and techniques of therapy and prevention, as well as information concerning the magnitude of disease problems.

8. *Health care,* per se. [U.S. DHEW, 1978c, p. 74]

These activities are conducted by a number of private as well as public institutions. At the federal level, the predominant institution is the National

TABLE 13-1 *Components of the National Institutes of Health, and Year of Founding*

Institute[a]	Year Founded
National Cancer Institute	1937
National Heart, Lung, and Blood Institute	1948
National Institute of Allergy and Infectious Diseases	1948
National Institute of Dental Research	1948
National Institute of Neurological and Communicative Disorders and Stroke	1950
National Institute of Arthritis, Metabolism, and Digestive Diseases	1950
National Institute of General Medical Sciences	1958
National Institute of Child Health and Human Development	1962
National Institute of Environmental Health Sciences	1966
National Eye Institute	1968
National Institute on Aging	1974

[a]*This table lists the current names of the institutes and the year of establishment of principal responsibility. There have been name changes over time and certain responsibilities have been shifted from one institute to another.*

Institutes of Health. Table 13-1 lists the number of different components of the Institutes as well as their founding year.

The various institutes engage in both intramural and extramural research activities. The majority of the funds are allocated to the National Cancer Institute, as well as to the National Heart, Lung, and Blood Institute. Through the Institutes, funds are allocated either through a contract or grant mechanism to various universities and private research organizations throughout the country.

Biomedical and health services research are not mutually exclusive. There are several areas in which there is a great deal of overlap. Perhaps this is best dramatized by the issues of technology transfer and technology assessment. The latter is concerned with the systematic measurement of the efficacy of technology developed; the question of technology transfer centers on the ability of the delivery system to assure that the latest technology is effectively applied at the local level. Since this activity has been gaining increased concern, attention within the health services research community and the biomedical community have attempted to deal with these questions.

Managerial Subsystem

The managerial subsystem cuts across the production, maintenance, and adaptive subsystems. Its function is to coordinate the various subsystems, assuring their overall effective operations. It is possible to identify two sets of activities which have the potential for fulfilling managerial functions within the health system: Health Systems Agencies and Professional Service Review organizations.

Health Systems Agencies

A national health planning program was created with the passage of Titles X and XIV—The National Health Planning and Resources Development Act of 1974. The legislation created a network of health system agencies (HSAs), State Health Planning and Development Agencies (SHPDAs), and Statewide Health Coordinating Councils (SHCCs) responsible for health planning and resources development throughout the country.

The emphasis of the legislation was on local health planning and it gave a great deal of authority and control to the respective HSAs. Essentially, the HSAs must (1) determine the need for *all* health services, (2) review and approve/disapprove all applications for a variety of federal health program funds, (3) review and approve/disapprove all building and program plans of health care institutions, and (4) conduct periodic reviews of the appropriateness of all institutional health services in their respective areas. The unique feature of the HSA is that it has the responsibility to both plan and implement programs.

Professional Service Review Organizations

Established in 1972, professional service review organizations (PSROs) are responsible for assuring that the services provided and paid for under Medicare, Medicaid, maternal and child health, and crippled children's programs are (1) medically necessary, (2) of a quality that meets professional standards, and (3) provided at the most economical level consistent with high-quality care (Goran, 1979).

To meet this objective, PSROs are operational in 195 PSRO geographic areas throughout the United States. These organizations are responsible for "utilizing the services of and accepting the findings of hospital committees which the PSRO feels are capable of conducting review effectively." The basic review system implemented by most PSROs consists of three interrelated components: concurrent review, medical care evaluation studies, and profile analysis.

- *Concurrent review:* review of admissions against physician-established criteria for medical necessity. Certified admissions are assigned an initial number of days according to local diagnosis (specific norms of care). Periods of hospitalization beyond the certified number of days are reviewed to determine whether there is continued need for hospitalization.

- *Medical care evaluation:* in-depth retrospective reviews to determine whether certain criteria thought to assure professionally accepted standards of care were met.
- *Profile analysis:* statistical analysis of aggregate patient care data conducted retrospectively after patient discharge. Emphasis is given to presenting patterns of health services utilization and patterns of care rendered to patients.

A recent evaluation of the current implementation status and effectiveness of the PSRO program reveals that the program has reduced Medicare hospital utilization and that overall, PSRO Medicare concurrent review activity pays for itself. In 1977, for example, it was estimated that PSRO saved the Medicare program $5 million more than it cost to run the concurrent review program. In 1978, the evaluation reports an estimated saving of $21 million over administrative costs (Health Care Financing Administration, 1980).

ENVIRONMENTAL FACTORS AFFECTING THE HEALTH SERVICES SYSTEM

Organizations and individuals composing the health services system operate within a larger environmental context. This context influences the basic structure and function of the health system and determines the feasibility of new programs and arrangements for providing health services.

The health services system described in the preceding section is characterized by a number of distinguishing features:

- Multiple financing mechanisms for funding health services.
- Emphasis on professional ethics in controlling physician behavior.
- Distinct health care programs for specific segments of the population.
- Embryonic nature of managerial activities within the overall health system.
- Constantly expanding technology and specialized skills, equipment, and facilities.
- Emphasis on curative medicine, with limited attention to primary prevention.

To provide an understanding as to why these particular features characterize the health services system in the United States, it is important to consider the basic economic and political values and legal constraints operating within the larger social system.

Economic and Political Values

The particular form society has developed to provide health services is conditioned by answers given to two basic questions (Darsky, 1968):

1. Who controls the system; that is, where is the authority located which decides and executes policy in health matters?

2. Under what terms shall health care be made available to the population; that is, what process shall govern the allocation of society's scarce resources into health, and under what terms shall these be distributed to sick persons?

Answers to both of these questions center around the basic values of society. The question of control is central to basic political values concerning the use of power and its regulation. In American society, a great deal of emphasis is placed on freedom from political constraint and on voluntary as opposed to formal authority.

The answer to the second question involves basic economic values and links the health system with the larger economic context. In American society, the allocation of scarce resources is governed by the concept of consumer sovereignty, as expressed in choices made in response to prices of goods and services in the marketplace. Although obvious departures occur in terms of welfare, medical care, veterans benefits, as well as other special arrangements, these are primarily residual and do not represent mainstream activities.

Individualism is thus a key value in determining the basic structure of the health services system and it provides an institutionally approved answer to questions of control and allocation of health services. Under this value, individuals are entitled only to that level of health, income, status, education, and general social well-being that results from their own individual efforts, actions, and abilities. Individualism emphasizes individual responsibility, minimal collective activity, and freedom from collective obligations except to respect the rights of other individuals.

The implications for the basic structure and function of the health services system are substantial. As described by Beauchamp (1976):

> the market ethic (individualism) obstructs the possibilities for minimizing death and disability, and alibies the need for structural change . . . through explanations for death and disability that "blame the victim" (Ryan, 1971). Victim blaming misdefines structural and collective problems of the victims. These behavioral explanations for public problems tend to protect the larger society and powerful interest from the burdens of collective action and instead encourage attempts to change the "faulty" behavior of victims.
>
> Market justice (individualism) is perhaps the major cause for over-investment and over-confidence in curative medical services. It is not obvious that the rise

of medical science and the physician, taken alone, should become fundamental obstacles to collective action to prevent death and injury. But the norms of market justice transform these scientific advances into an unrealistic hope for "technological short-cuts" (Etizoni and Remp, 1972) to painful social change. Moreover, the great emphasis placed on individual achievement in market justice has further diverted attention and interest away from primary prevention and collective action by dramatizing the role of the solitary physician-scientists, picturing them as our primary weapon and first line of defense against the threat of death and injury.

Individualism, however, is not unchallenged and must interface with society's humanitarian obligation to the well-being of its citizens as a whole. The history of our society is an increasing recognition of the principle of the common good. Under this value, disease is considered involuntary and individuals are entitled equally to the benefits of health protection, minimal standards of housing and income, as well as social well-being. The two values coexist, creating an uneasy balance. For example, the passage of Medicare and Medicaid provided financial resources to ensure a minimal level of care for most segments of the population. These funds, however, are used within a system guided by the values of individualism and characterized by the absence of formal controls on physician behavior and by the emphasis given to curative medical care. These two values have created arrangements that are contradictory in purpose and difficult to reconcile. These tensions are not confined to economic and political issues, but are also manifested in laws and regulations.

Legal and Legislative Factors

The economic and political values of society are in large measure reflected, and some would say enshrined, in its laws and constitutions. In order to implement or enforce values, we have devised various mechanisms to ensure that the majority of the population will know and observe them.

We expect most values to be self-evident and even self-enforcing. To a great extent this is true. For example, consider the moral principle that one should help a person in distress, sometimes referred to as the Good Samaritan Rule. Although this concept is probably felt by most Americans as a manifest Christian-Judeo precept, it is usually acted upon only if the would-be Samaritan feels competent to help or finds it convenient to do so. Frequently, for example, in the case of roadside accidents, this urge to help has been felt, but questions of ability or convenience have been raised, leading to reluctance to "get involved." In its political expression the question has taken the form of fear of undue liability. Therefore, legislative action was requested by some of the groups affected, such as medical societies and truckers' associations. Citing the difficulty of enforcing appropriate response by individual citizens, state legislatures in nearly every state during the

1960s enacted statutes which, rather than *requiring* samaritanship by all persons, simply promised immunity from legal liability for persons who stop and render first aid. Some statutes apply only to physicians and other medically trained persons. Policymakers assessed the attitude of the public as being willing to have at least some of its members officially encouraged to participate. They probably sensed that a mandatory value would be unpopular and patently unenforceable in actual practice. Therefore, the Good Samaritan Rule was codified but not made compulsory. There has been little public reaction to this legislative policy and even less evidence that it affected any group's values.

Not all laws, however, incorporate the prevailing opinions of society. Any close look at the laws affecting the delivery of health care quickly reveals that some are out of date, others inapplicable to new situations, and still others not indicative of demographic, social, economic, or political differences. The difficulty of keeping laws current, designing them to anticipate new developments, and making them generally applicable is apparent. The political process is expected to resolve contemporary problems and prevent or mitigate future ones, but the political process, being human-made, is imperfect. Nevertheless, many laws become enacted which do, at the time, accurately portray a snapshot of the prevailing political, economic, and social values of the population.

The danger, of course, is not allowing for those values to change with time and conditions. Although the law and legal process serve as a useful anchor against the shifting tides of fortune and fancy, its role as a conservator of values can on occasion be a hindrance to progress. Some would argue that the federal government's vigorous enforcement of the laws regulating the testing and marketing of new therapeutic drugs has prevented the beneficial adoption of several life- or pain-saving discoveries, at least for several years. Others would point out that the United States did not have any deformed babies caused by the precipitous use of thalidomide by pregnant women as was the case in many other countries in the world. Most observers agree, however, that the law is a conservative influence on society and is a persuasive force affecting living, working, and other endeavors. The law changes slowly and, in fact, is often difficult to change at all.

The Relationship of Policy to the Legal and Political Processes

Public policy is developed primarily and most ostensibly through legal and political processes. Although many identifiable policies are voluntary or nonenforceable (such as the functional prerequisite of formal education in business or health care administration for filling responsible management positions in hospitals), most of the major activities of the health care services field are affected directly or indirectly by government policies. Ranging from mechanisms for determining liability for accidents to requirements for forward planning for new construction, these policies are identified in the laws and regulations that are addressed to the promotion or protection of the health of the public. Government at all levels—federal, state, and local— is active in developing and enforcing health care policies.

In simplest terms, policy is created by the legislative process, implemented through the executive process, and enforced or tested through the judicial process. The rights of individuals and institutions are embodied in constitutions (federal and state) as well as in the court decisions interpreting constitutional provisions.

Both patients and providers find some measure of legal protection from unwarranted intervention in important areas. Patients have such personal rights as confidentiality and privacy. Hospitals, physicians, and other health care providers also have rights. For example, a group of physicians or nurses can expect not to be singled out for unfair regulation because they are protected by the rights of "due process" and "equal protection."

The other side of the "rights" issue naturally is "responsibilities." Since patients have the right to privacy, hospitals have the responsibility to protect patient's medical records from unjustified exposure. Because hospitals have the right not to be harassed by government, regulatory agencies (e.g., state health departments) must follow certain steps before taking any administrative actions, such as citing a hospital cafeteria for unsanitary practices.

The political and economic climate in recent years has promoted an increasing consciousness about legal rights by both individuals and institutions. Tension and confrontation are pervasive and administrators are often caught in the squeeze between adversaries. For example, hospital administrators may find themselves involved in litigation between an unhappy, injured patient and the hospital corporation. A medical clinic manager who has not been given adequate training or staff may be called to testify about the clinic's accounting practices if a government agency, such as the Medicare agency, challenges the clinic's billing practices for reimbursement purposes. A Health Service Agency (HSA) planner who has promised confidentiality to a client may be required under court order to disclose certain files to comply with a newspaper reporter's rights under a state freedom of information act. Examples arise daily in every health care setting.

Litigation has clearly become a major concern of health care administrators. Some of the new uses of the courts have been the result of temptations to shortcut or step up the policymaking process that slowly evolves in the legislatures or the ensuing implementation process followed by agencies. Most litigation, however, is the testing or vindication of legal rights. Rights are either privately created (e.g., in business contracts) or publicly based in legislation or constitutions.

The "rights" issues in the health care field are largely familiar because of their widespread media coverage: abortion, environmental protection, occupational health and safety, physician malpractice, program entitlement

(Medicare, Medicaid coverage; workers' compensation), hospital employee discrimination, antitrust violations, and numerous other issues particularly noticeable to those in the health care field.

The Impact of Regulations

While litigation and legislation are the legal and political mechanisms for forging overall policies, the practicing administrator is much more conscious of the day-to-day impact of the regulations and guidelines that implement those policies. As shown in Table 13-2, there has been an increasing number of regulations during the past 15 years. Much of the attention has been focused on the federal level, but states too, particularly the larger ones, have become more active and sophisticated in the regulation of health care services.

What are regulations? Broadly, regulations include principles, standards, guidelines, conditions, criteria, requirements, rules, or laws imposed by external authority for controlling or governing personal and institutional behavior; they are implemented by voluntary agreement or by governmental enforcement. But legally speaking, what are regulations? The official definition in the Federal Administrative Procedure Act* is helpful in answering the question, at least for most governmental purposes, since state administrative codes generally parallel the federal provisions. Simply put, the Act states that rules and regulations are agency statements of general or particular applicability and future effect, designed to implement, interpret, or prescribe law or policy, or describing the organization, procedure, or practice requirements of an agency. Note that there are two types of regulations: substantive and procedural. The former are exemplified by standards, guidelines, conditions, requirements, or similar measures for performance or

TABLE 13-2 *Pages of Regulations Published in the* Federal Register, *1950–1980*

Year	Number of Pages
1950	9,562
1960	14,479
1965	17,206
1970	20,036
1975	60,221
1980	87,012

SOURCE: *National Journal*, Sept. 25, 1976, p. 1361 (for 1950–1975). Personal communication with R. Kelly, Regulatory Information Service Center, Washington, D.C., Dec. 1, 1981 (for 1980).

---

*U.S. Code, Title 5, Chap. 5, Sec. 551.

compliance in order to gain approval, certification, or other privileges. The latter are characterized by both internal and external organizational rules, such as client reporting forms or deadlines and agency relationships or jurisdiction.

To a health administrator regulation is more than governmental. A typical health care institution or program is subject to surveillance by private agencies whose standards for accreditation, membership, or other purposes appear to be in the form of rules, both substantive and procedural. Table 13–3 illustrates the source and area of regulation affecting most institutions.

The net result of this level and scope of regulation is a multiplicity of authority and accountability. As noted by the AHA (1977),

> key decisions relating to patient care, terms of hospital payment, capital investment, and planning cannot be made without participation by a regulatory agency. . . . Reduction of managers' authority correspondingly limits their ability to determine the mix of factors used to produce health care services. . . . Within the hospital, increasing regulation has the effect of reducing the decision-making latitude of the administrator, the board of trustees, and the medical staff.

Other problems include the penalties or lack of incentives for certain administrative undertakings (such as shared services, because of tax policies) and cost shifting (such as Medicare nonreimbursement of community services).

It has become popular to decry the duplication and conflict in health regulations, as well as other defects and difficulties with the regulatory scheme affecting those involved in providing health care services. Federal deregulation of the airlines industry during the Carter Administration buoyed interest in finding ways to simplify or replace regulations in other fields. The proposed Regulation Reform Act of 1979 (HR 3263, S 262) recognized both the purposes and the problems of regulations in its findings that "in recent years, the use of regulation has increased—(a) in order to protect the environment and public health and safety; (b) to promote conservation of energy and other natural resources; (c) as a means of governing economic and commercial activity; (d) to enhance human rights; and (e) for other essential public purposes." To meet the problems of regulation frequently cited in the media as well as through congressional channels, the act states:

> The expanding impact of regulation on the economy, state and local governments, businesses, non-profit institutions, and individuals requires that—(A) the regulatory process be competently and sensitively managed to achieve the vital national objectives with which the process is entrusted; (B) the regulatory process be open to effective public participation; and (C) regula-

TABLE 13-3 *Regulations Affecting Health Facilities*[a]

Agency or Authority	Capital Construction	Cost and Charges for Service	Personnel Standards	Professional Performance (Peer Review)	Working Conditions	Training and Education	Patients' Rights	Accounting
Medicare	F	F	F	F	F	F	F	F
Medicaid	FS	FS	FS	FS	FS	FS	FS	FS
Public Health	SL		FSL		FSL			
JCAH	P		P	P			P	P
Blue Cross, intermediary, and private insurance	FSP	FSP	FSP	FSP				
State Insurance Commissioner	S	S			S			
State Licensing Agency	S		S		S			
Fire marshal	S							
Equal Opportunity Office			FS			FS		
National Labor Relations Board and State Department of Labor			FS		S			
State rate review	S	S						S
Internal Revenue Services		F						
Planning Agency	FSL							
PSRO				FSP				
AMA			P			P		
American College of Pathology			P					
AICPA								P
Office of Civil Rights							FS	

[a]F, federal; S, state; L, local; P, private or voluntary.

tory action be both fair and not unreasonably delayed; and (D) regulations be as clear and simple as possible, achieve statutory goals effectively and efficiently, and impose no unnecessary burdens on the public.

Former Secretary of the Department of Health and Human Services, Patricia Harris (1980), introduced procedures that required internal review of the costs of, and possible alternatives to, proposed regulations before they were developed. She wrote: "Every regulation is developed from a statutory base, and sometimes the statutes apply inconsistent requirements to the same health care providers. . . . Moreover, each regulation is usually supported by some interest group, and a regulation that appears unnecessary to one group may be essential to another." After noting that most health and safety regulations require conformance to certain standards and include sanctions for noncompliance, she suggested that a better regulatory scheme might provide rewards and positive incentives for compliance.

Havighurst (1977), on the other hand, has urged the replacement of regulations with marketplace incentives and controls, at least in the areas of planning, cost containment, and manpower development. He advocates the vigorous enforcement of federal antitrust laws to promote diversity, and thus competition, among providers. This view questions the dominance of the AMA, AHA, and large hospital systems in the market and suggests that price competition will be in the public interest. In effect, it requires the replacement of cost and quality regulatory controls with a different regulatory scheme: Federal Trade Commission surveillance of monopolistic practices in the health care industry. Adversly affected by such a policy would be shared services (e.g., cooperative laundry and computer services for groups of hospitals) and other multi-institutional arrangements.

Weiner (1980) says that "the role of regulation must be reexamined" and that regulation should be used creatively as a framework for free market-type innovations, just as the threat of regulation in the form of "cost caps" encouraged a voluntary cost-containment effort by the hospital industry in 1979-1980. An example of innovation is Weiner's proposal for "outcome-oriented regulations," which establish objectives or goals but leave the techniques to private decision makers. He concludes that "[t]he health care system is too diverse to force all decisions into predetermined channels and processes, or to sustain the assumption that only governmental agencies can make decisions that achieve desired regulatory objectives."

There are, of course, other viewpoints about the problems engendered by regulations in the health care system, and their solutions. Kinzer (1977) criticizes the existing web of state and federal regulations and recommends simplifications through federalization of some programs (e.g., Medicaid) and removing health controls from political pressures. Others contend that the real problem is defining the relationship between government and the private sector. "What we need is not a 'government takeover' but a rational division of labor between the public and private sectors; a cooperative effort aimed at benefiting the citizenry rather than aggrandizing either sector" (Jonas et al., 1977, p. 326).

In the end, however, the environment for the administrator of health care services will inevitably include both government and a multitude of quasi-government and private regulations. It will be imbued with the economic and political pluralism of values so evident in all the debates and decisions about health policy. Diversity within an ordered federal system is ensured by the legal and constitutional underpinnings of society, as well as the historical orientation of the American people toward individualism and the limited role of government paternalism.

CASE

A Patient's Confrontation with the Health System*

I would like to share with you the concerns of the family struggling with Alzheimer's disease. I feel I can best relate this to you by my own personal tragedy, not to exploit what happened to our family, but because it is typical of thousands of families who may be crying silently for help. I can tell you that it is like a funeral that never ends. My husband was a handsome, vital, athletic man, a civic leader, a public speaker, a highly respected business man. He was administrative vice president of his company. He is now a statistic. He is permanently hospitalized, not knowing his family or speaking a word in the past four years. He requires total care as the physical deterioration takes its toll. I have a husband, but I speak of him in the past tense. I am not a divorcee; I am not a widow; but where do I fit?

I began noticing eccentricities, withdrawal from society, disinterest, lack of communication about 12 years ago. In 1970, he was forced to retire. I excused, guided, and denied that this was happening. I found part-time employment, but each day it was more difficult to be away from him as he became more confused. We dipped into our savings, were managing on very little income, losing everything we had. I finally admitted we needed help. We had no neurologists in our area of South Dakota, so a daughter persuaded us to come to Minneapolis, where she could lend a hand. I decided to uproot (my husband could no longer make decisions). We left our home and friends of 32 years and moved to the city. There my husband was given complete neurological testing. I was given the diagnosis in a hospital waiting room filled with people. The doctor said, "Your husband has Alzheimer's disease, a progressive, irreversible, brain deterioration, for which there is no known cause or treatment. That's the way it is. You'll have to go on from there." He excused himself and left to see another patient. I have never seen that doctor again. I was given no explanation of what Alzheimer's disease is, what to expect, how I might learn to cope, nor was I directed to someone who might be able to direct me in the monumental problems ahead.

I was in a strange city, and I was not free to find employment. I tried work situations that might provide rent-free housing, but even that was impossible for me alone. We moved five times in 18 months, by necessity. That is, I moved. He came with me. We lived in an ever-diminishing world. His company of 25 years chose to terminate all of his benefits (disability, pension, insurance) because of this "early retirement." I was advised by an attorney not to fight it. I had moved to a different state, and the company had its own lawyers who could interpret the language the way they chose.

---

*Based on material presented at Senator Thomas Eagleton's Sub-Committee Hearing on Human Resources and HEW Appropriations, July 15, 1980, Washington, D.C.

I was unaware of VA assistance, and my husband could not communicate that information. I had accumulated living expenses, hospital costs, relocating costs, legal expenses, until we had no reserve. In this unreal world, I felt no sense of belonging. How could one explain this to strangers, and there were often embarrassing situations. People usually turned away. With the 24-hour vigil, I became totally exhausted—physically and emotionally. I felt I must be prepared for any emergency, night or day. It became frightening, living with this stranger who might push me or twist my arm, or throw things at the television set. The loving, gentle husband I once knew was no longer there.

This became an obsession with our entire family. I knew that we simply could not live that way any longer. We needed a care facility that could provide the necessary custodial care. We visited 20 nursing homes in one day, and finally found one that would take him. He was admitted the next day. The heavy guilt that the family endures is indescribable when this step is necessary at such an early age. We question if we are "copping out." I also wondered how long I could manage the costs, for insurance and Medicare neither one covers *this* problem. I inquired of Medical Assistance and was told that my car was too new for me to qualify. My husband stayed in the nursing home nearly three months, when I received a call that he had become violent and they refused to keep him, even overnight. In my opinion, they panicked, because of lack of training. They did not know how to care for this kind of patient. Most nursing homes are not equipped or staffed to handle this. At any rate, they sent him to a private hospital, where he remained for six days, before I could convince the hospital personnel to check his chart, which read: "This man has no insurance, no Medicare (he wasn't old enough). In an emergency, call the VA Hospital." They did, and he was admitted. Fortunately, he remains there. But many of our veterans, even career service men, are being turned away because they are suffering from an "untreatable" disease and there must be room for the "treatable" patients.

After my husband's admission to a permanent facility, and realizing that this meant a lifetime, I came home to my very small apartment feeling a despair that is impossible to put into words. I was suddenly alone and desolate. I do not wish to sound overly dramatic, but I am attempting to state facts so that you may better understand the effects of Alzheimer's disease on our families.

As for myself, I was becoming a nonperson and realized that my thinking must be turned around. My children were caring and supporting, again a blessing, for not all families find this to be true . . . some simply cannot deal with it and walk away. Acceptance is probably the most difficult step for our families, and there are thousands of us. For a long time we look for improvement and for things to get better. This is not true with Alzheimer's disease. The condition only worsens. We need guidance and research methods of helping these families find appropriate medical professionals who are knowledgeable about this unique problem that is not a "mental illness" but is indeed a physical condition.

We need assistance with the appropriate type of care as the disease progresses, whether it is day care, respite care, home care, or long-term care. One individual cannot survive very long when dealing with this around the clock. We must find ways to provide care facilities for our people who have no place to go. We need direction in business matters, for we must plan ahead, for when the afflicted individual is declared incompetent and will be unable to sign documents of any kind. The remaining spouse is usually the one who is the responsible party and may be untrained in such matters. Legal affairs may require attention, especially if there is property involved. The very real tragedy is for the younger family who is faced with the disease that will continue on for a period of many years. There are often young children who will need to be educated and cared for. There are many variables in patients, and therefore the duration of the illness varies also. Physical deterioration is usually a determining factor. In our family you will recall that it has been at least 12 years.

Education for the whole world is a top priority. We need to use every resource possible so that all will know what this strange word, Alzheimer's, is about. The general public needs to know, but most important, the medical community needs to know. In the beginning, I found it incredible that physicians and other medical professionals were not knowledgeable about Alzheimer's disease. It is indeed a happy surprise when we find some who are informed.

We have been advised to divorce, and some have. Some lose their homes and most material things, as I have. We have already lost a loved one in this slow, devastating process that diminishes one to a shell that simply breathes. We can do nothing for that victim at this time. Research is the hope for the future. We can help ourselves and do much to help others. This is the reason for my involvement today. I made a choice of helping drowning families in order that they might avoid some of the pitfalls I experienced. There was no one there when our family needed such a lift.

I now counsel families all across the nation and have established a "network" to provide necessary information and support. My files are filled with poignant letters from coast to coast. I personally answer every one and when necessary follow up with a telephone call. I have founded two separate kinds of family support groups. In our National Association for Alzheimer's Disease and Related Disorders, I am privileged to serve on the Board of Directors and also serve as National Chairman for Program Development. Since December 1979, we have established major groups in 15 states with four others awaiting acceptance. Many others are in the development process. Our families have lost, but we choose to continue. Perhaps our greatest loss is our spirit, for we have been degraded to a point of "begging for help" when we are already shattered.

Discussion Questions

1. *Identify the various health service organizations that (a) were involved and (b) should be involved in dealing with the problems confronting Mr. and Mrs. Glaze.*

2. *Suggest improvements that would enhance the actions as well as interactions of various health service organizations providing services to Mr. and Mrs. Glaze.*

FURTHER READING

BEGUN, J. W. *Professionalism and the Public Interest: Price and Quality in Optometry.* Boston: The MIT Press, 1981.

DONABEDIAN, A., S. J. AXELROD, and L. WYZEWIANSKI. *Medical Care Chart Book.* Ann Arbor, Mich.: Health Administration Press, 1980.

FALKSON, N. J. *HMOs and The Politics of Health System Reform.* Chicago: American Hospital Association, 1980.

FEDER, J., J. HOLAHAN, and T. MARMOR, eds. *National Health Insurance: Conflicting Goals and Policy Choices.* Washington, D.C.: Urban Institute, 1980.

LUFT, H. S. *Health Maintenance Organizations: Dimensions of Performance.* Wiley-Interscience. New York: Wiley, 1981.

MILLER, A. E. and M. G. MILLER. *Options for Health and Health Care: The Coming of Post-Clinical Medicine.* Wiley-Interscience. New York: Wiley, 1981.

RAFFEL, M. W. *The U.S. Health System: Origins and Functions.* New York: Wiley, 1980.

SMITH, D. B. *Long-term Care in Transition; The Regulation of Nursing Homes.* Ann Arbor, Mich.: Health Administration Press, 1981.

STARKWEATHER, D. B. *Hospital Mergers.* Ann Arbor, Mich.: Health Administration Press, 1981.

WILLIAMS, S. J. *Issues in Health Services.* New York: Wiley, 1980.

WILLIAMS, S., and P. TORRENS, eds. *Introduction to Health Services.* New York: Wiley, 1980.

14

The Future of Health Services Management

Explaining the past and describing the present are easier than predicting the future. Still, lessons from the past and present can point the way for future developments. The objective of this chapter is to consider some of the future trends and issues confronting the health system, the health service organizations within the larger system, and the health services manager.

THE HEALTH SYSTEM

Value Confrontation

Two basic values are critical in determining the future structure and function of health services. The first centers around the debate between individual and collective responsibility for health. Society has increasingly assumed the obligation of providing its citizens with a cleaner and healthier environment primarily through instituting controls on water, air, food products, and working conditions. In the name of protecting the community, public health measures have also been required which affect individuals more directly, such as vaccination and fluoridation. Now, some people are calling for an extension of these controls and measures that promote the health and safety of individuals. Seatbelts and motorcycle helmets are already required. Smoking bans, marijuana penalties, the laetrile controversy, and restrictive licensure of new professions (such as marital counseling) may lead to consideration of such imaginative schemes as mandatory exercise and weight-control programs for public employees. In response to what some people consider rampant government paternalism is the growing popularity of wholistic health groups, self-care activities, volunteer hospice organizations, and other evidence of individuals assuming the responsibility for their own health. Whatever form these developments take, public policy will have an important impact on the range and types of health care programs the government will be administering or regulating in the future.

The second issue relates to the first and is partially dependent on it: the debate between regulation and competition in the health care field. Successful deregulation of the airlines industry has contributed to extensive discussion in Congress and elsewhere about the pros and cons of allowing or promoting free-market forces in the health services field, as opposed to increasing government regulation. The outcome of these discussions will help determine the environment of tomorrow for the health care services administrator. Whether regulation is based at the federal, state, or local level is not as crucial as the extent of regulation. No one, however, seems to be predicting the absence of regulation. Regulation and litigation are bound to be facts of administrative life for the foreseeable future.

Disease Prevention and Health Promotion

The rediscovery of disease prevention and health promotion opens new avenues for the health system. Currently, the movement focuses on the individual's responsibility to improve and maintain his or her own health through the self-care/life-style reform/wholistic approach. Stemming from the civil rights and feminist movements of the 1960s and 1970s, this new and growing emphasis questions the authority of established institutions and the essential worth of the traditional approach to health care, and it proclaims the individual's duty to control his or her own destiny.

Some problems arise from this approach. Kronenfeld (1980) points out three major areas of difficulty:

1. The approach fails to account for structural factors beyond the individual's control. Although behaviors such as smoking, diet, and exercise are within the individual's province, other problems, such as air pollution and similar environmental hazards, demand action on a different level, one of structural change in our society.

2. Implicit in the self-help movement is the danger of developing a sophisticated "blame the victim" approach, that is, of accusing poor or uneducated individuals of not participating in the movement and thereby causing their own poor health.

3. To achieve meaningful change, the self-help movement must reach large numbers of people and must change multitudes of individual behaviors. At present, the movement is concentrated in the middle class and is therefore limited in scope.

Perhaps the most insidious failing of the self-help movement is that it reduces demand for more and better health services. The wholistic approach diverts attention from structural reforms and improvement in providing medical services (Salmon and Berliner, 1979).

Despite these problems, the movement has had a significant effect on legitimate health service activities. The recent formation of the U.S. DHEW Task Force on Disease Prevention and Health Promotion (1979) is a good illustration. This group focuses on three major areas—life-style, environment, and personal health—and on the major health problems of our society:

- Smoking and health
- Nutrition

- Alcohol abuse
- Exercise and fitness

- Hypertension
- Child health
- Adolescent pregnancy
- Environmental toxicology
- Occupational health
- Dental disease

- Drug abuse
- Hospital infection
- Sexually transmitted diseases
- Accidents
- Mental health

Cutting across these various problem areas, a number of recommendations have been formulated. They include:

1. Federal support for personal preventive health services through health insurance, as well as in departmental direct service delivery programs.

2. Efforts to strengthen the prevention capabilities of state and local health and education agencies, health planning agencies, and HMOs through both project and formula grants for carefully planned programs directed at high-priority problems.

3. More comprehensive authority to determine and enforce health and safety standards with respect to food and alcohol; better tailoring of research programs to regulatory needs in environmental and occupational health; and provision of a mechanism to ensure a prior HEW review of health-related decisions of the regulatory agencies.

4. Expanding the supply of prevention manpower in such key categories as epidemiology and environmental toxicology.

5. Provision of economic incentives for the delivery of preventive services through CHAP and HMOs.

6. Giving leadership to prevention activities through measures such as the issuance of a Surgeon General's Report on Prevention, the establishment of a Prevention Roundtable to coordinate federal prevention efforts, and the initiation of a National Health Promotion Program.

7. Expansion of the prevention knowledge base through community-based risk-reduction demonstration programs, the establishment of long-term prospective epidemiologic population studies, and studies on the childhood determinants of behavior, as well as a number of studies specific to the problems noted above. [US DHEW, 1979]

Whether these recommendations actually materialize remains to be seen, yet the rediscovery of health prevention and promotion will be an important factor in the future of health services.

Financial Arrangements:
The Case of National Health Insurance

The unrelenting debate on the role of national health insurance will no doubt continue through the 1980s. Past experience suggests, however, that it is unlikely that there will be any sweeping changes in the financing of health services, particularly in the passage of a comprehensive national health insurance program. Partly, this may be attributed to the continued opposition by the medical profession to such legislation. However, several other and perhaps more important factors are limiting passage of a national health insurance scheme (Burns, n.d.). First is the pervasive feeling that the country cannot afford the cost of such a program and that it is politically impossible to increase taxes for such an activity. A second inhibiting factor is the belief that resources currently devoted to health services are not capable of providing services promised within the national health insurance scheme. Third is the feeling that the health service system is "uncontrollable" and the constant revelations of mismanagement in Medicare and Medicaid tend to reinforce this general feeling. Finally, there is the polarization of values regarding basic social policy questions, including the role of private versus insurance carriers, eligibility, and cost sharing by the general population.

Although national health insurance is unlikely, various incremental modifications will be made in existing financial programs together with an ever-increasing set of controls and standards on all types of providers. As described by Stevens and Stevens (1974):

> Even without any form of national health insurance, the continuation of the present piecemeal approach to the funding of medical care will lead to stronger controls over providers, national standards of care and benefits, and greater administrative centralization. . . .
>
> Indeed, in the long run, the pragmatic, incremental approach to health legislation—extension of existing, programs and controls until a major rationalization is inevitable—may turn out to be more radical than that of the health insurance options now being suggested [because of the inequities caused without a rational plan] . . . .
>
> It may be, of course, that nothing approaching "equity" is possible in the provision of medical services. The problems of allocation (or tampering with the market, depending on your perspective) may be just so great, no matter how extensive the funding or how great the willingness to restructure providers, that equity is just not possible. . . .

Despite the failure to pass a national health insurance program, it is likely that the private sector will further expand its coverage options in a number of areas, including dental health and in health promotion and prevention activities.

Financial Arrangements:
The Case of Categorical Programs

Federal health programs are often described as a labyrinth of overlapping and often conflicting service activities. These have historically included a range of programs to help states or local communities establish mental health programs, run community health centers, provide maternal and child health services, as well as operate rate control, venereal disease, or immunization programs. The next few years are likely to see a major change in the allocation of federal funds supporting these various types of categorical programs. Under the change, separate categorical health programs that give grants to states and local agencies are likely to be gathered up into "block grants" given to the states; for example, basic health services block grants and preventive health services block grants. The block grants would give states a smaller proportion of the total of all FY81 current services level budget. Under this arrangement each state has discretion to allocate funds according to its own set of priorities. While states would not be able to allocate these funds for cash payments, for construction, or for the purchase of land and facilities, states are free to allocate funds to any particular program area and exclude others. The implications are substantial. Most obvious is the reduction of funds available for various service programs. Severe program cuts will be required to accommodate the reduction of dollars. Less obvious but perhaps more important is the shift of decision-making from Washington to 50 state capitals throughout the country. The shift will require the realignment of coalitions and pressure groups that heretofore were successful in the design and implementation of these various categorical programs. The ability of block grants to continue to truly meet the needs of state and local communities is contingent on the ability of local leaders to organize and assign priorities to health needs in accordance with the availability of funds (DeFriese et al., 1980).

Evaluation and Technology Assessment

New medical technology (defined as sets of techniques, drugs, equipment, and procedures used by health care professionals in the delivery of health services (Banta and Sanes, 1978) will continue to exert a profound influence in the 1980s. The major difference, however, will be greater emphasis on the evaluation of technological innovations. At the minimum, evaluation will focus on assuring the simple safety and efficacy of new technology. More likely, however, there will be an attempt to develop a comprehensive evaluation effort to examine costs, to consider the effects of providing technology on organizations and on the delivery of health services, and to assess the broader social and ethical implications of the new technology (Fineberg and Hiatt, 1979).

At present, few comprehensive evaluations exist, yet many studies have challenged much of current technology. For example, the development of intensive care units was a major technological advance and was estimated in 1974 to account for nearly 10% of all hospital costs. Since their implementation, several have cast serious doubt on the value of intensive care units for some types of patients. Similarly, the use of mass screening programs, various diagnostic tools such as Pap tests and chest x-rays, mass-immunization efforts such as swine flu inoculations, and the extensive use of life-support systems in the Karen Quinlan case, have all been challenged. Organ transplants and renal dialysis have drawn criticism since the common cold still defies modern science.

The development of a comprehensive evaluation effort will not be easy. Significant methodological and political obstacles must be overcome. Nevertheless, efforts toward evaluation and assessment will continue along the following lines (HSRC, 1979):

1. *Short-run studies of the existing regulatory process*
   - How do health systems agencies, PSROs, and other health regulatory agencies make decisions about medical technology?
   - What is the most useful way to present information about medical technology to these regulatory bodies?
   - What are the full costs associated with regulation of technology acquisition and who bears the cost?

2. *Long-run studies of environment and technology change*
   - To what extent can new methods of reimbursing health care providers affect patterns of adoption and use?
   - What characteristics of health maintenance organizations are important determinants of patterns of adoption and use?
   - How does government patent policy affect innovation in health care?
   - What effects can or will areawide limits on capital expenditure for health care have on the pattern of adoption?
   - What are the effects of competition, manpower specialization, and group practice on technological adoption, development, and use?
   - To what extent does the present system of medical injury compensation bias technology decisions in favor of overacquisition and overuse?

3. *Studies of social values affecting medical technology*
   - At what point in the rise of national expenditures for medical care does cost containment become a desirable, even primary, goal?
   - If application of resources to medical care must be constrained, what kinds of services should be curtailed and for whom?
   - What kind of rationing for availability of different kinds of technology are acceptable?

A final issue associated with the question of evaluation and assessment is the extent to which these findings can be translated into policy and actual practice in the delivery of health services. Evaluation and technology assessment have little value unless this information can be used by actual providers of health services.

THE HEALTH SERVICE ORGANIZATION

The Reality of Organizational Creation and Survival

The traditional view of health service organizations tends to focus on the ongoing operations and takes for granted the continued existence and survival of the organization. Yet there is a growing realization that organizations in general and health service organizations in particular follow life cycles similar to the biological models applied to living organisms (Kimberly et al., 1980). Organizational survival can no longer be taken for granted. For example, there was a steady increase in the number of hospital closures during the mid-1970s (McNeil and Williams, 1978). Other organizations have had similar experiences; for example, 25% of the medical group practices in operation in 1969 disbanded by 1975 (Todd and MacNamara, 1971). These trends are likely-to continue because of several environmental factors which affect the stability of organizations and thereby contribute to their ultimate demise. These environmental factors are (Hernandez and Kaluzny, 1982):

- *Inadequate reimbursement:* Medicaid and Medicare are often cited for contributing to the financial problems of many health service organizations.

- *Inconsistent reimbursement formulas:* those that disallow certain categories of expenses also contribute greatly to financial problems, particularly of hospitals. These inadequacies and inconsistencies often force the institutions to absorb costs above established ceilings.

- *Inflation:* The American Hospital Association estimates that total hospital expenditures rose 14.4% between January 1979 and January 1980. Reimbursement formulas by many hospitals have not kept pace with these expenses. Coupled with an aging or obsolete physical plant, inflation has forced the closure of many institutions.

- *Management problems:* Lack of management control manifested by poor accounting practices, inadequate collection efforts, and an inability to operate efficient staffing patterns has contributed to the poor financial conditions of many institutions as well as to the volatile nature of many of the group practice settings.

- *Social factors:* Basic population shifts from inner cities to suburbs have greatly affected service areas. Since these shifts are often accompanied by ethnic or racial redistributions, organizations often have a difficult time functioning within their given environments.

As the issue of survival has gained attention, so has the question of emerging organizations. New organizations are developing with increasing frequency. For example, new medical schools, HMOs, and consortia arrangements involving various types of health care facilities are continually emerging.

Although our understanding of these types of organizations is limited, the growth trend is likely to continue, and several factors facilitate this development. First is the growing disenchantment with existing organizational arrangements. Many health service organizations are becoming more complex and more formal, making it difficult for them to adapt to the changing needs and expectations of consumers. It is often easier to simply bypass these organizations and create new ones to meet specific needs and expectations within the community.

A second contributing factor is the allocation of federal funds for specific diseases. To the extent that these dollars are available, they facilitate the development of new organizational structures to provide services to meet specific categorical disease problems. As federal funds become available, they quickly attract a constituency to support the continuation of these categorical programs. This reinforces the basic structure developed to provide categorical services.

Humanistic Goals versus Bureaucratic Needs versus Professional Response

Health service organizations are currently under seige to develop managerial accountability and to ensure control, particularly cost/fiscal control within organizations. Unfortunately, in some cases accountability is being developed at the expense of a long-standing humanistic attitude toward both patients/clients and organizational personnel. While the attitude has been eroding over the past years, the push for accountability will accelerate the change if not complete the transition. The overall impact on organizations, efficiency remains to be determined. However, the immediate effects will be apparent to both personnel and patients.

The push for accountability will increase the likelihood of "burnout"— that is, the loss of the general feeling of job satisfaction resulting from the individual's ability to act in a caring and helpful way toward other individuals in need of help. Personnel, particularly the personnel involved with service delivery and midlevel managers within the organization who have much to do with the overall services provided by the organization, will be the first victims of increasing centralization and standardization of procedures.

Individuals functioning in this type of setting are forced to defend themselves against what often appear to be arbitrary administrative actions. Unionization among health providers (particularly service personnel) as well as the frequency of legal action against both professionals and institutions are expected reactions.

The particular tragedy is that patients as well as the health service worker are often the victims of the quest for accountability. Rules and regulations are arbitrarily applied and are usually inflexible to meet the varied and complex problems of providing health services.

Design Configurations

During the last decade, the traditional view of health service organizations has been drastically altered. For example, the idea of a "community hospital" —an institution solely operating within the community within which it is located—has been replaced with the idea of "multi-hospital systems." Under this arrangement, individual facilities participate through a consolidated or cooperative management structure. This approach to hospitals is likely to continue and may expand as many rural hospitals struggle to survive.

Perhaps more interesting is the development of various organizational forms involving other types of health service organizations. Although the future function of local health agencies remains in doubt, it is clear that these organizations will need to reorganize their basic structures in order to function even at their current level of operations. Presently, local health agencies operate in a fairly isolated county or city format. In the future, these organizations will consolidate into multi-county/city–county arrangements, to enhance access to resources and increase their political power.

The increasing complexity and dynamic nature of the environment within which health service organizations function will force basic design changes, particularly in the design of hospitals and health departments as major health service delivery organizations. One of the changes will be the development of adhocracies rather than traditional professional or bureaucratic structures. The adhocracy provides a structure that accommodates various disciplines relevant to meeting the changing health care needs of the community. Adhocracies are characterized as:

> Highly organic structures, with little formalization and behavior, high horizontal job specialization based on formal training, a tendency to group the specialists in a functional unit for housekeeping purposes but to employ them in small market-based project teams to do their work; a reliance on liaison devices to encourage mutual adjustment—the key coordinating mechanism— within and between these teams; and selected decentralization to and within these teams, which are located at various places in the organization and in-

volve various mixtures of line managers and staff and operating experts (Mintzberg, 1979).

The adhocracy is designed to undertake projects that serve specific clients and segments of the community. The development of teams mobilizes resources that reflect the interdisciplinary nature of many health care problems. Moreover, their ad hoc nature is consistent with the short time frame which resources are allocated to resolve specific problems. Coordination is maintained through an overall matrix format. However, the prime coordinating mechanism is mutual adjustment among organizational personnel.

Although both hospitals and local health agencies will be expanding their organizational structures to accommodate more adequately an ever-turbulent environment, the 1980s will also continue to see expansion of self-help-type organizations. These groups will continue to focus on specific social and economic problems faced by individuals with particular chronic conditions. These organizations supplement the function of the family in many respects. They provide individuals suffering from long-term chronic problems with the support mechanisms necessary to ensure their survival.

THE HEALTH SERVICES MANAGER

Management is viewed as an important component of the health care system and to many it is considered the panacea for a number of its problems.

Management Training*

The 1980s will see considerable changes in the manner and method of preparing health service managers. Several innovations need to be considered. First, given the obvious need for expertise in financial management, health care managers will have greater preparation in this area. In fact, the needs are so great that it is likely that specialized degrees will emerge (e.g., a master's in health care finance) to meet the needs of the field. This might suggest specialization with respect to specific functions within the overall management process (e.g., finance, operations research, or organizational development) rather than in the service area distinctions which have characterized the field (e.g., medical care, hospital administration, or community health services).

Moreover, this change may reflect maturation within the field itself. Academic programs are preparing managers for entry-level positions in various types of health service organizations. Entry-level positions will require specialized skills and a basic understanding of the unique qualities of health

---

*Based on material initially presented in Kaluzny (1980).

service organizations. Once individuals are within the organization, they will advance within the organization or within different types of health service organizations until they reach the chief executive officer position or their own level of aspiration. Advancement will be based on functional specialization rather than specialization in a particular health services area.

A second development will be the growing identity of academic programs around the generic idea of health administration as opposed to particular categorical areas such as hospital administration or medical care administration. As indicated, programs have traditionally been isolated within universities and divided into specific categorical program interests. These distinctions are no longer relevant, given the dynamic nature of health services and the recognition for greater functional rather than programmatic specialization.

A third development will center on a range of teaching modalities. These will include fairly specific changes in classroom instruction, such as programmed learning, case studies, and so on, but more important, a concentrated effort to meet Mintzberg's (1975) criticism that administrators need more than cognitive learning. The medical education model with its emphasis on basic and clinical sciences with associated faculty in each area provides a useful paradigm. Using this approach, practicing administrators will become more closely aligned with teaching programs and assume part-time academic positions as clinical faculty. Students will be assigned to work with these clinical professors following their basic academic course work. In a sense, the program will be divided between the basic sciences (i.e., the anatomy and physiology of health services) and clinical training in the intervention and management of health service organizations and programs. This division of activity will provide the opportunity to practice skills in a relatively controlled environment, providing feedback and ensuring mastery of the required skill.

Although this approach is similar to the existing idea of the administrative residency, it has some subtle differences which need emphasis. First, the practicing administrators are part of the basic academic program and share the content of that program. Under the traditional residency program, many administrators serving as preceptors either have no formal administrative training or had formal training early in the development of the field. Both conditions make it difficult if not impossible to create an opportunity to translate cognitive learning into skill learning. The field is now beginning to stabilize, and many administrators interested in teaching have had the basic cognitive learning. They will be able to demonstrate the application of this learning to field situations.

Second, the field itself has matured and there is a developing rapport between field sites and academic programs. Organizations are looking toward the academic programs for technical assistance in dealing with current organizational and administrative problems. These relationships provide the atmosphere and the facilities to enhance administrative training. Involvement of academic personnel in operational problems is an enriching experience for the academic as well as for the practitioner, and provides an important bridge from the academic to the practice world.

A final development will be the expanding role of continuing education and external degree programs. Although these are already in operation at several universities, their importance will increase as the programs attempt to meet the needs of the field. Moreover, these attempts will facilitate and strengthen relationships between the academic programs and operating agencies and provide the basis for a close and sustained interaction with practicing administrators.

The extent of curriculum innovation will be greatly influenced by the types of problems confronting health service administrators. Although the problems may vary, cost containment will probably be the single most important issue confronting most administrators in the foreseeable future. Moreover, the adequacy of the administrator will probably be judged solely on her or his ability to effectively deal with matters of organizational finance.

The ability of academic programs to prepare administrators to deal with financial problems will thus be their major challenge and provide the stimulus for academic innovation. Since the resolution of these problems will be difficult and highly visible to the external public, it will not be possible for the academic community to ignore the perceived discrepancy between how their graduates are performing and how relevant actors think they should be performing. This discrepancy will create a performance gap and will be the driving force for future curriculum innovation.

Managerial/Organizational Assessment

One of the major problems of management is the lack of any good indicator of organizational operations and performance. Although the area suffers from serious methodological as well as conceptual problems, systematic efforts are currently under way to develop measures of organizational operations that are useful guides for administrative decision making (Van de Ven and Ferry, 1980). These approaches are being applied to the systematic study of health service organizations (Kaluzny and Veney, 1980) and include efforts to develop indices of hospital performance (Griffith, 1978) as well as overall indicators of organizational design and process characteristics (AUPHA, 1981; AHA, 1980).

In the future, it is likely that managers will have at their disposal not only an array of managerial techniques and strategies but a set of tools to provide some indication of how well the organization is doing in terms of performance and operations. It is likely that these indicators will encompass all areas of organizational operations, with increasing emphasis on assessing the human aspects of organizations. Specifically,

> organizational assessment is the systematic measurement of organizational functioning from the perspective of the behavioral system, using scientific methods and procedures and characterized by the measurement of a range of variables encompassing the functioning of the total organizations, and making use of multiple methods of measurement over time. [Lawler et al., 1980, p. 10]

This information will be important to health service managers. For example, assessment data will provide valuable insight in job choice decisions (Lawler et al., 1980). Managers confronting new employment opportunities form opinions about the new organization on the basis of hearsay information or description of the situation by those with a vested interest in presenting a particular perspective. All these data are suspect. The availability of assessment data provides the new manager with a more realistic expectation about the new organization and increases his or her ability to perceive the situation correctly within a shorter time frame.

In addition, assessment data are particularly helpful in diagnosing problems involving the basic design components of the organization and in making decisions with respect to new organizational structures, pay systems, programs, and technologies. Unfortunately, most of these decisions are based on poor data and as a result, the solutions become the new problems; symptoms are perceived as causes and many problems simply go unnoticed. The availability of assessment data would enhance the manager's ability to diagnose problems and derive appropriate solutions to these problems.

In addition, the systematic diagnosis of organizational problems has a significant effect on the ability to produce and evaluate organizational change. The availability of ongoing assessment data provides a benchmark and thus permits an opportunity to assess the impact of change on various aspects of organizational operations. This would require a shift in focus by health service managers. Instead of advocating a particular solution, the manager needs to present solutions as a series of options and use assessment data to evaluate these options as they affect the community as well as the organization. In essence, this approach requires a

> shift from the advocacy of a specific reform to the advocacy of the seriousness of the problem and hence to the advocacy of persistence in alternative reform efforts should the first one fail. The political stance would become "this is a serious problem." We propose to initiate policy "A" on an experimental basis. And if after five years there has been no significant improvement we should shift to policy "B." And making explicit that a given problem solution is only one of several that the administrator or party could in good conscience advocate and by having already a plausible alternative, the administrator could afford honest evaluation of outcomes. Negative results,

the failure of the first program, would not jeopardize his job for his job
would be to keep after the problem until something was found and worked.
[Campbell, 1969, p. 410]

Although it is likely that these types of management tools will be available, a remaining question is the extent to which they will be effectively and creatively used within the health service organization. There is the obvious time lag between the development of technology and its ultimate implementation and adoption within the organization. As attention has been given to the manner in which the physician adopts new technology, similar attention must be given to the role of the health manager and his or her adoption of managerial technology.

The Role of Management

The past decade has witnessed the growth of management; it now plays a significant role in health service organizations. To some extent, this growth has been accompanied by a set of expectations that far exceed the potential of management. Nevertheless, expansion of management will continue, partly because managers are increasing their ability to deal with relevant problems facing health service organizations. Expansion is also a function of default. That is, the increased differentiation of organizations will facilitate more centralized administrative control. Other groups will have less interest in the total operation of the organization and will be less willing to spend the resources and efforts necessary to control the organization (Pfeffer and Salancik, 1978).

Although the expansion of the managerial role will continue, this expansion is likely to be accompanied by a better understanding of what managers actually do in both substantive and symbolic terms. In substantive terms, management will continue as a processor and responder to the demands and constraints confronting the organization. In this role, the manager will determine how to adapt the organization to meet the constraints of its environments and will implement the adaptations.

An increasingly important role of managers is to take action to modify the environment within which the organization functions. In this role, rather than simply dealing with the problem of using resources, the major focus is on the problem of acquiring resources. Managerial activities focus on altering the system of constraints and dependencies confronting the organization. As described by Pfeffer and Salancik (1978):

> What happens in an organization is not only a function of the organization, its structure, its leadership, its procedures, or its goals. What happens is also a consequence of the environment and the particular constituencies and constraints deriving from that environment.

In addition to an increased understanding of the substantive content of the managerial role, there will be an increasing recognition of the symbolic role of management. Again as described by Pfeffer and Salancik (1978):

> In creating the symbolic role of the manager, the organization also creates a mechanism for dealing with external demands. When external demands cannot be met because of constraints on the organization, the administrator can be removed. Replacing the leadership, who has come to symbolize the organization to the various interest groups, may be sufficient to release pressures on the organization. As long as all believe that the administrator actually affects the organization, then replacement signals a change taken in response to external demands. The change communicates an intent to comply and this intent may be as useful as actual compliance for satisfying external organizations (p. 264).

Although not a new or particularly novel idea, the recognition that managers play symbolic roles provides an opportunity to place the managerial role in a more realistic perspective. That is, many of the organizational activities and problems are purely a function of the larger external environment in which the organization functions. Management is able to influence only a small portion of these activities and is often expendable in attempts to realign design with environmental changes. The realization of this symbolic role of managers provides them with an opportunity to gain insight into larger events, of which they are often victims. Through this insight managers will have an opportunity to intervene more effectively, thereby influencing the larger events.

EXERCISE

The Future of Health Services

Step 1: Assessment of Individual Values

Below is a listing of a series of statements regarding various aspects of the health services system and organizations within that system. Please indicate on the scale from 1 to 5 the extent to which you agree or disagree with the following statements.*

Statement	Strongly Agree • • • Strongly Disagree
1. The age structure of the population will continue to shift toward an older population; the median age will continue to increase, and	

---

*Statements 1 to 33 are adapted in part from "Environmental Assessment of the Hospital Industry, 1979." Chicago: American Hospital Association, 1979.

Statement	Strongly Agree	•	•	•	Strongly Disagree
a larger proportion of the population will be concentrated in the over-65 group.	1	2	3	4	5
2. Population shifts will continue producing local changes in demand for health services.	—	—	—	—	—
3. Public interest in and concern about health and health care activities will persist. Attitudes toward personal fitness, diet, nutrition, and preventive services will remain favorable and will be sustained by leisure activities and continued emphasis on personal fulfillment.	—	—	—	—	—
4. Business and industry will increasingly attempt to intervene in decisions about health care delivery because of the costs of health insurance, and will experiment increasingly with sponsorship or health programs for employees in the future.	—	—	—	—	—
5. The direction of national health policy is toward reducing the capacity of the inpatient sector of the hospital industry in relation to population in order to control costs. National health planning guidelines and planning agencies will be increasingly influential in shaping the structure of the industry of the future.	—	—	—	—	—
6. Health service organizations will increasingly compete with each other and with new organizational entities to maintain or increase their share of various market segments.	—	—	—	—	—

Statement	Strongly Agree	•	•	•	Strongly Disagree
7. An important consequence of increased competition will be the continued growth of multi-institutional and shared services arrangements.	—	—	—	—	—
8. The number of investor-owned hospitals and beds will continue to increase, although less rapidly than in the recent past.	—	—	—	—	—
9. The number of specialized limited-purpose institutions providing services for a particular patient population will increase dramatically, especially ambulatory and home care services.	—	—	—	—	—
10. Because of the gradually aging population, nursing and convalescent homes will have an increasingly large population to serve between 1980 and 2000.	—	—	—	—	—
11. Greater sensitivity to the special needs of the terminally ill patient will provide for continuing interest in hospices, but shortages of trained personnel to staff them and uncertainties as to their cost will retard adoption of hospices by many institutions.	—	—	—	—	—
12. The financing of hospital operations will continue to be the focal point of two countervailing forces. On the one hand are the steadily increasing pressures to contain costs. On the other are					

Statement	Strongly Agree • • •	Strongly Disagree

the growing financial requirements of institutions. The
forces will affect individual
hospitals differently.
     —   — — —   —

13. Feeling the pressure of tax-
payer concern, state and local
governments will respond with
proposals to cut spending for
health programs, along with
public hospitals and other
governmental services. This
may take the form of closure
of institutions, increasing the
time required for determining
eligibility, and slowing the pace
of payments to vendors, as
well as intensifying traditional
health care cost-containment
programs. States experiencing
financial difficulties may also
subject hospitals to similar
payment restrictions, due to
the states' financial status
rather than to explicit cost-
containment concerns. In
some instances, state and
local governments may lay
off employees (e.g., teachers).
As a result, private health
insurance coverage for these
employees may lapse.
     —   — — —   —

14. Financing the capital requirements of the hospital
will continue to be a focal
point of long-run cost-
containment strategies,
creating conflicts with the
industry's need for increasing amounts of capital to
meet community needs and
governmental requirements.
     —   — — —   —

Statement	Strongly Agree	•	•	•	Strongly Disagree
15. Regulation of the health care industry will increase and intensify, despite renewed interest in competition as an alternative to regulation and attempts to reduce the costs of regulation.	—	—	—	—	—
16. The expansion and proliferation of regulatory agencies will generate new requirements for data and analysis. Agency staffs will be more technically sophisticated and more capable of detailed analysis.	—	—	—	—	—
17. State and federal legislation will continue to increase, without any greater coordination between them; legislation will be one of the primary external sources of industry change. At the same time, however, the industry will gain experience in influencing legislation and will be more able to exploit the lack of firm support for many pieces of legislation, particularly those with controversial aspects. Consequently, the industry will increasingly be in a position to favorably affect legislative proposals.	—	—	—	—	—
18. The hospital industry will increasingly be involved in litigation focusing on a widening array of subjects: reimbursement, staff privileges, privacy, entitlement, licensure, product liability, malpractice, antitrust.	—	—	—	—	—

Statement	Strongly Agree	•	•	•	Strongly Disagree

19. The major controversies related to human resources will be linked to the issues of supply, demand, qualifications, and distribution. The hospital industry, presenting its concerns about a present and future shortage of personnel in many professions and in many areas of the country, will favor expansionary manpower policies. The direction, at least of federal government policy, if not checked, will be toward a curtailment or restriction of growth in the health professions in relation to population because of concerns about cost and supply-induced demand. — — — — —

20. The area of "employee relations" will be greatly altered as changes in society gradually spill over into the workplace. Traditional modalities of providing patient care will be influenced by changes in the population and in the manner of training health care professionals, and by less conventional employee attitudes about work. — — — — —

21. The role of the health care delivery system will be defined increasingly in terms of prevention and maximizing the ability of the individual to maintain or improve

Statement	Strongly Agree	•	•	•	Strongly Disagree
health. This trend will include increased emphasis on less in-trusive and costly therapies.	—	—	—	—	—
22. Continuing concern about the value of technology, both in terms of economic costs and social values, will stimulate new efforts to con-trol or channel the processes of technological diffusion and application. Although concern has been expressed primarily about capital-intensive technology, non-capital-intensive technology and techniques will attract greater attention as equally important sources of higher expenditures.	—	—	—	—	—
23. Clinical practice will be in-creasingly differentiated according to the patterns of physician organization. Different types of medical organization will experiment with physician skills, technol-ogies, and protocols of care to produce a broader range of utilization patterns.	—	—	—	—	—
24. Clinical innovation and research will continue to be plagued by the basic/applied research problem.	—	—	—	—	—
25. The entire area of clinical practice will be surrounded increasingly by controversies about ethics and moral choice.	—	—	—	—	—
26. In addition to their present legal liability for all that					

	Statement	Strongly Agree	•	•	•	Strongly Disagree
	occurs in hospitals, governing boards will increasingly be viewed as being directly accountable to the public or community which the hospital serves. The structure of governance and management will continue toward reorganization along corporate lines. In response to new responsibilities the composition of boards will change accordingly.	—	—	—	—	—
27.	The growth of multi-hospital arrangements will pose challenges to traditional notions of governance. In arrangements where strong central control is exerted, significant governance activity will shift from the boards of individual institutions to the central board. Where such arrangements are formed only for specific projects and in shared service organizations, individual boards will be more able to maintain their independence.	—	—	—		—
28.	The role and responsibility of the chief executive officer will continue to develop along patterns generally found in business organizations.	—	—	—	—	—
29.	The management staff of hospitals will become increasingly more specialized and sophisticated.	—	—	—	—	—
30.	Contract management of hospitals will continue to grow, stimulated by the					

Statement	Strongly Agree	•	•	•	Strongly Disagree
need for specialized management skills and for sophisticated information systems.	—	—	—	—	—
31. The traditional clinical prerogatives and organizational practice preferences of physicians will be altered by increases in the supply of physicians, regulatory mechanisms, and changes in payment systems.	—	—	—	—	—
32. Increases in the overall supply of physicians, and particularly of specialists, will lead to increasing applications for admission to medical staffs, including nonphysician practitioners, who have traditionally been denied privileges.	—	—	—	—	—
33. Pressure will continue to be applied by government to hospitals as a vehicle for controlling the physician-related component of increased health care expenditures.	—	—	—	—	—
34. AHA will be seen less as an ally of hospitals and more as a "puppet" of government policies.	—	—	—	—	—
35. Blue Cross/Blue Shield will become "captured" and cease to exist as an independent third-party payer, instead serving as a quasi-government agency setting rates through reimbursement mechanisms.	—	—	—	—	—

Statement	Strongly Agree	•	•	•	Strongly Disagree
36. JCAH will become dependent on government support and cease to be an independent organization.	—	—	—	—	—
37. HSAs will replace all other planning organizations and exercise more power than the state planning agency.	—	—	—	—	—
38. HMOs will dominate urban health care delivery systems but fail in most rural areas.	—	—	—	—	—
39. Physicians will come to prefer salaried positions on hospital staffs rather than fee-for-service practice.	—	—	—	—	—
40. Emergency rooms will become primary care clinics in nearly all hospitals.	—	—	—	—	—
41. Room rates will rise to $500 per day by 1985.	—	—	—	—	—
42. Most persons will be able to sign up with a family physician and be assured of prepaid care by 1985.	—	—	—	—	—
43. New hospitals will cease to be built, except in rapidly expanding population areas and new towns.	—	—	—	—	—
44. Average salaries for health service managers will be $50,000 by 1985.	—	—	—	—	—
45. VA hospitals will be phased out by 1985.	—	—	—	—	—
46. By 1985, health administrators will be required to be licensed in most states.	—	—	—	—	—

Step 2: Small-Group Discussion of Individual Judgments

Divide class into small groups. Each person should take a few minutes to think out loud and share with the group how he arrived at his particular assessment. What factors led to his agreement or disagreement with the given statements? The objective of this discussion is for each individual to become more clear about his or her own personal assessment of the future of health services.

Step 3: Identify Potential Conflicts

Following an individual presentation of their assessments, the groups should identify areas in which there is particular disagreement. These should be noted and discussed in detail within the group.

Step 4: Sharing of Small-Group Output

Representatives from each of the groups should list the particular areas of greatest disagreement. The objective of this session is not to resolve these areas of disagreement but through total class participation to permit a clear identification and ensure an understanding as to the reasons why there is disagreement on the various statements.

SUGGESTED READING

BROOK, R., K. WILLIAMS, and A. AVERY. "Quality Assurance Today and Tomorrow: Forecast for the Future." *Annals of Internal Medicine* 85(6) (Dec. 1976): 809–817.

DYE, T. R. *Understanding Public Policy.* Englewood Cliffs, N.J.: Prentice-Hall, 1972.

LEVEY, S., and T. McCARTHY, eds. *Health Management of Tomorrow.* Philadelphia: J. B. Lippincott, 1980.

NEUHAUSER, D. "The *Really* Effective Health Service Delivery System." *Health Care Management Review* 1 (1) (Winter 1976): 25–32.

REINHARDT, U. E. "Proposed Changes in the Organization of Health Care Delivery: An Overview and Critique." *MMFQ—Health and Society* 51(2) (Spring 1973): 169–222.

RELMAN, A. "The New Medical-Industrial Complex." *New England Journal of Medicine* 303(17) (Oct. 23, 1981): 963–970.

ROGERS, D., and R. BLENDON. "The Academic Medical Center: A Stressed American Institution." *The New England Journal of Medicine* 298(17) (Apr. 27, 1978): 940–950.

Glossary

These are commonly used abbreviations and acronyms in the community of health administrators, policymakers, and bureaucrats. Although many come and go as issues are posed and answers proposed, some are more durable and remain in the vocabulary.

AA: Alcoholics Anonymous

AAFRC: American Association of Fund Raising Council

AAMC: Association of American Medical Clinics, Association of American Medical Colleges

ACHA: American College of Hospital Administrators

ADA: American Dental Association

ADAMHA: Alcohol, Drug Abuse, and Mental Health Administration

AFDC: Aid to Families with Dependent Children

AGPA: American Group Practice Association

AGMA: Association of Group Medical Administrators

AHA: American Hospital Association

AHEC: area health education center

AHPA: American Health Planning Association

AICPA: American Institute of Certified Public Accountants

AIP: annual implementation plan

AMA: American Medical Association

AMPAC: American Medical Political Action Committee

ANA: American Nurses Association

AOA: American Optometric Association, American Osteopathic Association

APA: Administrative Procedures Act

APhA: American Pharmaceutical Association

APHA: American Public Health Association, American Protestant Hospital Association

APTD: aid to the permanently and totally disabled

ASAHP: American Society of Allied Health Professions

ASTHO: Association of State and Territorial Health Officials

AUPHA: Association of University Programs in Health Administration

BCA: Blue Cross Association

BCBS: Blue Cross/Blue Shield

BHI: Bureau of Health Insurance

Blue sheet: Drug Research Reports

CAT scanner: computerized axial tomography

CBO: Congressional Budget Office

CCU: coronary care unit

CD: certificate of deposit

CDC: Center for Disease Control (formerly the Communicable Disease Center)

CHAMPUS: Civilian Health and Medical Program of the Uniformed Services

CHIP: Comprehensive Health Insurance Plan

CHP: comprehensive health planning

CON: certificate of need

CPA: certified public accountant

CPI: Consumer price index

DD: developmental disability

DDS: doctor of dental surgery

DEA: Drug Enforcement Administration

DO: doctor of osteopathy

DOA: dead on arrival

DVM: doctor of veterinary medicine

ECF: extended care facility

ECFMG: Educational Commission for Foreign Medical Graduates

EEOC: Equal Employment Opportunity Commission

EMS: emergency medical services

EPA: Environmental Protection Agency

EPSDT: early and periodic screening, diagnosis, and treatment

ER: emergency room

ERISA: Employment Retirement Income Security Act

EST: earliest starting time

FASB: Financial Accounting Standards Board

FDA: Food and Drug Administration

FICA: Federal Insurance Contributions Act

FLEX: Federal Licensing Examination

FMG: foreign medical graduate

FNP: family nurse practitioner

FTC: Federal Trade Commission

FY: fiscal year

GAAP: Generally Accepted Accounting Principles

GHAA: Group Health Association of America

GP: general practitioner

HEW: Department of Health, Education, and Welfare (until 1980)

HHS: Department of Health and Human Services (since 1980)

HIBAC: Health Insurance Benefits Advisory Council

HMO: health maintenance organization

HRA: Health Resources Administration

HSA: health service area; Health Services Administration; Health Systems Agency

HSRC: Health Services Research Center

ICDA: International Classification of Diseases, Adapted

ICF: intermediate care facility

ICU: intensive care unit

IOM: Institute of Medicine of the National Academy of Sciences

IPA: individual practice association

JCAH: Joint Commission on Accreditation of Hospitals

JUA: joint underwriting association

LHD: local health department

LIFO: "last in, first out" (inventory pricing method which assumes that the last goods in are the first goods out)

LOS: length of stay

LPN: licensed practical nurse

LST: latest starting time

LVN: licensed vocational nurse

MAC: maximum allowable cost

MAP: medical audit program

MBO: management by objectives

MCAT: Medical College Admission Test

MCH: maternal and child health

MD: Doctor of Medicine

MEDLARS: Medical Literature and Analysis Retrieval System

MR: mentally retarded

NACo: National Association of Counties

NAIC: National Association of Insurance Commissioners

NCHS: National Center for Health Statistics

NCHSR: National Center for Health Services Research

NCOAHE: National Commission on Allied Health Education

NHI: national health insurance

NHSC: National Health Service Corps

NIH: National Institutes of Health

NIMH: National Institute of Mental Health

NLN: National League for Nursing

NLRB: National Labor Relations Board

NMA: National Medical Association

NP: nurse practitioner

NPRM: notice of proposed rulemaking

OAA: old age assistance

OASDHI: Old Age, Survivors, Disability and Health Insurance Program

Ob-gyn: obstetrics-gynecology

OEO: Office of Economic Opportunity

OMB: Office of Management and Budget

OPD: outpatient department

OR: operating room, operations research

OSHA: Occupational Safety and Health Act

OT: occupational therapy or therapist

OTA: Office of Technology Assessment

OTC: over-the-counter drug

PA: physician assistant; professional association

PAS: Professional Activities Survey

PC: professional corporation

PDR: *Physicians' Desk Reference*

PERT: program evaluation and review technique

PHS: U.S. Public Health Service

PMA: Pharmaceutical Manufacturers Association

POMR: problem-oriented medical record

PPBS: program planning budgeting system

PRRB: Provider Reimbursement Review Board

PSRO: professional standards review organization

PT: physical therapy or therapist

QAP: quality assurance program

RFP: request for proposal

RN: registered nurse

RVS: relative value scale or schedule

SHA: state health agency

SHCC: statewide health coordinating council

SHPDA: state health planning and development agency

SMSA: standard metropolitan statistical area

SNF: skilled nursing facility

SSI: supplemental security income

T-bill: Treasury bill

Title IV of the Social Security Act (42 U.S.C. § 601 et seq.): Grants to States for Aid and Services to Needy Families with Children and for Child-Welfare Services

Title V of the Social Security Act (42 U.S.C. § 701-716): Maternal and Child Health and Crippled Children's Services

Title XVIII: Medicare

Title XIX: Medicaid

UCR: usual, customary, and reasonable

UR: utilization review

USP: *United States Pharmocopeia*

USPHS: United States Public Health Service

VNA: visiting nurse association

WHO: World Health Organization

References

AARON, H. J. *Politics and the Professors: The Great Society in Perspective.* Washington, D.C.: The Brookings Institution, 1978.

ADAMS, S. J. "The Structure and Dynamics of Behavior in Organizational Boundary Roles." In M. D. Dunnette, ed., *Handbook of Industrial and Organizational Psychology.* Chicago: Rand McNally, 1976, pp. 1175–1199.

ADIZES, I. "Organizational Passages—Diagnosing and Treating Lifecycle Problems of Organizations." *Organizational Dynamics* (Summer 1979): 3–25.

AGGARWAL, R., and HAHN, D. B. "More Emphasis Should Be on Working Capital Management." *Hospital Financial Management* (Dec. 1979): 13–80.

ALDRICH, H. E. *Organizations and Environments.* Englewood Cliffs, N.J.: Prentice-Hall, 1979.

ALLISON, G. *Essence of Decision: Explaining the Cuban Missile Crisis.* Boston: Little, Brown, 1971.

ALSDURF, W. H. "Improving Inventory Records Now Becoming More Important." *Hospital Financial Management* (June 1980): 62–63.

ALTMAN, S. H., and BLENDON, R. *Medical Technology: The Culprit Behind Health Care Cost?* Washington, D.C.: U.S. Department of Health, Education, and Welfare, 1979.

AMA CENTER FOR HEALTH SERVICES RESEARCH AND DEVELOPMENT. *Profile of Medical Practice 1978.* Chicago: American Medical Association, 1979.

AMERICAN ASSOCIATION OF FUND RAISING COUNCIL, INC. *Giving USA 1977: A Compilation of Facts and Trends on American Philantrophy for 1976.* New York: AAFRC, 1977, pp. 35–37.

AMERICAN HOSPITAL ASSOCIATION. *Budgeting Procedures for Hospitals.* Chicago: American Hospital Association, 1971.

AMERICAN HOSPITAL ASSOCIATION. *The Practice of Planning in Health Care Institutions.* Chicago: American Hospital Association, 1973.

AMERICAN HOSPITAL ASSOCIATION. *Hospital Regulation: Report of the Special Committee on the Regulatory Process.* Chicago: American Hospital Association, 1977.

AMERICAN HOSPITAL ASSOCIATION. "The Nation's Hospitals: A Statistical Profile." *Hospital Statistics.* 1975, 1979 edition, Chicago.

AMERICAN HOSPITAL ASSOCIATION. "Environmental Assessment of the Hospital Industry, 1979." Chicago, 1979.

AMERICAN HOSPITAL ASSOCIATION. *Federal Regulation: Hospital Attorney's Desk Reference.* Chicago, 1980.

AMERICAN HOSPITAL ASSOCIATION. *Program for Institutional Effectiveness Review.* Chicago: American Hospital Association, 1980.

AMMER, D. S. *Purchasing and Materials Management for Health Care Institutions.* Lexington, Mass.: Lexington Books, 1975.

ANNAS, G. *The Rights of Hospital Patients, The Basic ACLU Guide to a Hospital Patient's Rights.* New York: Avon, 1975.

ANTHONY, R. N., and HERZLINGER, R. *Management Control in Non-Profit Organizations.* Homewood, Ill.: Richard D. Irwin, 1975.

ARNOLD, M., et al. *Health Program Implementation Through PERT.* San Francisco: Western Regional Office, APHA, 1966.

ASCH, S. E. *Social Psychology.* New York: Prentice–Hall, 1952.

ASSOCIATION OF STATE AND TERRITORIAL HEALTH OFFICIALS. *Comprehensive NPHPRS Report: Services, Expenditures, and Programs of State and Territorial Health Agencies, Fiscal Year 1977.: ASATHO, 1979.*

ASSOCIATION OF UNIVERSITY PROGRAMS IN HEALTH ADMINISTRATION, Health Management Appraisal Methods Program, Washington, D.C., 1981.

ASSUNTA, SISTER MARY. "Credit Granting—A Way of Life for Hospitals." *Managing the Patient Account.* Chicago: Hospital Financial Management Association, 1970.

ATWATER, J. B. "Must Local Health Officers Be Physicians?" *American Journal of Public Health* 70(11) (Jan. 1980):11.

BACHARACH, S. B., and LAWLER, E. J. *Power and Politics in Organizations.* San Francisco: Jossey-Bass, 1980.

BALDWIN, L. E. "An Empirical Study: The Effect of Organizational Differentiation and Integration on Hospital Performance." *Hospital Administration* 17(4) (Fall 1972): 52–71.

BALES, R. F. "Task Roles and Social Roles in Problem-Solving Groups." In E. Maccoby, T. M. Newcomb, and E. L. Hartley, eds., *Readings in Social Psychology.* New York: Holt, Rinehart and Winston, 1958, pp. 437–446.

BANTA, H. D., and SANES, J. R. "Assessing the Social Impacts of Medical Technologies." *Journal of Community Health* 3(3) (Spring 1978):245–258.

BANTA, H. D., and THACKER, S. "The Premature Delivery of Medical Technology: A Case Report." Unpublished paper of the Office of Technology Assessment, U.S. Congress, Washington, D.C., n.d.

BATES, R. T. "How the Materials Manager Affects Cash Flow." *Hospital Financial Management* (May 1979):40–45.

BEAUCHAMP, D. E. "Public Health as Social Justice." *Inquiry* 13 (Mar. 1976):3-14.

BEGUN, J. W. *Professionalism and the Public Interest: Price and Quality in Optometry.* Boston, Mass.: The MIT Press, 1981.

BELLIN, L. E. "Local Health Departments: A Prescription Against Obsolescence." In A. Levin, ed., *Health Services: The Local Perspective,* Vol. 32, No. 3. Montpelier, Vt.: The Academy of Political Science, Capital City Press, 1977, pp. 42-52.

BELLIN, L., and WEEKS, L. eds. *Challenge of Administering Health Services.* Ann Arbor, Mich.: Health Administration Press, 1980.

BERMAN, H. J., and WEEKS, L. E. *The Financial Management of Hospitals,* 3rd ed. Ann Arbor, Mich.: Health Administration Press, 1976.

BERMAN, J., and WEEKS, L. E. *The Financial Management of Hospitals,* 4th ed. Ann Arbor, Mich.: Health Administration Press, 1979.

BLACK'S LAW DICTIONARY, 5th ed. St. Paul, Minn.: West, 1979.

BLENDON, R. J. "The Prospects for State and Local Governments Playing a Broader Role in Health Care in the 1980s." *American Journal of Public Health,* 71 (Suppl.) (Jan. 1981):9-14.

BLOOM, J. R. "Team Care: Solution for Hospital Oncology Units." *Health Care Management Review* 4(4) (Fall 1979):23-30.

BOERGADINE, L. C. "Prudent Buyer." *Hospital Financial Management* (Feb. 1978): 44-46.

BOWERS, D. G. "OD Techniques and Their Results in 23 Organizations: The Michigan ICL Study." *Journal of Applied Behavioral Science* 9(1) (1973):21-43.

BOWERS, D. G., and FRANKLIN, J. L. "Survey-Guided Development: Using Human Resources Measurement in Organizational Change." *Journal of Contemporary Business* (Summer 1972):43-55.

BOWERS, D. G., and FRANKLIN, J. L. *Survey-Guided Development I: Data-Based Organizational Change.* La Jolla, Calif.: University Associates, 1977.

BRAGG, J. E., and ANDREWS, I. "Participative Decision Making: An Experimental Study in a Hospital." *Journal of Applied Behavioral Science* 9(6) (1973):727-733.

BRESLAU, N. "The Role of the Nurse Practitioner in a Pediatric Team: Patient Definitions." *Medical Care* 15(12) (Dec. 1977):1014-1023.

BROOK, R., WILLIAMS, K., and AVERY, A. "Quality Assurance Today and Tomorrow: Forecast for the Future." *Annals of Internal Medicine* 85(6) (Dec. 1976):809-817.

BROOK, R. H., DAVIES-AVERY, A., GREENFIELD, S., HARRIS, L. J., LELAH, T., SOLOMON, N. E., and WARE, J. E., JR. "Assessing the Quality of Medical Care Using Outcome Measures: An Overview of the Method." *Medical Care* 15(9) (Sept. 1977):Suppl.

BROWN, M. "Multi-Hospital Systems: Trends, Issues and Prospects." Paper presented at the Hospital Research and Educational Trust Invitational Conference on Multi-Hospital Systems, Washington, D.C., Mar. 1980.

BROWN, M., and MONEY, W. H. "Contract Management: Is It for Your Hospital?" *Trustee* 29(2) (Feb. 1976):12–16.

BROWN, C. R., and UHL, H. S. M. "Mandatory Continuing Education: Sense or Nonsense." *JAMA* 213(10) (Sept. 7, 1970):1660–1668.

BROWN, M., et al. "Trends in Multi-Hospital System: Resulting from the 1979 AHA Survey on Multi-Hospital Systems." *Hospital* (in press).

BUCHER, R., and STELLING, J. G. *Becoming Professional*, Vol. 46. Sage Library of Social Research. Beverly Hills, Calif.: Sage, 1977.

BUCHER, R., and STRAUSS, A. "Professions in Process." *American Journal of Science* 66 (January 1961):325–334.

BURNS, E. "Rethinking Public Policies on Health Care." Manuscript, Columbia University, New York, n.d.

CAMERON, C., and KOBYLARZ, A. "Nonphysician Directors of Local Health Departments: Results of a National Survey." *Public Health Reports* 95(4) (July–Aug. 1980): 386–391.

CAMPBELL, D. T. "Reforms as Experiments." *American Psychologist* 24(4) (Apr. 1969): 409–429.

CAMPBELL, J. P. "On the Nature of Organizational Effectiveness." In P. S. Goodman, J. Penning, and associates, eds., *New Perspectives on Organizational Effectiveness*. San Francisco: Jossey-Bass, 1977.

CAMPBELL, J. P., DUNNETTE, M. D., LAWLER, F. E., and WEICK, K. E. *Managerial Behavior, Performance, and Effectiveness*. New York: McGraw-Hill, 1970.

CARTWRIGHT, D. "Influence Leadership and Control." In *Handbook of Organizations*, J. D. March, ed. Chicago: Rand McNally, 1965.

CASCIO, W. F. *Applied Psychology in Personnel Management*. Reston, Va.: Reston, 1978.

CHARNS, M., and SCHAEFER, M. *Managing the Dynamics of Health Care Organizations*. Englewood Cliffs, N.J.: Prentice-Hall, 1981.

CHASE, G. "Implementing a Human Service Program: How Hard Will It Be?" *Public Policy* 27(4) (Fall 1979):385–435.

CHILD, J. "Organizational Structure, Environment and Performance: The Role of Strategic Choice." *Sociology* 6(1) (Jan. 1972):1–22.

CHURCHMAN, C. W. *The Systems Approach*. New York: Dell. 1968.

CLEAVERLY, W. O. *Essentials of Hospital Finance*. Germantown, Md.: Aspen Systems Corp., 1978.

COCHRANE, A. *Effectiveness and Efficiency*. London: The Nuffield Provincial Hospitals Trust, 1972.

COOPER, P. D. *Health Care Marketing*. Germantown, Md.: Aspen Systems Corp., 1979.

COOPERATIVE INFORMATION CENTER FOR HOSPITAL MANAGEMENT STUDIES. *Abstracts of Hospital Management Studies,* Ann Arbor, Mich.: Health Administration Press, 1970-1982.

CORLEY, R. N., R. L. BLACK, and O. L. REED, *The Legal Environment of Business,* 5th ed. New York: McGraw-Hill, 1981.

COUNCIL OF WAGE AND PRICE STABILITY. "The Complex Puzzle of Rising Health Care Costs: Can the Private Sector Put It Together?" Washington, D.C.: Executive Office of the President, 1976.

DARSKY, B. "Some Aspects of the Institutional and Social Structure of the American Medical Care System." Paper presented at the School of Public Health, University of North Carolina, Chapel Hill, N.C., 1968.

DARSKY, B., and METZNER, C. "Health Organizations in American Society." University of Michigan, Ann Arbor, Mich., mimeographed, n.d.

DAVIS, S., and LAWRENCE, P. *Matrix.* Reading, Mass.: Addison-Wesley, 1977.

DAVIS, S. M., and LAWRENCE, P. R. "Problems of Matrix Organizations." *Harvard Business Review* 56(3) (May-June 1978):131-142.

DEEGAN, A. X. *Management by Objectives for Hospitals.* Germantown, Md.: Aspen Systems Corp., 1977.

DeFRIESE, G. H. *et al.* "The Program Implications of Administrative Relationships Between Local Health Departments and State and Local Government." *American Journal of Public Health* 71 (10) (Oct. 1981), 1109-1115.

DELBECQ, A. L., VAN de VEN, A. H., and GUSTAFSON, D. H. *Group Techniques for Program Planning.* Glenview, Ill.: Scott, Foresman, 1975.

DeVRIES, R. A. "Strength in Numbers." *Hospitals JAHA* 52 (Mar. 16, 1978):81-84.

DILLON, R. D. *Zero Based Budgeting for Health Care Institutions.* Germantown, Md.: Aspen Systems Corp., 1979.

DITTMAN, D. A. and OFER, A. R. "The Impact of Reimbursement on Hospital Cash Flow." *Topics in Health Care Financing* 3(1) (Fall 1976):27-31.

DONABEDIAN, A. "Evaluating the Quality of Medical Care." *Milbank Memorial Fund Quarterly* 44(3) (Part 2) (July 1966):166-206.

DONABEDIAN, A. *The Definition of Quality and Approaches to Its Assessment,* Vol. 1. Ann Arbor, Mich.: Health Administration Press, 1980.

DONABEDIAN, A., AXELROD, S. J., and WYZEWIANSKI, L. *Medical Care Chart Book.* Ann Arbor, Mich.: Health Administration Press, 1980.

DOWNS, A. *Inside Bureaucracy.* Boston, Mass.: Little, Brown, 1967.

DOWNS, G. W., and MOHR, L. B. "Conceptual Issues in the Study of Innovation." *Administration Science Quarterly* 21 (Dec. 1976):700-714.

DUFF, R. S., and HOLLINGSHEAD, A. B. *Sickness and Society.* New York: Harper & Row, 1968.

DYE, T. R., *Understanding Public Policy*. Englewood Cliffs, N. J.: Prentice-Hall, 1972.

DYCK, F. J., MURPHY, F. A., et al. "Effect of Surveillance on the Number of Hysterectomies in the Province of Saskatchewan." *New England Journal of Medicine* 296(23) (June 1977):1326-1328.

ELMORE, R. F. "Organizational Models of Social Implementation." *Public Policy* 26(2) (Spring 1978):185-228.

EMREY, R., WILSON-SCOTT, D., BERNHART, M. H., and FALLOW, C. E. *New Methods for Assessing Developing Country Health Services Management Needs*. Wash., D.C.: Association of University Programs in Health Administration, July 1979.

ETZIONI, A., and REMP, R. "Technological 'Shortcuts' to Social Change." *Science* 175 (1972):31-38.

FALKSON, J. *HMOs and the Politics of Health System Reform*. Chicago: American Hospital Association, 1980.

FEDER, J., HOLAHAN, J., and MARMOR, T., eds. *National Health Insurance: Conflicting Goals and Policy Choices*. Washington, D.C.: Urban Institute, 1980.

FELDMAN, D. C. "A Contingency Theory of Socialization." *Administrative Science Quarterly* 21(3) (Sept. 1976):433-452.

FELDMAN, D. C. "Organizational Socialization of Hospital Employees: A Comparative View of Occupational Groups." *Medical Care* 15(10) (Oct. 1977):799-813.

FELDSTEIN, P. J. *Health Associations and the Demand for Legislation: The Political Economy of Health*. Cambridge, Mass.: Ballinger, 1977.

FIEDLER, F. E. "Style or Circumstance: The Leadership Enigma." In F. E. Kast and J. E. Rosenzweig, eds., *Contingency Views of Organization and Management*. SRA, Inc., 1973, pp. 229-237.

FINEBERG, H. V., and HIATT, H. H. "The Evaluation of Medical Practices." *New England Journal of Medicine*, 301(20) (Nov. 15, 1979):1086-1091.

FLOOD, A. B., and SCOTT, W. R. "Professional Power and Professional Effectiveness: The Power of the Surgical Staff and Quality of Surgical Care in Hospitals." *Journal of Health and Social Behavior* 19(3) (Sept. 1978): 240-254.

FORREST, C. R., and JOHNSON, A. C. "A Comparative Analysis of Task Activities of Hospital and Mental Health/Human Services Administrators." Paper presented at 1979 Meeting AUPHA, Toronto, Canada, May 1980.

FORRESTER, J. W. *Industrial Dynamics*. Cambridge, Mass.: MIT Press, 1961.

FOTTLER, M. D., and PINCHOFF, D. M. "Acceptance of Nurse Practitioner: Attitudes of Health Care Administrators." *Inquiry* 13(3) (Sept. 1976):262-273.

FRANK, C. W. *Maximizing Hospital Cash Resources*. Germantown, Md.: Aspen Systems Corp., 1978.

FREELAND, M., et al. "Projections of National Health Expenditures, 1980, 1985 and 1990." *Health Care Financing Review* (Winter 1980):1-27.

FREIDSON, E. *Profession of Medicine: A Study of the Sociology of Applied Knowledge.* New York: Dodd, Mead, 1970.

FREIDSON, E. *Doctoring Together: A Study of Professional Social Control.* New York: Elsevier, 1975.

FRENCH, J. R. P., and RAVEN, B. "The Basis of Social Power." In D. Cartwright and A. Zander, eds., *Group Dynamics.* Evanston, Ill.: Row, Peterson, 1960, 607-623.

FRESHNOCK, L. J., and GOODMAN, L. J. "Medical Group Practice in the United States: Patterns of Survival Between 1969 and 1975." *Journal of Health and Social Behavior* 20(4) (Dec. 1979):352-362.

GALBRAITH, J. *Designing Complex Organizations.* Reading, Mass.: Addison-Wesley, 1973.

GALBRAITH, J. *Organization Design.* Reading, Mass.: Addison-Wesley, 1977.

GEORGOPOULOS, B. S. *Hospital Organization Research: Review and Source Book.* Philadelphia: W. B. Saunders, 1975.

GERSTENFELD, A. "MBO Revisited: Focus on Health Systems." *Health Care Management Review* 2(4) (Fall 1977):51-57.

GIBSON, R. M. "National Health Expenditures, 1978." *Health Care Financing Review* 1(1) (Summer 1979):1-36.

GIBSON, J. L., IVANCEVICH, J. M., and DONNELLY, J. H., JR. *Organizations: Behavior, Structure, Processes.* Dallas, Tex.: Business Publications, Inc., 1976.

GOODMAN, L. J., BENNETT, E. H., and ODEM, R. J. *Group Medical Practice in the U.S.* Chicago: American Medical Association, 1976.

GORAN, M. J. "The Evolution of the PSRO Hospital Review System." *Medical Care* 17(5) (Suppl.) (May 1979):1-47.

GOSS, M. E. W. "Influence and Authority Among Physicians in an Outpatient Clinic." *American Sociological Review* 26(1) (1961):39-50.

GOULDNER, A. W. *Patterns of Industrial Bureaucracy.* Glencoe, Ill.: Free Press, 1954.

GRAD, F. P. *Public Health Law Manual.* Washington, D.C.: American Public Health Association, 1973.

GREEN, R. *Assuring Quality in Medical Care: The State of the Art.* Cambridge, Mass.: Ballinger, 1976.

GREER, A. L. "Advances in the Study of Diffusion and Innovation in Health Care Organizations." *Milbank Memorial Fund Quarterly, Health and Society* 55 (Fall 1977):505-532.

GREER, A. L. "Technology, Assessment, Diffusion, and Implementation." *Journal of Medical Systems* 5(1):1981.

GREINER, L. E. "Evolution and Revolution as Organizations Grow." *Harvard Business Review* 50(4) (July-Aug. 1972):37-46.

GRIFFITH, J. R. *Quantitative Techniques for Hospital Planning and Control.* Lexington, Mass.: D. C. Heath, 1972.

GRIFFITH, J. R. *Measuring Hospital Performance. An Inquiry Book.* Chicago: Blue Cross Association, 1978.

GRIFFITH, J. R., HANCOCK, W. M., and MUNSON, F. *Cost Control in Hospitals.* Ann Arbor, Mich.: Health Administration Press, 1976.

HAGE, J. *Communication and Organizational Control: Cybernetics in Health and Welfare Settings.* New York: Wiley, 1974.

HAGE, J. *Theories of Organizations: Form, Process, and Transformation.* New York: Wiley-Interscience, 1980.

HAGE, J. and DEWAR, R. "Elite Values Versus Organizational Structure in Predicting Innovation." *Administrative Science Quarterly* 18(3) (Sept. 1973):279–290.

HALL, R. W. "Merger of the City and County Health Department in a Rural Midwestern State." In J. O. Hepner, ed., *Health Planning for Emerging Multihospital Systems.* St. Louis, Mo.: C. V. Mosby, 1978, pp. 258–261.

HAMNER, W. C., and ORGAN, D. W. *Organizational Behavior: An Applied Psychological Approach.* Dallas, Tex.: Business Publications, Inc., 1978.

HANFT, RUTH S. "Health Manpower." In S. Jonas, ed., *Health Care Delivery in the United States.* New York: Springer, 1977, pp. 67–95.

HANLON, J. J. *Public Health Administration and Practice.* St. Louis, Mo.: C. V. Mosby, 1974.

HARDIN, G. "The Tragedy of the Commons." *Science* 162 (1968):1243–1248.

HARE, V. C. *Systems Analysis: A Diagnostic Approach.* New York: Harcourt Brace & World, 1967.

HARRIS, L. G. "Potential for Conflict—An Application from a Doctor of Osteopathy for Medical Staff." A case report in hospital administration prepared for the Committee on Credentials in partial fulfillment of the requirements for fellowship, American College of Hospital Administrators, Chicago, 1979a.

HARRIS, L. G. "The Role of an Administrative Physician." A case report in hospital administration. Prepared for the Committee on Credentials in partial fulfillment of the requirements for fellowship, American College of Hospital Administrators, Chicago, 1979b.

HARRIS, P. R. "Further Dialogue on Health Care Regulations." *American Journal of Law and Medicine* 5(4) (Winter 1980):343.

HASENFELD, Y., and ENGLISH, R. A., eds. *Human Service Organizations.* Ann Arbor, Mich.: University of Michigan Press, 1977a.

HASENFELD, Y., and ENGLISH, R. A. "Human Service Organizations: A Conceptual Overview." In Y. Hasenfeld and R. English, eds., *Human Service Organizations.* Ann Arbor, Mich.: University of Michigan Press, 1977b.

THE HASTINGS CENTER. "The Concept of Health." *The Hastings Center Studies* 1(3) (1973).

HAVIGHURST, C. "Controlling Health Care Costs: Strengthening the Private Sector's Hand." *Journal of Health Politics, Policy and Law* 1(4) (Winter (1977):471–498.

HAYT, HAYT, and GROESCHEL. *Law of Hospital, Physician, and Patient.* Berwyn, Ill.: Physicians Record Co., 1972.

HEALTH CARE FINANCING ADMINISTRATION, OFFICE OF RESEARCH. "Demonstration and Statistics, Professional Standards Review Organization; 1979 Program Evaluation." U.S. Depart. of Health and Human Services, Baltimore, Md., May 1980.

HEALTH INSURANCE INSTITUTE. *Source Book of Health Insurance,* 1978-79. New York.

HEALTH INSURANCE INSTITUTE. *The Adequacy of Private Health Insurance Coverage.* Washington, D.C.: Health Insurance Institute, 1980.

HEALTH SERVICES RESEARCH 11(4) (Winter 1976). Special Issue: "Health Status Indexes—Work in Progress."

HEALTH SERVICES RESEARCH CENTER. Research Proceeding/Medical Technology, Sept. 1979.

HENNING, W. "The Financial Impact of Materials Management." *Hospital Financial Management* (Feb. 1980):36–42.

HERKIMER, A. G., JR. *Understanding Hospital Financial Management.* Germantown, Md.: Aspen Systems Corp., 1978.

HERNANDEZ, S. R., and KALUZNY, A. D. "Hospital Closure: A Review of Current and Proposed Research." *Health Services Research,* (Summer 1982).

HILLIER, F. S. and LIEBERMAN, G. J. *Operations Research.* San Francisco: Holden-Day, 1974.

HIRSCH, P. M. "Organizational Effectiveness and the Institutional Environment." *Administrative Science Quarterly* 20(3) (Sept. 1975):327–344.

HORNGREN, C. T. *Introduction to Management Accounting,* 4th ed. Englewood Cliffs, N.J.: Prentice-Hall, 1978.

HOSPITAL FINANCIAL MANAGEMENT ASSOCIATION. *Managing the Patient Account.* Chicago: HFMA, 1970.

HOSPITAL FINANCIAL MANAGEMENT ASSOCIATION. *Patient Account Management Techniques.* Chicago: HFMA, 1976.

HOUSE, R. J. "A Path Goal Theory of Leader Effectiveness." *Administrative Science Quarterly* 16(3) (Sept. 1971):321–338.

HOUSE, R. J., and MITCHELL, T. R. "Path-Goal Theory of Leadership." *Journal of Contemporary Business* 3(4) (Autumn 1974):81–97.

HOUSER, R. "How to Build and Use a Flexible Budget." *Hospital Financial Management* (Aug. 1974):12–20.

HUGHES, J. F. "Why Your Hospital Should Convert to Periodic Interim Payment." *Hospital Financial Management* (Feb. 1972):13–18.

IVANCEVICH, J. M. "Changes in Performance in a Management by Objectives Program." *Administrative Science Quarterly* 19(4) (Dec. 1974):563–575.

JOHNS, C. A. "Long-Range Facility Planning: An Initial Attempt by a Community Hospital." In J. O. Hepner, ed., *Health Planning for Emerging Multi-Hospital Systems.* St. Louis, Mo.: C. V. Mosby, 1978, pp. 53–57.

JOINT COMMISSION ON ACCREDITATION OF HOSPITALS. *Accreditation Manual for Hospitals—1980 Edition.* JCAH, 1979.

JONAS, S., BANTA, D., and ENRIGHT, M. "Government in the Health Care Delivery System." In S. Jonas, ed., *Health Care Delivery in the United States.* New York: Springer, 1977, pp. 289–328.

The Journal of Applied Behavioral Sciences, 14(3) (July–Aug.–Sept. 1978). Special Issue: "Towards Healthier Medical Systems: Can We Learn from Experience?"

KAISER, D. L., VENEY, J. E., and KALUZNY, A D. "Classifying Administrative Roles." Unpublished manuscript, University of North Carolina, School of Public Health, Chapel Hill, N.C., 1980.

KALUZNY, A. "Curriculum Innovation: The Case of Health Administration." In S. Levey and T. McCarthy, eds., *Health Management for Tomorrow.* Philadelphia: J. B. Lippincott, 1980.

KALUZNY, A., and KONRAD, T. "Organizational Design and the Provision of Primary Care Programs." In G. Bisbee, ed., *Innovation in Ambulatory Primary Care.* Chicago: Hospital Research and Educational Trust, 1981.

KALUZNY, A. D., and VENEY, J. E. "Who Influences Decisions in the Hospital? Not Even the Administrator Really Knows." *Modern Hospital* (Dec. 1972):52–53.

KALUZNY, A. D., and VENEY, J. E. *Health Service Organizations: A Guide to Research and Assessment.* Berkeley, Calif.: McCutchan, 1980.

KALUZNY, A. D., and VENEY, J. E. "Types of Change and Hospital Planning Strategies." *American Journal of Health Planning* 1(3) (Jan. 1977):13–19.

KALUZNY, A. D., VENEY, J. E., GENTRY, J. T., and SPRAGUE, J. B. "Scalability of Health Services: An Empirical Test." *Health Services Research* 6(3) (Fall 1971): 214–223.

KASTELER, J., KANE, R. L., OLSEN, D. M., and THETFORD, C. "Issues Underlying Prevalence of 'Doctor-Shopping' Behavior." *Journal of Health and Social Behavior* 17(4) (Dec. 1976):328–339.

KATZ, A. H., and BENDER, E. I. "Self-Help Groups in Western Society: History and Prospects." *Journal of Applied Behavioral Science* 12(3) (July–Aug.–Sept. 1976): 265–282.

KATZ, D., and KAHN, R. L. *The Social Psychology of Organizations.* New York: Wiley, 1966.

KATZ, D., and KAHN, R. L. *The Social Psychology of Organizations,* 2nd ed. New York: Wiley, 1978.

KEISO, D. E. and WEYGANDT, J. J. *Intermediate Accounting.* New York: Wiley, 1977.

KELMAN, H. C. "Compliance, Identification and Internalization: Three Processes of Attitude Change." *Journal of Conflict Resolution* 2(1) (Mar. 1958):51-60.

KEYNES, J. M. *The General Theory of Employment, Interest and Money.* London: Macmillan, 1936.

KILMANN, R. *Social Systems Design.* New York: North-Holland, 1977.

KIMBERLY, J. R. "Hospital Adoption of Innovation: The Role of Integration into External Informational Environment." *Journal of Health and Social Behavior* 19(4) (Dec. 1978):361–373.

KIMBERLY, J. R., MILES, R. H., and ASSOCIATES. *The Organizational Life Cycle.* San Francisco: Jossey-Bass, 1980.

KINTNER, E. W. *An Antitrust Primer: A Guide to Antitrust and Trade Regulation Laws For Businessmen,* 2nd ed. New York: Macmillan, 1973.

KINZER, D. M. *Health Controls Out of Control: Warnings to the Nation from Massachusetts.* Chicago: Teach'em, Inc., 1977.

KIRKMAN-LIFF, B. L. "A Simulation of Primary Care Delivery by Public Health Departments." Unpublished Dr. P. H. dissertation, School of Public Health, University of North Carolina, Chapel Hill, N.C., 1980.

KOTLER, P. *Marketing for Non-Profit Organizations.* Englewood Cliffs, N.J.: Prentice-Hall, 1975.

KOTTER, J. P. "The Psychological Contract: Managing the Joining-Up Process." *California Management Review* 15(3) (Spring 1973):91-99.

KOVAR, M. G. "Uses of National Data in Planning." National Conference on Assessment and Evaluation Strategies in Aging: People, Population and Programs, Asheville, N.C., May 1977.

KOVNER, A., and NEUHAUSER, D., eds. *Health Services Management: Readings and Commentary.* Ann Arbor, Mich.: Health Administration Press, 1978.

KRONENFELD, J. "Self Care as a Panacea for the Ills of the Health Care System: An Assessment." *Social Science and Medicine* 13 (1980):263-267.

KUHL, I. K. *The Executive Role in Health Service Delivery Organizations.* Washington, D.C.: AUPHA, Office of Applied Research, August 1977.

LANDAU, M., and STOUT, R. "To Manage Is Not to Control: Or the Folly of Type II Errors." *Public Administrative Review* 39(2) (Mar.-Apr. 1979):148-156.

LAW, S. *Blue Cross: What Went Wrong?* New Haven, Conn.: Yale University Press, 1976.

LAWLER, E., III, NADLER, D., and CAMMANN, C., eds. *Organizational Assessment: Perspectives on the Measurement of Organizational Behavior and the Quality of Work Life.* New York: Wiley-Interscience, 1980.

LAWRENCE, P. R., and LORSCH, J. W. *Developing Organizations: Diagnosis and Action.* Reading, Mass.: Addison-Wesley, 1969a.

LAWRENCE, P. R., and LORSCH, J. W. *Organization and Environment.* Homewood, Ill.: Richard D. Irwin, 1969b.

LAWRENCE, R. S., et al. "Physician Receptivity to Nurse Practitioners: A Study of the Correlates of the Delegation of Clinical Responsibility." *Medical Care* 15(4) (Apr. 1977):298–310.

LEAVITT, H. J. "On the Design Part of Organizational Design." In R. H. Kilmann, L. R. Pondy, and D. P. Slevin, eds., *The Management of Organization Design: Strategies and Implementation,* Vol. 1. New York: North-Holland, 1976.

LEMBCKE, P. A. "Medical Auditing by Scientific Methods: Illustrated by Major Female Pelvic Surgery." *JAMA* 162(7) (1956):646–655.

LEVEY, S., and LOOMBA, N. P. *Health Care Administration: A Managerial Perspective.* Philadelphia: J. B. Lippincott, 1973.

LEVEY, S., and McCARTHY, T., eds. *Health Management for Tomorrow.* Philadelphia: J. B. Lippincott, 1980.

LEVIN, R. I., and KIRKPATRICK, C. A. *Quantitative Approaches to Management.* New York: McGraw-Hill, 1975.

LEVY, L. H. "Self-Help Groups: Types and Psychological Processes." *Journal of Applied Behavior Science* 12(3) (July–Aug.–Sept. 1976):310–322.

LIKERT, R. *New Patterns of Management.* New York: McGraw-Hill, 1961.

LIKERT, R. *The Human Organization.* New York: McGraw-Hill, 1967.

LINK, M. J. "A Wage and Salary Program Changes from Traditional Merit Based Program to a Program Based on Cost of Living, Job Market Factor and 'Getting the Most' Out of Your Merit Increases." A case report in hospital administration prepared for the Committee on Credentials in partial fulfillment of the requirements for fellowship, American College of Hospital Administrators, 1979.

LONGEST, B. "The Contemporary Hospital Chief Executive Officer." *Health Care Management Review* 3(2) (Spring 1978):43–84.

LONGEST, B. B. "A Response Theory of Organizational Strategy Formulation: The Case of Community Hospitals." Working Paper 24, Center for Health Services and Policy Research, Northwestern University, Evanston, Ill., 1979.

LOOMBA, N. P. *Management: A Quantitative Approach.* New York: Macmillan, 1978.

LORSCH, J. W. "Introduction to the Structural Design of Organizations." In G. W. Dalton, P. R. Lawrence, and J. W. Lorsch, eds., *Organizational Structure and Design.* Homewood, Ill.: Richard D. Irwin, 1970, pp. 1–16.

LORSCH, J. W. "Environment, Organization and the Individual." In A. R. Negandhi, ed., *Modern Organization Theory.* Kent, Ohio: Kent State University Press, 1973.

LUFT, H. S. *Health Maintenance Organizations: Dimensions of Performance.* Wiley-Interscience. New York: Wiley, 1981.

MAIER, N. R. F. *Principles of Human Relations.* New York: Wiley, 1952.

McAULIFFE, W. E. "Studies of Process–Outcome Correlations in Medical Care Evaluations: A Critique." *Medical Care* 16(11) (Nov. 1978):907–930.

McCARTHY, T. "Medical Technology Assessment." In S. Levey and T. McCarthy, eds., *Health Management for Tomorrow.* Philadelphia: J. B. Lippincott, 1980, pp. 271–280.

McCOOL, B., and BROWN, M. *The Management Response: Conceptual, Technical and Human Skills of Health Administration.* Philadelphia: W. B. Saunders, 1977.

McNEIL, D., and WILLIAMS, R. "Wide Range of Causes Found for Hospital Closures." *Hospitals* 52(23) (Dec. 1, 1978):76–81.

MECHANIC, D. "Sources of Power of Lower Participants in Complex Organizations." *Administrative Science Quarterly* 7(3) (Dec. 1962):349–364.

MERTON, R. K. *Social Theory and Social Structure,* rev. ed. Glencoe, Ill.: Free Press, 1957.

MEYER, M. W. "Introduction: Recent Developments in Organizational Research and Theory." In M. W. Meyer and associates, eds., *Environments and Organizations.* San Francisco: Jossey-Bass, 1978.

MILES, D. *Health Team Effectiveness in Health Status in Laurence County, Alabama: Terminal Progress Report.* National Center for Health Services Research, July 25, 1977.

MILLER, A. E. and M. G. MILLER. *Options for Health and Health Care: The Coming of Post Clinical Medicine.* Wiley-Interscience. New York: Wiley 1981.

MILLER, C. A., BROOKS, E. F., DeFRIESE, G. H., GILBERT, B., JAIN, S. C., and KAVALER, F. "A Survey of Local Public Health Departments and Their Directors." *American Journal of Public Health* 67(10) (October 1977):931–939.

MINTZBERG, H. *The Nature of Managerial Work.* Englewood Cliffs, N.J.: Prentice-Hall, 1973.

MINTZBERG, H. "The Manager's Job: Folklore and Fact." *Harvard Business Review* (July–Aug. 1975):49–61.

MINTZBERG, H. *The Structuring of Organizations: A Synthesis of the Research.* Englewood Cliffs, N.J.: Prentice-Hall, 1979.

MOHR, L. B. "The Concept of Organizational Goal." *American Political Science Review* 67(2) (June 1973):470–481.

MOREHEAD, M. *Quality of Medical Care Provided by Family Physicians as Related to Their Education, Training and Methods of Practice.* New York: Health Insurance Plan of New York, 1958.

MUNSON, F. C. "Crisis Points in Unit Management Programs." *Hospitals, JAHA* 47 (July 16, 1973):122–136.

MURDICK, R. G., and ROSS, J. E. *Information Systems.* Englewood Cliffs, N.J.: Prentice-Hall, 1975.

NADLER, D. A. *Feedback and Organization Development: Using Data-Based Methods.* Reading, Mass.: Addison-Wesley, 1977.

NATHANSON, C. A., and BECKER, M. H. "Control Structure and Conflict in Outpatient Clinics." *Journal of Health and Social Behavior* 13(3) (Sept. 1972):251–262.

NATIONAL CENTER FOR HEALTH CARE TECHNOLOGY. "Health Care Technology Assessment: Research Grants Programs." Rockville, Md., 1980.

NATIONAL CENTER FOR HEALTH STATISTICS. *Data Systems of the National Center for Health Statistics.* n.d.

NATIONAL COMMISSION FOR THE PROTECTION OF HUMAN SUBJECTS OF BIO-MEDICAL AND BEHAVIORAL RESEARCH. *Appendix to Report and Recommendations: Institutional Review Boards.* DHEW Publ. No. (OS)78-0009. Washington, D.C.: DHEW, 1978a.

NATIONAL COMMISSION FOR THE PROTECTION OF HUMAN SUBJECTS OF BIO-MEDICAL AND BEHAVIORAL RESEARCH. *The Belmont Report: Ethical Principles and Guidelines for the Protection of Human Subjects of Research.* Appendix Vols. 1 and 2. DHEW Publ. No. (OS)78-0013. Washington, D.C.: DHEW, 1978b.

NATIONAL COMMISSION ON ALLIED HEALTH EDUCATION. *The Future of Allied Health Education.* San Francisco: Jossey-Bass, 1980.

NATIONAL LEAGUE FOR NURSING. *Nursing Data Book.* New York: NLN, 1978.

NATIONAL PUBLIC HEALTH PROGRAM REPORTING SYSTEM. *The Association of State and Territorial Health Officials. Comprehensive NPHPRS Report: Services, Expenditures and Programs of State and Territorial Health Agencies—Fiscal Year 1976.* Washington, D.C.: ASTHO-SPHPRS Publ. No. 39, Apr. 1978.

NATIONAL RESEARCH COUNCIL, INSTITUTE OF MEDICINE. *Medical Technology and the Health Care System.* Washington, D.C.: National Academy of Sciences, 1979.

NEELY, G. "Affirmative Action: Reflections on the Issues Raised from a Social Psychological Perspective." Monograph Series for American Society for Training and Development. Madison, Wis., 1978.

NEUHAUSER, D. "The *Really* Effective Health Service Delivery System." *Health Care Management Review* 1(1) (Winter 1976):25–32.

NEUHAUSER, D., and ANDERSON, R. "Structural Comparative Studies in Hospitals." In B. S. Georgopoulos, ed., *Organization Research in Health Institutions.* Ann Arbor, Mich.: University of Michigan, Institute for Social Research, 1972.

NEUHAUSER, D. and A. KOVNER (eds). *Health Services Management: Readings and Commentary.* Health Adminstration Press, 1978.

OLDHAM, G. "The Motivational Strategies Used by Supervisors: Relationships to Effectiveness Indicators." *Organizational Behavior and Human Performance* 15 (1976): 66–86.

OSBURN, R. N., and HUNT, J. G. "Environment and Organizational Effectiveness." *Administrative Science Quarterly* 19(2) (June 1974):231–246.

PALMER, R. H., and REILLY, M. C. "Individual and Institutional Variables Which May Serve as Indicators of Quality of Medical Care." *Medical Care* 17(7) (July 1979): 693–717.

PAYNE, B. C., et al. *The Quality of Medical Care: Evaluation and Improvement.* Chicago: Hospital Research and Educational Trust, 1976.

PERROW, C. "Three Types of Effectiveness Studies." In P. S. Goodman, J. M. Penning, and associates, eds., *New Perspective on Organizational Effectiveness.* San Francisco: Jossey-Bass, 1977.

PFEFFER, J. *Organizational Design.* Arlington Heights, Ill.: AHM Publishing Co., 1978.

PFEFFER, J., and SALANCIK, G. R. "Organizational Context and the Characteristics and Tenure of Hospital Administrators." *Academy of Management Journal* 20 (1977): 79–88.

PFEFFER, J., and SALANCIK, G. R. *The External Control of Organizations: A Resource Dependence Perspective.* New York: Harper & Row, 1978.

POPOLI, A. F. "A Hospital Consortium." In J. O. Hepner, ed., *Health Planning for Emerging Multi-Hospital Systems,* St. Louis, Mo.: C. V. Mosby, 1978, pp. 321–326.

POZGAR, N. *Legal Aspects of Health Care Administration.* Germantown, Md.: Aspen Systems Corp., 1979.

PRICE, J. L. and O. W. MUELLER. *Professional Turnover: The Case of Nurses.* Jamaica, N.Y.: Spectrum Publications, 1981.

PYHRR, P. A. "Zero-Based Budgeting." *Harvard Business Review* (Nov.–Dec. 1970): 111–121.

PYLE, W. W., WHITE, J. A., and LARSON, K. D. *Fundamental Accounting Principles,* 8th ed. Homewood, Ill.: Richard D. Irwin, 1978.

RAFFEL, M. W. *The U.S. Health System: Origins and Functions.* New York: Wiley, 1980.

RAKICH, J. S., LONGEST, B. B., and O'DONOVAN, T. R. *Managing Health Care Organizations.* Philadelphia: W. B. Saunders, 1977.

REINHARDT, U. E. "Proposed Changes in the Organization of Health Care Delivery: An Overview and Critique." *Milbank Memorial Fund Quarterly—Health and Society* 51(2) (Spring 1973):169–222.

RELMAN. A. "The New Medical-Industrial Complex." *New England Journal of Medicine* 303(17) (Oct. 23, 1981):963–970.

REYNOLDS, J., and STUNDEN, A. E. "The Organization of Not-for-Profit Hospital Systems." *Health Care Management Review* 3(3) (Summer 1978):23–36.

RHEE, S. "Factors Determining the Quality of Physician Performance in Patient Care." *Medical Care* 14(9) (Sept. 1976):733-750.

RHEE, S. "Relative Importance of Physicians' Personal and Situational Characteristics for the Quality of Patient Care." *Journal of Health and Social Behavior* 18(1) (Mar. 1977):10-15.

RISING, E. *Design for Improved Patient Flow.* Ambulatory Care Systems, Vol. 1. Lexington, Mass.: Lexington Books, 1977.

ROBERTSON, J. C. *Auditing.* Dallas, Tex.: Business Publications, Inc., 1976.

ROEMER, M. I. "A Realistic System: Health Maintenance Organizations in a Regionalized Framework." In R. Roemer, C. Kramer, and J. E. Frink, eds., *Planning Urban Health Services from Jungle to System.* New York: Springer, 1975, pp. 253-287.

ROEMER, M. I., and FREIDMAN, J. W. *Doctors in Hospitals: Medical Staff Organization and Hospital Performance.* Baltimore, Md.: Johns Hopkins Press, 1971.

ROGERS, D., and BLENDON, R. "The Academic Medical Center: A Stressed American Institution." *New England Journal of Medicine* 298(17) (Apr. 27, 1978):940-950.

ROGERS, E. M., and SHOEMAKER, F. F. *Communication of Innovation: A Cross-Cultural Approach.* New York: Free Press, 1971.

ROMM, F. J., and HULKA, B. S. "Developing Criteria for Quality of Care Assessment: Effects of the Delphi Technique." *Health Services Research* 14(4) (Winter 1979): 309-312.

RUBIN, I. M., and BECKHARD, R. "Factors Influencing the Effectiveness of Health Teams." *Milbank Memorial Fund Quarterly, Health and Society* 50(3) Part 1 (July 1972).

RUBIN, I., PLOVNICK, M., and FRY, R. "Initiating Planned Change in Health Care Systems," *Journal of Applied Behavioral Science* 10(1) (1974):107-124.

RUBIN, I. M., FRY, R. E., and PLOVNICK, M. S. *Managing Human Resources in Health Care Organization: An Applied Approach.* Reston, Va.: Reston, 1978.

RUHE, C. H. W. "Medical Education in the United States 1978-1979." *JAMA* 243(9) (Mar. 7, 1980):841-866.

RUSSELL, L. B. *Technology in Hospitals: Medical Advances and Their Diffusion.* Washington, D.C.: The Brookings Institution, 1979.

RYAN, W. *Blaming the Victim.* New York: Vintage Books, 1971.

SALMON, J. W., and BERLINER, H. S. "Health Policy Implications from the Holistic Health Movement." *Journal of Health Politics, Policy, and Law* (forthcoming) (1979).

SCHEIN, E. H. *Organizational Psychology.* Englewood Cliffs, N.J.: Prentice-Hall, 1970.

SCHLAG, D. "Cash Surpluses Can Produce Income." In William Cleaverly, *Financial*

Management of Health Care Facilities. Germantown, Md.: Aspen Systems Corp., 1976, pp. 203–204.

SCHRAMM, C. J. "Hospital Consolidation: Lessons from Other Industries." The Johns Hopkins Center for Hospital Finance and Management. Prepared for delivery at the AHA/HRET Conference on Multi-Hospital Systems, Washington, D.C., Mar. 18, 1980.

SCOTT, W. R., FORREST, W. H., and BROWN, B. W. "Hospital Structure and Post-Operative Mortality and Morbidity," In S. Shortell and M. Brown, eds., *Organizational Research in Hospitals.* Chicago: Blue Cross Association, 1976.

SEAWELL, L. V. *Hospital Financial Accounting, Theory and Practice.* Chicago: Hospital Financial Management Association, 1975.

SEEMAN, M., and EVANS, J. "Stratification and Hospital Care: The Performance of the Medical Intern." *ASR* 26(1) (Feb. 1961):67–80.

SELZNICK, P. *T.V.A. and the Grass Roots,* University of California Press, Berkeley, 1949.

SHANNON, R. E. *Systems Simulation.* Englewood Cliffs, N.J.: Prentice-Hall, 1975.

SHEPS, C., ed. *Higher Education for Public Health: A Report of the Milbank Memorial Fund Commission.* New York: Prodist, 1976.

SHEPS, C. G. "The Role of Health Services Research in the Veterans' Administration—And Beyond." *Journal of Medical Systems* 5(1) (1981).

SHONICK, W., and PRICE, W. "Reorganizations of Health Agencies by Local Government in American Urban Centers: What Do They Portend for 'Public Health'?" *Milbank Memorial Fund Quarterly, Health and Society* 55(2) (Spring 1977):233–271.

SHORTELL, S. M. "Organizational Theory and Health Service Delivery." In S. M. Shortell and M. Brown, eds., *Organizational Research in Hospitals.* Chicago: Blue Cross Association, 1976, pp. 1–12.

SHORTELL, S. M. "The Role of Environment in a Configurational Theory of Organizations." *Human Relations* 30(3) (1977):275–302.

SHORTELL, S. "Measuring Hospital Medical Staff Organization Structure." *Health Services Research* 14(2) (Summer 1979).

SHORTELL, S., and BROWN, M., eds. *Organizational Research in Hospitals. An Inquiry Book.* Chicago: Blue Cross Association, 1976.

SHUMAN, L. J., SPEAS, R. D., and YOUNG, J. P., eds. *Operations Research in Health Care: A Critical Analysis.* Baltimore, Md.: Johns Hopkins University Press, 1975.

SIMON, H. *The Sciences of the Artificial.* Cambridge, Mass.: MIT Press, 1969.

SKINNER, K. "Burn-Out: Is Nursing Dangerous to Your Health?" *Journal of Nursing Care* 12(12) (Dec. 1979).

SMEJDA, H. "How You Can Comply with the Fair Debt Collection Practices Act." *Hospital Financial Management* (April 1978):22–28.

SMITH, D. B. *Long-Term Care in Transition: The Regulation of Nursing Homes.* Ann Arbor, Mich.: Health Administration Press, 1981.

SMITH, D. B., and KALUZNY, A. D. *The White Labyrinth: Understanding the Organization of Health Care.* Berkeley, Calif.: McCutchan, 1975.

SMITH, H. L., SHORTELL, S. M., and SAXBERG, D. O. "An Empirical Test of the Configurational Theory of Organization." *Human Relations* 32(8) (Aug. 1979): 667–688.

SNELLING, D. "Short-Term Investment of Excess Cash." In William Cleaverly, *Financial Management of Health Care Facilities.* Germantown, Md.: Aspen Systems Corp.. 1976, pp. 206–214.

SOUTH, J. C. "The Performance Profile: A Technique for Using Appraisals Effectively." *Journal of Nursing Administration* 8(1) (1978):27–31.

SOUTHWICK, A. *Law of Hospital and Health Care Administration.* Ann Arbor, Mich.: Health Administration Press, 1978.

SPEIGEL, A. D., and HYMAN, H. H. *Basic Health Planning Methods.* Germantown, Md.: Aspen Systems Corp., 1978.

STAMPS, P. L., DUSTON, T. E., RISING, E. J., ALLEN, D., and BONDY-LEVY, M. "How Consumers Exercise Control Through Their Bill-Paying Patterns." *Inquiry* 15 (June 1978):151–159.

STARKWEATHER, D. B. *Hospital Mergers.* Ann Arbor, Mich.: Health Administration Press, 1981.

STEERS, R. M. "Problems in the Measurement of Organizational Effectiveness." *Administrative Science Quarterly* 20(4) (Dec. 1975):546–558.

STETTLER, H. F. *Auditing Principles,* 4th ed. Englewood Cliffs, N.J.: Prentice-Hall, 1977.

STEVENS, R., and STEVENS, R. *Welfare Medicine in America: A Case Study of Medicaid.* New York: Free Press, 1974.

STOGDILL, R. M., and COONS, A. E. *Leader Behavior: Its Description and Measurement.* Bureau of Business Research, Ohio State University 1957.

SWEENY, M. "Implementation of a Management Objectives Program in a Major Medical Center." A case report in hospital administration prepared for the Committee on Credentials in partial fulfillment of the requirements for fellowship, American College of Hospital Administrators, Chicago, 1977.

TANNENBAUM, A. S. *Control in Organizations.* New York: McGraw-Hill, 1968.

TELLER, E. "The Hydrogen Bomb Program." In F. Kast and J. Rosenzweig, eds., *Science, Technology and Management.* New York: McGraw-Hill, 1963.

TERRIS, M. "The Epidemiologic Revolution, National Health Insurance and the Role of

Health Departments." *American Journal of Public Health* 66(12) (Dec. 1976): 1155–1164.

TICHY, N. M. *Organizational Design for Public Health Care: The Case of the Dr. Martin Luther King Health Center.* New York: Praeger, 1977.

TODD, C., and MACNAMARA, M. E. *Medical Groups in the U.S., 1969.* Chicago: American Medical Association, 1971.

TOSI, H., HUNTER, J., CHESSER, R., TARTER, J. R., and CARROLL, S. "How Real Are Changes Induced by Management by Objectives?" *Administrative Science Quarterly* 21(2) (June 1976):276–306.

TRACY, G. S., and GUSSOW, Z. "Self-Help Groups: A Grass Roots Response to a Need for Services." *Journal of Applied Behavioral Science* 12(3) (July–Aug.–Sept. 1976): 381–396.

THE URBAN INSTITUTE. *Medical Technology: Research Priorities.* Proceedings of the Urban Institute Conference, West Palm Beach. Fla, Dec. 1978.

U.S. BUREAU OF THE CENSUS. *Statistical Abstracts of the United States,* 1969, 1979 ed.

U.S. CONGRESS, OFFICE OF TECHNOLOGY ASSESSMENT. "The Computer Topography (CT) Scanner Adds Simplification for Health Policy." Draft, Sept. 1976.

U.S. CONGRESS, OFFICE OF TECHNOLOGY ASSESSMENT. "Assessing the Efficacy and Safety of Medical Technologies." Washington, D.C.: U.S. Government Printing Office, 1978.

U.S. DEPARTMENT OF HEALTH, EDUCATION AND WELFARE. *Improving Health Care Through Research and Development.* Report of the Panel on Health Services Research and Development of the President's Advisory Committee, Washington, D.C., 1972.

U.S. DEPARTMENT OF HEALTH, EDUCATION AND WELFARE. "Protection of Human Subjects." *Federal Register* 39(105) (Part 2) (May 30, 1974):18914–18920.

U.S. DEPARTMENT OF HEALTH, EDUCATION AND WELFARE. *DHEW Publ. No. (OS)78-0014.* Washington, D.C.: DHEW, 1978a.

U.S. DEPARTMENT OF HEALTH, EDUCATION AND WELFARE, NATIONAL CENTER FOR HEALTH SERVICES RESEARCH. *NCHSR: Research Priorities.* Nov. 1978b.

U.S. DEPARTMENT OF HEALTH, EDUCATION AND WELFARE. *Special Study: Implications of Advances in Biomedical and Behavioral Research.* DHEW Publ. No. (OS)78-0015. Washington, D.C.: DHEW, 1978c.

U.S. DEPARTMENT OF HEALTH, EDUCATION AND WELFARE. *Supply of Optometrists in the U.S., Health Manpower References* (October, 1978), Publication No. (HRA) 79-80.

U.S. DEPARTMENT OF HEALTH, EDUCATION AND WELFARE, OFFICE OF THE ASSISTANT SECRETARY FOR HEALTH. *Disease Prevention and Health Promo-*

tion: Federal Programs and Prospects. Washington, D.C.: U.S. Government Printing Office [(PHS) Publ. No. 79-55071B], 1979.

U.S. DEPARTMENT OF HEALTH, EDUCATION AND WELFARE, BUREAU OF HEALTH MANPOWER. *Schools of Public Health: Educational Data Project, 1974–1979.* Mar. 1980a.

U.S. DEPARTMENT OF HEALTH, EDUCATION AND WELFARE, BUREAU OF HEALTH MANPOWER. *A Report on Public and Community Health Personnel.* Apr. 1980b.

U.S. EQUAL EMPLOYMENT OPPORTUNITY COMMISSION. *Affirmative Action and Equal Employment: A Guidebook for Employers,* Vol. 1. Washington, D.C.: U.S. Equal Employment Opportunity Commission, Jan. 1974.

U.S. NATIONAL CENTER FOR HEALTH STATISTICS. *Health Resource Statistics, 1976–1977.* Public Health Service Publication No. 79-1509.

VALINSKY, D. "Simulation." In L. Shuman, R. Speas, Jr., and J. Young, eds., *Operations Research in Health Care.* Baltimore Md.: Johns Hopkins University Press, 1975.

VANAGUNAS, A. "Quality Assessment: Alternate Approaches." *Quality Review Bulletin* 5(2) (Feb. 1979):7–10.

VAN de VEN, A., and FERRY, D. *Measuring and Assessing Organizations.* New York: Wiley-Interscience, 1980.

VAN de VEN, A., and MORGAN, M. "A Revised Framework for Organizational Assessment." In E. Lawler, D. Nadler, and C. Cammann, eds., *Organizational Assessment: Perspectives on the Measurement of Organizational Behavior and Quality of Work Life.* New York: Wiley-Interscience, 1980.

VAN HORNE, J. C. *Fundamentals of Financial Management,* 3rd ed. Englewood Cliffs, N.J.: Prentice-Hall, 1977.

VARELA, J. *Psychological Solutions to Social Problems,* New York: Academic Press, 1971.

VAUGHN, J. C., and JOHNSON, W. L. "Educational Preparation for Nursing–1978." *Nursing Outlook* 27(9) (Sept. 1979):608–614.

VENINGA, R. *Health Administration: Interpersonal Effectiveness.* Englewood Cliffs, N.J.: Prentice-Hall, forthcoming (1981).

VRACIU, R. A. "Programming, Budgeting and Control in Health Care Organizations: The State of the Art." *Health Services Research* 14(2) (Summer 1979):126–149.

WAGNER, H. M. *Principles of Operations Research.* Englewood Cliffs, N.J.: Prentice-Hall, 1979.

WALSH, J. L., and ELLING, R. H. "Professionalism and the Poor–Structural Effects and Professional Behavior." *Journal of Health and Social Behavior* 9(1) (Mar. 1968):16–28.

WARNER, D. M., and HOLLOWAY, D. C. *Decision Making and Control for Health Administration.* Ann Arbor, Mich.: Health Administration Press, 1978.

WARREN, D. G. *Problems in Hospital Law.* Germantown, Md.: Aspen Systems Corp., 1978.

WASHINGTON REPORT ON MEDICARE AND HEALTH. "HEW Civil Rights Drive Aimed at Health." 34(1) (Jan. 7, 1980).

WEAVER, J. L. *Conflict and Control in Health Care Administration,* Vol. 14. Sage Library of Social Research. Beverly Hills, Calif.: Sage, 1975.

WEBBER, J., and DULA, M. "Effective Planning Committee for Hospitals." *Harvard Business Review* (May-June 1974):133-142.

WEICK, K. E. *The Social Psychology of Organizing.* Reading, Mass.: Addison-Wesley, 1969.

WEICK, K. E. "Educational Organizations as Loosely Coupled Systems." *Administrative Science Quarterly* 21(1) (Mar. 1976):1-19.

WEINER, S. M. "Health Care Policy and Politics: Does the Past Tell Us Anything About the Future?" *American Journal of Law and Medicine* 5(4) (Winter 1980):331-341.

WEISBORD, M., LAWRENCE, P., and CHARNS, M. "The Dilemmas of Academic Medical Centers." *Journal of Applied Behavioral Science* (July-Aug.-Sept. 1978).

WEISS, H., BECKARD, R., RUBIN, I., and KYTE, A. *Making Health Teams Work.* Cambridge, Mass.: Ballinger, 1974.

WENNBERG, J. E., BLOWERS, L., PARKER, R., and GITTLSOHN, A. M. "Changes in Tonsillectomy Rates Associated with Feedback and Review." *Pediatrics* 59(6) (June 1977):821-826.

WIELAND, G., ed. *Improving Health Care Management: Organization Development and Organization Change.* Ann Arbor, Mich.: Health Administration Press, 1980.

WILLIAMS, S. J. *Issues in Health Services.* New York: Wiley, 1980.

WILLIAMS, S., and TORRENS, P., eds. *Introduction to Health Services.* New York: Wiley, 1980.

WILLIAMSON, J. W. *Assessing and Improving Health Care Outcomes: The Health Accounting Approach to Quality Assurance.* Cambridge, Mass.: Ballinger, 1978a.

WILLIAMSON, J. W. "Formulating Priorities for Quality Assurance Activity." *JAMA* 239(7) (Feb. 13, 1978b):631-637.

WILLIAMSON, J. W., BRASWELL, H. R., HORN, S. D., and LOHMEYER, S. "Priority Setting in Quality Assurance: Reliability of Staff Judgments in Medical Institutions." *Medical Care* 16(11) (Nov. 1978):931-940.

WILLIAMSON, J. W., BRASWELL, H. R., and HORS, S. D. "Validity of Medical Staff Judgments in Establishing Quality Assurance Priorities." *Medical Care* 17(4) (Apr. 1979):331-346.

WILLIS, W. R., JR. "Can Incident Reports be Used as Evidence for the Plaintiff?" The Hospital Medical Staff. Chicago: AHA, 1979.

WILSON, J. Q. "Innovation in Organization: Notes Toward a Theory." In J. D. Thompson, ed., *Approaches to Organization Design*, Pittsburgh, Pa.: University of Pittsburgh Press, 1966.

WING, K. R. *The Law and the Public's Health.* St. Louis, Mo.: C. V. Mosby, 1976.

WOODWARD, J. *Industrial Organization: Theory and Practice.* London: Oxford University Press, 1965.

ZALTMAN, G., and DUNCAN, R. *Strategies for Planned Change.* New York: Wiley-Interscience, 1977.

ZALTMAN, G., DUNCAN, R., and HOLBEK, J. *Innovations and Organizations.* New York: Wiley, 1973.

ZELTEN, R. A. "Alternative HMO Models." National Health Care Management Center, University of Pennsylvania, Issue Paper No. 3, Apr. 1979.

ZUCKERMAN, H. S. "Multi-Institutional Systems: Promise and Performance." *Inquiry* 16(4) (Winter 1979):291–314.

ZUCKERMAN, H. and WEEKS, L. *Multi-Institutional Hospital Systems*, Chicago: Hospital Research and Educational Trust, 1979.

Index

PERT, 173–179
    COST analysis, 178-179
    critical path, 176, 178-179
    EST, 174-177
    Gantt chart, 177
    LST, 174-177
    slack time, 176-177
    subpath, 177
Pfeffer, J., 26, 51, 68, 415, 416
Phasing perspective, of design, 85
Physical protection of assets, 205
Physicians, 369-371
Pinchoff, D., 93
Placement of personnel, 298
Plaintiff, 326
Planning:
    budgeting and, 103-126
    controls, 292-293
    design and, 8-9, 68-93
    financial management and, 103-104
    long-range facility, 20-23
    phase of managerial process, 8-9
    quantitative model, 131, 139-154
    resource, 103-154
        acquisition, 103-126
        allocation, 131-154
Plant, in financial management, 204-205
Plovnick, M., 272
Poisson model, 145-146
Policies and procedures, in relation to control, 294-295
Political process, relationship to policy, 391-393
Political values, effect on health services system, 389-390
Popoli, A., 58
Population, diseases affecting, 356, 358, 361
Position, within an organization, 32, 36
Power, 84-85, 225-227, 230, 246-247
Pozgar, N., 350
Practitioners, 369-372
    financing, 373
    HMO, 370-372
    independent, 369-370
Predictive validity, 286
Preferred stock, 197
Prevention, 363
Price, J., 42, 272
Price variance, 312
Primary attribute, of change, 212
Privacy, right of, 324, 346
Private carriers, 381-382
Private sources of funds, 192-198
    bonds, 195-196
    contracts, 192
    credit, 192-195
        loans, 193
        trade credit, 193-195
    donations, 197-198
    equity financing, 196-197
    grants, 192
Proactive planning, 104
Procedural regulations, 393-394
Procedure decision, 160-161, 164-167
Procedures and policies, in relation to control, 294-295
Process consultation, as type of facilitative strategy, 223-224

Process measures, of quality, 30
Production subsystem, 32, 39, 358-375
    definition, 39
    hospitals, 364, 367-369
    practitioners, 369-372
    public health, 359-366
    self-help groups, 372-375
Productivity, 29-30
Professional:
    associations, 375-376
    care, financing, 372
    component of environment, 107
    control, 247
    force in health service organizations, 56
    schools, 376-380
        allied health, 379-380
        medical, 376-377
        nursing, 379
        public health, 378
    structure, 45-50
Profile analysis, in PSRO, 388
Profit, 192, 296
Profit center, 115
Pro forma financial statement, 124-126
Programming, 110-113, 292-293
Promotion, of personnel, 300
Property, in financial management, 204-205
Protocol, in risk management, 338-339
PSRO, 258, 387-388
Psychological contract, 262-263
Public funds, 188-190
    appropriation, 188-190
    contract, 190
    grant, 190
    loan, 190
    reimbursement, 190
Public health, 359-366, 378
    constituencies served by, 362
    definition, 359
    financing, 363-364
    future possibilities for, 362-363
    schools, 378
    services, 359, 361
    structure, 363-364
Public policy, 391-393
Pyhrr, P., 111, 124
Pyle, W., 302

Quality:
    assurance, 70, 227-229, 253-255, 259
        bi-cycle approach, 253-254
        design and, 70
        nominal group technique, 255
    control, and risk management, 340
    measurement of, 29-30
Quantitative control, 274-287
    conditions for success, 277-279
    framework, 274-277
    measurement, 279-286
Quantitative method of trend analysis, 138
Quantitative planning model, 131, 139-154
    application, 152-154
    choice of type of model, 152-154
    complex, 146-151
    simple, 139-146
Queueing model, 147-150